The Antibody Molecule

Oxford Medical Histories Series

This series of Oxford Medical Histories is designed to bring to a wide readership of clinical doctors and others from many backgrounds a short but comprehensive text setting out the essentials of differing areas of medicine. Volumes in this series are written by doctors and with doctors, in particular, in mind as the readership.

History describes the knowledge acquired over time by human beings. It is a form of storytelling, of organizing knowledge, of sorting and giving impetus to information. The study of medical history, just like the history of other human endeavours, enables us to analyse our knowledge of the past in order to plan our journey forward and hence try to limit repetition of our mistakes — a sort of planned process of Natural Selection, described as being in the tradition of one of the most famous of medical historians, William Osler. Medical history also encourages and trains us to use an academic approach to our studies which thereby should become more precise, more meaningful and more productive. Medical history should be enjoyable too, since that is a powerful stimulus to move forward, a fun thing to do both individually and in groups.

The inspiring book that led to this series introduced us to clinical neurology, genetics, and the history of those with muscular dystrophy. Alan and Marcia Emery explored *The History of a Genetic Disease*, now often styled Meryon's disease rather than Duchenne Muscular Dystrophy. The first to describe a disease process is not necessarily the owner of the eponym but the Emerys are helping put that right for their subject, Edward Meryon. The second book in the series, on radiology, took us on a journey round a world of images.

Thus future volumes in this series of Oxford Medical Histories will continue the journey through the history of our bodies, of their relationship to our environment, of the joyful and the sad situations that envelope us from our individual beginnings to our ends. We should travel towards other aspects of our humanity, always leaving us with more questions than answers since each new discovery leads to more questions, exponential sets of issues for us to study, further thoughts and attempts to solve the big questions that surround our existence. Medicine is about people and so is history; the study of the combination of the duo can be very powerful. What do you think?

Christopher Gardner-Thorpe, MD, FRCP, FACP
Series Advisor, Oxford Medical Histories

The Antibody Molecule

From Antitoxins to Therapeutic Antibodies

by

Anthony R. Rees

Principal
Rees Consulting AB,
Uppsala, Sweden

and

Professor Emeritus,
University of Bath, UK

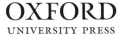

OXFORD
UNIVERSITY PRESS

OXFORD
UNIVERSITY PRESS

Great Clarendon Street, Oxford, OX2 6DP,
United Kingdom

Oxford University Press is a department of the University of Oxford.
It furthers the University's objective of excellence in research, scholarship,
and education by publishing worldwide. Oxford is a registered trade mark of
Oxford University Press in the UK and in certain other countries

© Oxford University Press 2015

The moral rights of the author have been asserted

First Edition published in 2015

Impression: 1

Published in the United States of America by Oxford University Press
198 Madison Avenue, New York, NY 10016, United States of America

British Library Cataloguing in Publication Data

Data available

Library of Congress Control Number: 2014944571

ISBN 978–0–19–964657–9

Printed and bound by
CPI Group (UK) Ltd, Croydon, CR0 4YY

For my wife Marianne and Melissa, Emma, Charlotte, Madeleine,
Lucy, Bruno, and Margo
And in memory of my dear mother

"... *every effect is a distinct event from its cause ... In vain, therefore,
should we pretend to determine any single event, or infer any cause and
effect, without the assistance of observation and experience*".

Reproduced from David Hume, *Enquiries concerning the human understanding and concerning
the principles of morals.*, Reprinted from the 1777 edition and edited by L.A. Selby-Bygge,
2nd Edn. 1902, Impression of 1970. Oxford University Press.

Foreword

'Another antibody book' was the subject line of the email I received from Tony Rees almost a year ago with a request that I consider writing the foreword. From his self-deprecating email one would have thought that Tony was adding to the ponderous pile of texts that have focused on this well-studied and even better documented molecule, texts that range from those purely methodological to those purely didactic. Was there a need for yet another treatise on the antibody? Probably not. However, knowing Tony's work on antibody modelling and engineering as I did, and his intimate association with antibody-based technologies, I suspected something more interesting must have been brewing. Indeed it was. Tony set out to record an historical account of the antibody molecule, from its first description in the late-nineteenth century to our current infatuation with it as a therapeutic entity. What Tony succeeded in doing was to capture a snapshot of the world of immunology and of the personalities that drove the field, moving it from one purely descriptive to one based on molecular principles. His account reads like a mystery novel, with all the drama that can be found with personality clashes, false starts and, at the end, resolution and clarity.

Several themes emerge from this historical perspective of immunology as glimpsed through the antibody molecule. Immunology is, at its heart, a discipline inseparable from the physiology of the organism. It interacts in a dynamic way with every organ system, balancing its protective features with the unavoidable collateral damage that accompanies the inflammatory response. Maintaining this equilibrium is key to survival of the organism; perturbations inexorably lead to pathology. To understand the immune response one needed a holistic approach, a fact widely appreciated by its early practitioners, but eclipsed during periods of reductionist fervour. The pendulum swung up and back throughout the history of the antibody molecule, from *in vitro* dissection to *in vivo* biology, coming to rest in this century at a synthesis of the two approaches, with the advent of methods that permitted reductionism at the whole animal level through the use of recombinant DNA technology and the use of genetically modified organisms. Detailed molecular dissection of the antibody molecule, the pathways that generate its remarkable diversity, and the systems that are recruited to mediate its *in vivo* responses could be manipulated, engineered, and re-introduced into the organism to interrogate the outcome. And with these tools came insights into genetics, cell biology, and structural biology that continue to captivate not only immunologists but also the wider community of scientists.

I was witness to this sea change in antibody research that began in the mid-1970s as molecular biologists began to wield their formidable tools to approach the problem of antibody diversity. The problem was clearly recognized-how could the organism encode the required diversity of antibody molecules, on the order of trillions of different proteins, if one accepts the prevailing viewpoint that each gene encodes only one protein.

The genome is far too small to accommodate this genetic diversity. Remarkably clever ideas were put forward to resolve this paradox by formidable intellects unaccustomed to being challenged, yet which remained untestable and thus equally tenable. Enter the gene cloners. They managed, in a few frenetic years, to bury elegant theories while elevating others, revealing the power of combinatorial diversity inherent in the unique organization of the antibody genes. As a young postdoctoral fellow in Phil Leder's lab at the NIH I had a front row seat to the spectacle, working at a time where each new sequencing gel contained a result worth publishing, revealing V regions, J and D segments, recombination signal sequences, switch regions, and alternative splice sites. The novelty of the genetic mechanisms that had evolved to generate the antibody repertoire was breathtaking. The competition was fierce and the atmosphere charged, with each new journal article, conference report, or casual discussion revealing one group now pulling ahead, now falling behind. Tony's book took me back to those remarkable days, capturing the excitement of discovery and the eureka moments that can still bring a chill to my spine. It's fair to say that your never forget your first eureka.

Fortunately for those of us who have never gotten over our infatuation with this remarkable molecule, its final history has not been written. Tony's book has shown us where we started and taken us to the point where we can glimpse where we might be headed, but the inevitable twists and turns are certain to reveal new and unexpected landscapes in biology.

Jeffrey Ravetch
The Rockefeller University
New York, NY

Preface

Immunology is one of the oldest of the medical sciences with a history that has seen chemists, physicists, biologists, and clinicians alike seeking to unravel the most complex system in the human body outside the brain. In this book I have not been so bold as to try to replicate the erudition and breadth of immunology history in classics such as those of Arthur Silverstein or Pauline Mazumdar. My objective was to take a chronological approach since for an amateur historian this was the easiest path along which I could explore the byways of research in different fields that impacted our understanding of this family of molecules. In doing so, I have uncovered what for me were many surprises, having been raised on the traditional science history found in most standard textbooks and scientific reviews. Where I express that 'surprise' in the text I have tried to be as objective as possible but also not shy away from stating my personal interpretation where I believed it was justified.

While this has been a long journey of discovery it has also been one that has produced dilemmas. With a limit on the size of the book I decided to exclude areas that may be considered by some to be of equal historical importance. For example, I do not discuss in any great depth the tolerance debate, nor do I include to any great extent the development of antibody control mechanisms. The T-cell receptor and major histocompatibility antigens and their roles in antigen processing have barely a mention except *en passant*. The fledgling field of epigenetics is perhaps too young to be able to draw any meaningful conclusions as yet. To have expanded the story to include these and other subjects would have opened a Pandora's Box of quasi-relevant topics that are best addressed in another place. I hope the reader will understand my rationale but at the same time be excited and sometimes surprised by the beauty of antibody history, created in its early years by giants of scientific endeavour and now exploited by a multitude of scientists for the good of human health.

ARR

Uppsala 2014

Acknowledgements

When beginning to write this book I had no idea what I had taken on. Two years later I now have a much better appreciation of the daily routine of Hercules. During this time I have had enormous help and cooperation from many sources. Firstly I would like to thank Tim Berners-Lee and Robert Cailliau along with Larry Page and Sergey Brin for bringing 200 years of the world's literature to the desktop. Of course, without the cooperation of the world's library archives this would not have been possible. To be able to print original papers, or communications to learned societies, of Pasteur, Ehrlich, Koch, and others from the Deutsche Mediscinsche Wochenschrift or Compte Rendus of the French Academy of Sciences from the mid-to-late nineteenth century is a miracle of twenty-first-century communication. There are many persons to thank without whose help the search for original material would have been a truly enormous task. My thanks go to Paul Carter, Robin Snyder and Charles Eigenbrot of Genentech, Claire Smith of *Nature* magazine, Jane Beattie of the University of Melbourne Archives and Elizabeth Dexter (daughter of McFarlane Burnet), Juliet Ralph of the Bodleian Library for her remarkable sleuthlike tracking down of nineteenth-century manuscripts, Kornelia Grundman of the Emil von Behring Bibliothek, Marburg, Irma Gigli of the University of Texas, Ivan Sutherland for also pointing out the dangers of assuming photos on the web are authentic, Annette Faux of the MRC LMB Archives, Jo Hopkins of the Royal Society, London, Allegra Grevelius of Nobel Media, Neils Strandberg Pedersen of the Statens Serum Institute, Denmark, Lee Vucovich of the UAB Lister Hill Library, USA, Caroline Morley of the Wellcome Trust, and Jennifer Einstein of The Rockefeller University. Of the many academic colleagues who have helped me in various ways or provided personal photographs and memories I would like to thank Alen Perelsen, Martin Weigert, David Baltimore, David Davies, Roberto Poljak, Tasuku Honjo, Susumu Tonegawa, Greg Winter, Richard Lerner, Robert Huber, Axel Ullrich, Brad Guild, Robert Stroud, Gerald Edelman, and Donald Capra. My special thanks go to Florian Rüker, Jim Huston, Neil Simister, Andrew Martin, and with a heavy heart to the late Michael Neuberger, all of whom read various portions of the text and provided me with immeasurably helpful comments. For his pointed suggestions and for agreeing to write the Foreword I say a massive thanks to Jeff Ravetch. I would also like to pay tribute to the many names unmentioned, except perhaps in references, that in all honesty probably carried out the key experiments for those whose names were more well known. I salute these unsung heroes of immunology. For much-needed help with sourcing photographs I would like to thank Anna-Lena Ståhl of Ink Republic and for help with some of the more difficult French translations to my colleague and friend, Michel Kaczorek. I would also like to acknowledge the enormous contribution access to the University of Bath on-line library has made to the research for this book. For her forbearance during my numerous communications, for her valuable advice, and for politely accepting my frequently delayed submissions I would like to say a big thanks to Caroline Smith, my editor at OUP. It would not be complete without acknowledging the enormous influence the history of science treatises of Arthur Silverstein, Pauline Mazumdar, and Joseph Fruton have had on me during this journey through antibody history.

Contents

Abbreviations

ADCC	antibody-dependent cellular toxicity		LFA	lymphocyte function antigen
AEV	avian erythroblastosis virus		MAR	matrix association region
AID	activation-induced cytidine deaminase		mRNA	messenger RNA
			NBCC	National Breast Cancer Coalition
ARD	average relative displacement		NCI	National Cancer Institute
BBB	blood–brain barrier		NK	natural killer
CAMAL	combined antibody modelling algorithm		PC	phosphorylcholine
			PCR	polymerase chain reaction
CCA	chimpanzee coryza agent		PDGF	platelet-derived growth factor
CD	cardiac dysfunction		PIGS	prediction of immunoglobulin structure
CDR	complementarity-determining regions		RAG1	recombinase active gene 1
CEA	carcinoembryonic antigen		RAG2	recombinase active gene 2
CHARMM	Chemistry at HARvard Molecular Mechanics		RIGS	radioimmunoguided surgery
			RSV	respiratory syncytial virus
CHD	congenital heart disease		RSV	Rous sarcoma virus
CSR	class switch recombination		SDM	site-directed mutagenesis
DC-CK1	dendritic cell cytokine 1		SHM	somatic hypermutation
DNP	dinitrophenyl		SRBC	sheep red blood cells
DSB	double-stranded breaks		SSV	Simian sarcoma virus
EGF	epidermal growth factor		TdT	terminal deoxynucleotidyltransferase
Fv	fragment variable			
GM-CSF	granulocyte monocyte colony stimulating factor		TNF	tumour necrosis factor
			TNFα	tumour necrosis factor alpha
HAT	hypoxanthine, aminopterin, and thymidine		TPP	thrombotic thrombocytopenic purpura
HPRT	hypoxanthine-guanine phosphoribosyltransferase		UNG	uracil-DNA glycosylase
			VHH	variable heavy domain of heavy chain antibodies
IFNγ	interferon gamma			
Ig	immunoglobulin		WAM	web antibody modelling
IL	interleukin			
IVIG	intravenous pooled immunoglobulin			

Chapter 1

Antibody pre-history: The emergence of empirical immunology

Early foundations

Our journey starts in the small town of Berkeley in Gloucestershire, a little known and quiet corner of England, except perhaps for two extraordinary events in its history. In 1327 Edward II was murdered (reputedly) in Berkeley Castle. Apart from his legacies to Oxford and Cambridge—Oriel College and Kings Hall—the life of Edward achieved little to be remembered for. Five hundred years later, in 1749, the birth of the boy Edward to Stephen Jenner, the Vicar of Berkeley, was set to change the treatment of human disease for all time.

By the time he was 14, Jenner was in training as a surgeon, and at 23 he was a practicing physician, already dedicated to understanding how to control the high mortality due to the smallpox (*variola*) virus.

His use of the technique of 'variolation', in which live samples of this *variola* virus were used as inoculants and already practiced in many areas of the world despite the high death rate (10–30%) associated with the procedure, was taken by Jenner from phenomenology to empirical science over the next 40 years. His acute observational skills and extensive knowledge of animal and plant biology led him to question why cow maids exposed to cowpox virus believed they were protected from smallpox infection. In the now famous example (see Fig.1.1), the local boy James Phipps was inoculated with 'matter' from the cowpox secretions of cow maid Sarah Nelms and subsequently challenged with the smallpox virus. By this early clinical trial Jenner demonstrated beyond doubt that exposure of humans to a related but benign virus (cowpox) could substantially reduce the risk of later encounter with a more virulent cousin (smallpox).

As Jenner observed (some of Jenner's early anecdotal reports submitted to the Royal Society were rejected as being too preliminary. He privately funded the publication and printing of his early findings in book form, entitled *The Inquiry*):

> In order to ascertain whether the boy, after feeling so slight an affection of the system from the cow-pox virus, was secure from the contagion of the smallpox, he was inoculated the 1st of July following with variolous matter, immediately taken from a pustule. Several slight punctures and incisions were made on both his arms, and the matter was carefully inserted, but no disease followed. The same appearances were observable on the arms as we commonly see when a patient has had variolous matter applied, after having either the cow-pox or smallpox. Several months afterwards he was again inoculated with variolous matter, but no sensible effect was produced on the constitution.[1]

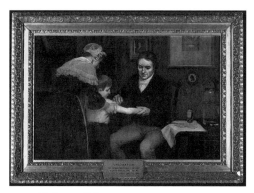

Fig. 1.1 Edward Jenner with James Phipps.
Reproduced courtesy of the Wellcome Library, London.

The term virus as used by Jenner and others later should not be confused with the modern understanding of viruses. At this time the term was used to describe an infectious agent that was extremely small and not visible in the ordinary light microscope, as in the Latin *virus* and *virulentus* which referred to poisons or toxins that cause disease or illness. Although used somewhat indiscriminately during the 1700s and 1800s, it was not until 1898 that Martinus Willem Beijerinck, working in Delft, properly identified the first virus, tobacco mosaic virus, and coined the name, although he thought viruses were liquid in nature. Their particulate nature was confirmed early in the 1900s, notably by the work of Paschen who asserted that the 'elementary bodies' he identified microscopically in cells were the infectious agent of *vaccinia* infection, supported by Negri's work which demonstrated that lymph containing the *vaccinia* virus particles remained infectious after filtration.[2]

By 1780 more than 6000 individuals (that Jenner was aware of through his many colleagues also using his methods) had been inoculated with the cowpox *vaccinae* procedure, with none showing serious reaction to the second stage smallpox challenge. Unknown to Jenner, but providing the foundation for later hypotheses on infection and immunity, the initial challenge with the cowpox virus would have triggered a primary response leading to low-affinity antibodies that were capable of cross-reacting with the smallpox virus. To gain extended protection against smallpox however, the individual had to be subsequently challenged with the smallpox virus itself. This critical insight of Jenner separated him from the variolation 'folklore'. We now know this second inoculation would have invoked a secondary antibody response and an associated antibody affinity maturation process that would have targeted specific smallpox antigens, along with the production of memory B cells, events that were necessary for conferring early protection from the life-threatening smallpox virus and for ensuring lifelong immunity.

It is not the purpose of this example to discuss the complete immunological backdrop to Jenner's experiments, but we do know that the immune responses in Jenner's two-stage vaccinations in 23 different individuals would not have been mediated solely by antibody responses. The description of a pregnant woman who herself had immunity through variation and the presence of smallpox in the infant at birth, which later claimed its life, was a striking example that at any given time scientific knowledge is bounded. The following observation was made on this case, reported by a surgeon colleague and forming part of Jenner's published work:

> In addition to the circumstances the mother conveying the variolous infection to her unborn child, without feeling any indisposition from its action on her own constitution...[3]

This suggested Jenner and his contemporaries could understand that the infectious smallpox virus could be passed to the unborn child by the mother, but the question of why the child was not protected by the same mechanism that protected the mother was outside his comprehension. As John Locke observed:

> No man's knowledge can go beyond his experience.[4]

By the 1930s, it would be shown that 'globulin' is passed from mother to offspring in mammals via the placenta (or yolk sac) and/or via the mother's milk. By the 1950s Brambell and others would demonstrate that the mother's immunoglobulin G (IgG) repertoire is transported by a receptor-mediated mechanism, providing *pari passu* a donor antibody repertoire to combat disease. For the highly virulent smallpox virus this maternal antibody was insufficient to protect the infant in Jenner's patient. The development of the various elements of the cell-mediated immune system, barely developed in the newborn, was later shown to be a critical key component of such anti-viral responses.

Infectious disease and causality

Non-human studies

As so often happens in science, simultaneous discovery propels the body of knowledge forward in leaps rather than small steps. In the nineteenth century the size of the leaps was no less great than the advances of today, but the dissemination of information was much less effective, and peer review not well developed, so that advances were often considered 'misinformed' rather than ground-breaking. Occasionally, significant publications were not seen by contemporaries for some time, as in the scathing attack by Koch on Pasteur in 1881, which took many months after its publication before Pasteur was aware of, or made aware of, its content.[5]

An example of what we now consider a landmark advance, made in the period 1830–40 by the entomologist Alessandro Bassi in Lodi, was not widely appreciated at the time, and in fact had to wait until its rediscovery by Pasteur, whose scientific credentials were better accepted. With hindsight, it is clear that Bassi's work in attributing disease in silkworms to a microorganism made a critical contribution to the demise of spontaneous generation as an explanation of infection. Nonetheless, at the time, his discoveries were treated with severe scepticism, so much so, that in order to convince his peers he agreed to expose his work to public academic review by describing and demonstrating his findings experimentally in front of members of the faculties of medicine and philosophy at the Royal Imperial University of Pavia.[6]

In Berlin, Jakob Henle and his student and later Nobel-Prize-winning scientist Robert Koch were developing an understanding of causative factors in certain animal diseases. Koch's discoveries resulted in a series of cause and effect postulates appearing in his publications in various forms between 1878 and 1884. The 'Koch postulates' provided the foundation for infectious disease aetiology for the next 100 years. Similar studies were being conducted by Pasteur in Paris, although we will return to the special advances made by Pasteur a little later and the conflictual environment in which he and Koch exchanged views on the credibility of their various scientific claims.

It is unlikely that Bassi and Henle or Koch were aware of each other's work, and the further developments that led to the 'Koch postulates' came well after Bassi's death in 1856. So, what was it that was so ground-breaking about Bassi's work and further, why is the work of Koch that much better remembered and acknowledged that that of Bassi? The answer may lie in the fact that Bassi's target was a particular fungal disease of the silkworm known as *muscardine*, of immense importance to the Italian silk industry but of little relevance to the human condition, while Koch's focus was on the study of pathogenic organisms in animals. A further defect in the technical armory of Bassi was that in numerous other studies on diseases of importance in agriculture, Bassi failed to achieve the prime objective for establishing causality, namely that of proving infectivity with a 'pure' preparation of the infectious agent where adventitious carryover of associated material (e.g. virus or soluble toxins) had been eliminated. Despite the shortcomings, the revolutionary procedures to prevent the fungal disease, dictated by Bassi to silkworm farmers in his 1836 *Practica* monograph, had a major impact on the Italian silk industry:

1. Disinfect silkworm (*Bombyx mori*) eggs with calcium chloride, alcohols, or nitric acid.
2. Disinfect containers brought in from outside the farm in a similar way and destroy them.
3. Only use fresh uninfected mulberry leaves as food.
4. Disinfect with boiling water or flames all instruments/implements used in the nursery.
5. The nursery should be kept dust-free and workers should take hygienic measures.
6. If infection arises, destroy the infected silkworms and disinfect all instruments and clothing that have come into contact with the diseased silkworms.[7]

If the above reads like a set of procedures that in modified form could apply to a modern hospital, this only confirms the precocity of Bassi's work.

Infectious diseases in animals—early causality studies

Among some of the most virulent and prevalent diseases in the nineteenth century were cholera, typhus, typhoid fever, anthrax, smallpox, and rabies. Of those, the zoonotic anthrax and rabies were essentially untreatable, with close to 100% mortality. The economic impact on the European farming community of large numbers of sheep and cattle deaths and the ease with which the infection spread to neighbouring herds demanded an understanding of anthrax biology and more importantly, measures for its prevention or cure. In the early 1800s the aetiology of this disease was essentially unknown.

The first recorded identification of 'rod-like' bodies in the blood of sheep was made in 1838 by Onésime Delafond, a veterinary professor at the Ecole d'Alfort (Val-de-Marne). While this was the first description of the 'bacillus', Delafond appears to have failed to understand its importance, as René Valléry-Radot observes in his *Life of Pasteur*:[8]

> *Bien qu'un professeur d'Ecole d'Alfort, M. Delafond montrât à ses élèves dès l'année 1938 qu'il y avait dans le sang charbonneux des petits bâtonnets, comme il les appelait, ce n'était alors pour lui et ses élèves qu'une **sorte de curiosité sans importance scientifique**.*[8] (Author's emphasis.)

> In 1938, Monsieur Delafond, a professor from the Ecole d'Alfort, showed his students the presence of small rods in anthrax-infected blood, which for both him and his students was considered only a curiosity of no scientific importance. (Translated by the author.)

> Text extract reproduced with permission from *La Vie De Pasteur*, René Vallery-Radot, Coll. Acteurs de la Science, p.372, Copyright © Editions l'Harmattan 2009.

The confirmation of Delafond's observation came when Casimir Davaine and Pierre Francois Olive Rayer (in 1850) showed that the blood from infected sheep contained 'small filiform bodies having about twice the length of a blood corpuscle'.[9] Davaine failed to follow this up due to other commitments until 13 years later when, having been presented with blood samples from infected sheep by a local physician, he saw the same 'bodies' which he named *bacteridia*. His conclusion that these were the cause of anthrax was published,[10] but failed attempts by others to repeat his work by innoculation of rabbits with infected blood placed his results in doubt within the scientific community. After all, this was the first suggestion that a living microorganism was responsible for an animal disease!

In Berlin, Robert Koch saw the results of Davaine,[11] and based on his own work with mice, guinea pigs, and rabbits, concluded there was no doubt that *bacillus anthracis* was the causative agent. Despite observations that injection of 'uninfected blood' could also cause anthrax, which Koch explained on the basis of anthrax 'spores' that would be difficult to detect but could ferment in the host blood, and the rather extraordinary view later expressed by Brauell[12] that, even though his own observations supported Davaine's conclusions, all the evidence pointed *against bacteridia* as responsible for the disease, Koch took the position that causality had been established and proposed the now famous 'postulates' in his 1878 paper.[13] The three Koch postulates stated the following (this version is taken from Codell Carter;[14] there are various versions of the postulates and some authors state there are four postulates):

1. The microorganism must be exhibited in all cases of the disease;

2. The distribution of the microorganism must correlate with and explain the disease phenomenon;

3. The microorganism must be distinguishable in some way from organisms that are associated with other diseases.[14]

Of course there were objections to the validity of the postulates, which Koch intended to be general and not just providing a causality basis for anthrax. For example, it was known that in certain circumstances animals were able to carry a given bacillus *asymptomatically* ('carriers'), thus potentially opening to question postulate 2—Koch may not have known about healthy carriers until somewhat later, despite Jenner's observations. In addition, one of Koch's major causation arguments seemed to be that injection of bacilli unrelated to anthrax did not cause the disease in contradistinction from his pure anthrax preparations which did (postulate 3). This latter position had many agnostics since Koch's criterion of 'purity' was based on microscopy—virus particles adhering to the bacilli would obviously not have been visible and smaller 'toxic' soluble substances would certainly have been unidentifiable.

Here was a moment in scientific history in which spontaneous generation was about to be convincingly buried, but it would not go down without a fight from the conservative scientific community. As an example of the nineteenth century spontaneous generation 'fundamentalism' Koch was up against, the famous chemist Leibig's attack on the 'yeast is a plant' theory of fermentation from Schwann (1837) took the form of a satirical article[15] in which he shows Schwann's yeast cell as an animal shaped like a distillation apparatus with sugar going in at the mouth and alcohol coming out of the anus, with carbonic acid exiting from the genitals. It has been said that this attack essentially ruined Schwann's later scientific career.

While Davaine and Koch's explanations were a step forward, the hypothesis would remain unproven until the 'accessory substance' issue had been laid to rest, as Pasteur would do a year after Koch's 1876 paper. In defending his position Koch himself believed it was impossible to make a preparation of anthrax pure enough to dispel the doubts of the scientific establishment, a position he continued to take even as late as 1881 in his public attack on Pasteur's work.[16]

Further questions about the causality model for anthrax, giving some additional fuel to the anti-Koch lobby, arose when Paul Bert published results in 1877[17] that seemed to invalidate the whole concept of 'disease by bacilli'. Bert was a professor of physiology in Paris and an expert on hypoxia (he demonstrated the first barometric chamber to study the effects of oxygen-enhanced air at pressures equivalent to those experienced by balloonists and mountaineers, which paved the way for high-altitude survival procedures). Bert exposed anthrax bacilli to oxygenation (under pressure) and then re-introduced the treated bacilli into animals. The disease was triggered but no *bacteridia* (rods) could be detected in the blood of the exposed animals. As Bert concluded:

> … bacteridia are neither the cause nor necessary effect of splenic fever (anthrax) which must be due to a virus.[17]

The paris approach

Just south-east of the Champs Elysée, other events were taking place. Louis Pasteur, now at the Ecole Normale Supérieur in rue d'Ulm, Montparnasse, began his journey into anthrax studies, prompted by the work of Davaine, Bert, and others. Pasteur's interest in infectious diseases must have been partly driven by the heart-rending loss of three of his children to typhoid fever. The choice of anthrax as his focus was likely to have also been influenced by the outbreak of the disease in sheep and cattle in 1876–7, with its threat to debilitate the French agro-economy.

As often happens in science, unresolved problems where some base understanding has already been established can be attractive targets for those who believe their own creativity and original thinking can provide 'the answers'. The uncertainty of whether anthrax bacillus was the cause of the disease or whether it was due to adhered virus, secreted toxins from the bacilli, or some other co-fermenting bacillus, was still the key question at issue. The experiments of Bert further confused the situation.

So, how did Pasteur lay the ghost and convince the scientific establishment, remembering of course that he was already famous for his discoveries in chemistry (chiral properties using polarized light), the introduction of 'pasteurization' in wine and beer to avoid microbial contamination, and his extension of Bassi's work on microorganism-infected silkworms? His approach was to perform a succession of *in vitro* experiments that were cleverly designed and at the same time scrupulously executed. Dilutions of the anthrax bacillus in successive culture media (dropwise transfer from bottle to bottle of sterile urine) were carried out. After the *n*th dilution, the ability of the final culture to cause the disease was as virulent as the initial preparation. Pasteur's attempt to carry out the defining experiments that would determine once and for all that the anthrax bacillus was the causative agent were described in a key publication in 1877.[18] He recounted the experiment in the paper 'Germ theory and its application to medicine and surgery', published in 1878[19] (reproduced here in the original French):

> *Pour affirmer expérimentalement qu'un organisme microscopique est réellement agent de maladie et de contagion, je ne vois d'autre moyen, dans l'état actuel de la Science, que de soumettre le microbe… à la méthode des cultures successives, en dehors de l'économie. Notons que par douze cultures, chacune d'un volume de 10 centimètres cubes seulement la goutte originelle est diluée autant que si elle l'avait dans un volume liquide égal au volume de la terre. C'est précisément le genre de preuves auquel nous avons soumis la bactéricidie charbonneuse, M. Joubert et moi. Apres l'avoir cultivée un grand nombre de fois dans un liquide prive de toute virulence, chaque culture ayant pour semence une gouttelette de la culture précédente, nous avons constaté que le produit de la dernière culture était capable de se multiplier et d'agir dans le corps des animaux en leur donnant le charbon avec tous les symptômes de cette affection. Telle est la preuve, suivant non indiscutable, que **le charbon est la maladie de la bactéricidie**.[19]* (Author's emphasis.)

To establish experimentally that a microscopic organism is actually the infectious agent, I see no other means in the present state of science, than to submit the microbe… to the method of successive cultures. After one dozen of such successive cultures, the volume of 10cc from the first culture would have been diluted into a volume equal to the volume of the earth. This is precisely the type of proof M. Joubert and I have obtained with anthrax. After cultivation of a highly virulent sample a large number of times, each successive culture containing a droplet from the previous culture was able to multiply in the animal and cause anthrax with all the symptoms of the infection. That is the incontestable proof that the anthrax disease derives from a bacterium. (Translated by the author.)

Pasteur's method was serial dilution of the original anthrax-containing solution until the final infecting solution was so dilute it was as if the original solution had been dissolved in a volume the size of the earth. The volume of the earth is ~10^{24}L. Pasteur's drop size is unknown, but assuming it was ~50µL, each transfer into 10mL would have been a 200x dilution. There were 12 successive dilutions (12 cultures), giving an effective dilution volume of 200^{12} or 10^{27} mL. So, Pasteur's dilution would have been equivalent to suspending his original drop in a volume of 10^{24}L. Voila!

In the 1878 paper Pasteur addressed the fact that in his view Koch had not established causality with anthrax but that he, Pasteur, had demonstrated for the first time and beyond doubt that nothing other than the *bacillus anthracis* could be responsible for the disease, including the elimination of any virus aetiology. As he observed in his concluding comments to this paper:

> … *la bactéridie peut se multiplier dans les liquides artificiels, indéfiniment, sans perdre son action sur l'économie, et il est impossible d'admettre que, dans ces conditions, elle soit accompagnée d'une substance soluble on d'un virus, partageant avec elle la cause des effets du sang de rate ou de la maladie charbonneuse…*[18]

> … the bacteria are capable of multiplying in an artificial medium indefinitely, without loss of their activity, so that it is impossible to accept that, under these conditions, a soluble factor such as a virus shares with the bacterium the cause and effect of splenic fever or anthrax… (Translated by the author.)

The explanation of Bert's observations, provided by Pasteur, lay in the fact that exposure of anthrax to oxygen (under pressure) had destroyed the vegetative form of the bacillus but not the spore form, the latter of which was both infective and undetectable with the methods of the time. Pasteur speculated that Bert's animals had probably died of some other bacterial infection, the most likely of which was septicaemia. Bert subsequently acknowledged Pasteur's explanation in a statement to the Academy of Sciences.[20]

In seeking to gain a further score for French science, Pasteur observed[21] that he had been the first person to unequivocally identify the spore form of bacteria when studying the silkworm diseases in the early 1860s, clearly disputing the claim of Koch.[22] Scientific competitiveness, sometimes given to acerbic expression, was neither new nor unusual. In this instance, the Franco-Prussian war of 1870–1 and its ignition of nationalist tendencies among French and German scientists, already the subject of much historical discussion elsewhere, would certainly have played its part. Koch and Pasteur demonstrated their national allegiances with some vigour, Koch expressing his in a somewhat unprovoked attack on the veracity of Pasteur's work, stating 'Only a few of Pasteur's beliefs about anthrax are new, and they are false…'[23] while Pasteur penned letters to Germany denouncing Prussian militarism and, with a more dramatic statement, returned his honorary MD degree awarded in 1868 by the University of Bonn.

We shall not digress here to describe the gifted further work of Robert Koch as he unravelled the aetiology of tuberculosis and proposed measures for its clinical management, for which he received the Nobel Prize in 1905. The stage was now set for the genesis of 'pre-molecular immunology' on which great actors, such as Metchnikoff, Ehrlich, von Behring, Kitasato, and others (all students or collaborators with Koch) would play their parts.

From disease causality to disease prevention

It is perhaps unfair to label the extraordinary advances in the aetiology of infectious diseases during the 1800s as 'phenomenology' since, although microbiology in this period was still embryonic, its great innovators employed the logical methods of hypothesis and analysis to arrive at conclusions about disease causation, what Karl Popper later called the 'hypothetico-deductive' method. Pasteur's work on wine, silkworms, and beer was an example of this scientific approach at work: observation, interpretation, hypothesis, and testing. It was this methodology that led to the redefinition of 'vaccination', and with it an unprecedented impact on human health.

In his laboratory in Paris Pasteur had *observed* that samples of cholera virus (fowl cholera), a 'microscopic parasite', when cultured in a chicken culture broth exhibited unchanged virulence if the intervals between transfer was relatively short. As the intervals increased, virulence was attenuated until at very long intervals (many months) the cultures, when injected into chickens, failed to cause disease. Extraordinarily, when the same chickens were then challenged with the virulent form, they did not develop the cholera disease but were 'protected'.[24] His *interpretation* was that something had happened to the 'virus' to attenuate its virulence, even though, as he described it, this was still a 'live vaccine'. Exposure to air was one *hypothesis*. To *test* this he made parallel cultures in either open or sealed flasks and carried out virulence tests. Only those preparations exposed to oxygen were attenuated. The essential tenet of Pasteur's view of the protective mechanism was that an attenuated organism would have lost its virulent character due to some alteration induced by oxygen exposure but that when injected into the host it would continue to multiply (i.e. it would still be 'alive') and deplete the host of essential nutrients that would be in limited availability. When the untreated, virulent form of the same organism was then injected it would face a limiting nutrient environment and be inhibited from multiplication. This view of the vaccine effect was consistent with his understanding of the earlier work of Jenner, where he presumed that the non-virulent and virulent forms of his cholera preparations were, by analogy, equivalent to Jenner's non- (or weakly) virulent *vaccinia* (cowpox) preparation and the more virulent *variola* (smallpox) preparation respectively.

Pasteur published his findings in 1880, the year in which he received the Nommé Grand-Croix de la Légion d'Honneur for his contributions to science. Whatever his understanding of the mechanism of attenuation Pasteur had resurrected Jenner, but now the non-virulent but protective agent was derived from a purified preparation rather than a crude extract of skin lesions as in Jenner's *vaccinia* experiments. The implication of attenuation for effective vaccination in the prevention of human disease epidemics was clear to Pasteur as he made his February 1881 presentation to the French Academy of Sciences:[25]

> Truly, there is more here than an isolated fact. We are in possession of a general principle. One may hope that there may be an action inherent in atmospheric oxygen, a natural force always present which will enable us to perform similar attenuations on other viruses.[25]

It was not until October of the same year that Pasteur commented further on the details of his cholera attenuation approach in a short communication to the Academy.[26] Some historians have asserted that he was afraid of competition or that others would not be able to repeat his results. Whatever his motive for holding back some of the details, the results stood head-and-shoulders above those of all others in the field at the time.

When Pasteur referred to 'other viruses', it was an obvious next step for Pasteur to attempt the same treatment on that most virulent of diseases, anthrax. His own assumption that attenuation of the cholera agent was related to its exposure to oxygen now seems like a lucky strike given that the cholera bacillus is in fact an aerobic organism. Nevertheless, this success prompted Pasteur to explore the same approach with the anthrax bacillus. Here, he ran into difficulties since the same treatment would not have destroyed the anthrax spores. At the time, Toussaint, a veterinary professor in Toulouse, had found that attenuation of anthrax could be achieved by treatment at 55°C for ten minutes, a treatment that would have killed the bacillus and inhibited spore formation. Subsequent vaccination by Toussaint of dogs and sheep against controls firmly established a 100% protective effect of the temperature-treated bacilli. The effect on Pasteur, when in August 1880 he received the news from a colleague at the Academy of Sciences, was devastating. Here was a 'dead' microbe giving a protective effect against a highly virulent bacillus when Pasteur's assumptions to date had been that 'attenuated but *live*' preparations were essential to give protection. As he put it in a letter to Toussaint:

> It overturns all the ideas I had on viruses, vaccines etc. I no longer understand anything. Ten times yesterday, I had the idea of taking the train to Paris. I really cannot believe this surprising fact until I've seen it, seen it with my own eyes, though the observation that establishes the fact makes me want to confirm it to my own satisfaction.[27]

From Gerald Geison, The Private Science of Louise Pasteur,
Copyright ©1995 Princeton University Press.
Reprinted by permission of Princeton University Press.

Pasteur's own experiments on attenuation of anthrax appeared to be having limited success using oxygen exposure, probably due to spore resistance to this treatment. Nevertheless, he carried out vaccination studies in sheep, supposedly using the oxygen attenuation method. In parallel with his own work Chamberland, a colleague at the same institute, had demonstrated some success with a variation of Toussaint's approach, who had also attempted Lister's carbolic acid as a method of attenuation, by killing the anthrax organism using chemical treatment with potassium bichromate (a strong oxidising agent that would have had a more drastic effect than oxygen).

As news of Pasteur's small-scale anthrax vaccine experiments in sheep broke, he was offered a challenge by the veterinarian Rossignol in what is probably the most famous public set of experiments ever conducted. The account of the vaccinations at Pouilly-le-fort in May/June 1881[28] demonstrated that of the sheep and cows treated with the attenuated anthrax and then challenged with the unmodified anthrax bacilli, none died, while all the controls either died or showed severe debilitating effects. Pasteur's conclusions were:

> In summary, we now possess a vaccine of anthrax which is capable of saving animals from this fatal disease; a virus vaccine that is itself never lethal; a live vaccine, one that can be cultivated at will and transported without alteration. Finally, this vaccine is prepared by a procedure that we believe can be generalized since, the first time around, this was the method we used to develop a fowl cholera vaccine. Based on all the conditions that I list here, and by looking at everything only from a scientific point of view, the development

of a vaccination against anthrax constitutes significant progress beyond the first vaccine developed by Jenner, since the latter had never been obtained experimentally.[29]

Text extract reproduced from 'Summary Report of the Experiments Conducted at Pouilly-le-Fort, Near Melun, on the Anthrax Vaccination', with permission from *Yale Journal of Biology & Medicine*, Volume 75, pp. 59–62, Copyright © 2002. Originally published in *Comptes Rendus de l'Academie des Science*, Volume 92, pp. 1378–1383, June 13, 1881 by Louis Pasteur (with the collaboration of Mr. Chamberland and Mr. Roux) and translated by Tina Dasgupta, Yale School of Medicine, Original Contributions Editor, *Yale Journal of Biology and Medicine*.

There is some doubt[30] whether the vaccine used at Pouilly-le-Fort was the preparation developed by Pasteur himself, employing oxygen attenuation but not yet refined enough for Pasteur to be sure of its efficacy, or the chemically-attenuated (potassium bichromate) preparation of Chamberland (see Fig. 1.2). Maurice Cassier observes:

Pasteur's laboratory notebooks studied by Cadeddu (1987), and Geison (1995) show that the vaccines used at Pouilly-le-Fort were prepared according to a method of attenuation of microbes by addition of a chemical compound, borrowed from Toussaint, and not the attenuation method by atmospheric oxygen that had been developed by Pasteur. It is nevertheless believed that the commercial vaccines prepared after Pouilly-le-Fort were produced by Pasteur's method which was gradually fine-tuned, as attested by Pasteur's correspondence, Chamberland's writings in 1883–, and Roux's notebooks from 1885 and 1889 (Archives de l'Institut Pasteur, Fonds E. Roux; ROU.4, 'Notes sur le charbon et la vaccination charbonneuse' ('Notes on anthrax and the anthrax vaccine'), document 10612, and 'Vaccines charbonneux: Semences et manipulation' ('Anthrax vaccines: Seeds and manipulation'), document 10611).[31]

Gerald Geison is more explicit, stating:

In his published accounts of the Pouilly-le-Fort trial, Pasteur wrote with the casual assurance of one who had never for a moment doubted the safety or efficacy of the vaccine used

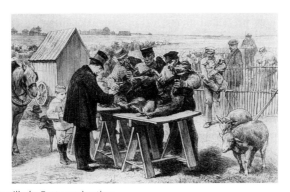

Fig. 1.2 The Pouilly-le-Fort vaccination.
Reproduced with permission of SPL and IBL Bildbyrå, Sweden.

there. Those same public accounts not only failed to disclose but actively misrepresented the nature of the vaccine actually used at Pouilly-le-Fort.[32]

From Gerald Geison, *The Private Science of Louise Pasteur*, Copyright ©1995 Princeton University Press. Reprinted by permission of Princeton University Press.

This doubt was publicly compounded by Robert Koch's attribution of the first proper anthrax 'vaccination' to Toussaint and his continued denigration of Pasteur's contribution.[33] Notwithstanding these criticisms, the results obtained by Pasteur were the first examples of a publicly validated vaccination programme using a purified, attenuated organism. This was truly the beginning of 'immunological' intervention in disease, albeit so far only with farm animals.

The treatment of rabies

During the years 1882 to 1885, Pasteur carried out extensive animal studies on the rabies 'virus' using rabbits to *passage* the virus. In arguably the most important medical advance of the nineteenth century his studies culminated in 1885 in treatment of rabies in man with resounding success.

By passaging in rabbits and using the spinal cord in a series of infections in dogs (up to 90 passages at the time of communicating the 1885 paper), Pasteur had established two features of rabies behaviour. Firstly, removing the spinal cords and exposing them to air for varying periods attenuated the virulence (the longer the exposure, the less virulent or, as Pasteur postulated, the fewer the virus particles remaining in the cord tissue—a further demonstration of Pasteur's belief in the oxygen attenuation theory). Secondly, he established a stable incubation period of eight days in rabbits for the early passages, dropping to seven days for the later passages. By introducing extracts of the rabbit spinal cords intradermally into dogs in a series of innoculations, starting with the least virulent (longest exposure to air) and progressing on to the most virulent, up to 50 dogs had been rendered refractory to the disease. In some instances, dogs already exposed to rabies before 'innoculation' also became protected, facts which Pasteur had already communicated to the French Commission on Rabies and which would have become widely known.

On the 6th July 1885 an extraordinary event occurred. Three people who had been bitten by rabid dogs presented themselves in Pasteur's laboratory. One of these and the most at risk was a 9-year-old boy, Joseph Meister, who had been bitten two days before (see Fig. 1.3). In a decision that would be unethical today, Pasteur decided to test his 'dog procedure' on the boy. He inoculated the boy via an intradermally implanted syringe in the hypochondrium (upper abdominal region) daily over a period of ten days with rabbit cord material that had been exposed to air for 15 days (first inoculation) down to one day (last inoculation). Three months and three weeks later Pasteur presented his findings to the Academy of Sciences.[34] The boy was alive and healthy.

There are a number of interesting features of this story, only possible to elaborate with hindsight. Firstly, and a misnomer not new to us, the rabies infectious

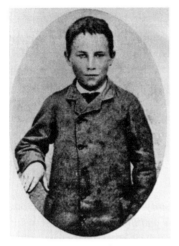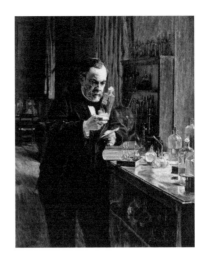

Fig. 1.3 Joseph Meister and Henry Pasteur.
Reproduced with permission of SPL and IBL Bildbyrå, Sweden.

agent was not a microorganism but a neurotropic RNA virus and the air treatment would have affected its viability through the oxidation/aerobic effects on the host nerve cells, the virus itself, or both. Secondly, the *rhabdovirus*, being neurotropic, travels to the brain via the nerve axons from the point of infection. Only when it enters the brain are the encephalitic and associated effects initiated. Thus, in Pasteur's rabbits with relatively short neuronal paths, the incubation period of seven to eight days would have reflected the transit time to the brain. In humans, symptoms may take a month or two to appear, reflecting the considerably longer neuronal path lengths (the speed of axonal transport in humans is about 3mm/hour). Thus, when Pasteur was uncertain about the effectiveness of his procedure for a man who had been bitten some six days previously, he had presumed the rabbit incubation period applied. The man appears to have been protected. Was it luck or simply as Pasteur himself had earlier observed, 'Dans les champs de l 'observation le hasard ne favorise que les esprits préparés', conventionally rendered as 'Chance favours the prepared mind' (quotation from Louis Pasteur's speech at Douai on 7 December, 1854 on the occasion of the formal inauguration of the Faculty of Arts at Douai and of the Faculty of Sciences at Lille (Université Lille Nord de France).

In fact, the boy Joseph Meister would have had ample time to generate his own antibody response, and with the high number of innoculations involved, would almost certainly have generated a high-affinity response of perhaps exceptional effectiveness. Today, rabies post-exposure vaccination is still employed, although normally supplemented by passive immunization with human anti-rabies IgG (from vaccinated human donors) in the early days after presentation.[35]

Reprise

From Jenner to Pasteur, an extraordinary scientific road had been cut into the rocks of ignorance with the help of other giants of innovation, such as Henle, Koch, Davaine, Toussaint, Chamberland, and others. While their advances were impressive even by today's metrics, the one element missing from their work that was about to be unravelled was an explanation of *how* vaccination worked and what changes occurred in the host that led to its protection. In short, *mechanism* was needed, an absence that was soon to be addressed by the application of chemistry and cell biology.

Acknowledgements

Text extracts reproduced from *Studies in History and Philosophy of Science Part C: Studies in History and Philosophy of Biological and Biomedical Sciences*, Volume 36, Issue 4, Cassier, M., Appropriation and commercialization of the Pasteur anthrax vaccine, pp. 722–742, Copyright © 2005, with permission from Elsevier, http://www.sciencedirect.com/science/journal/13698486

References

1. **Jenner, E.** (1798). *An Inquiry into the Causes and Effects of the Variolae Vaccinae, a Disease discovered in some of the Western Counties of England, particularly Gloucestershire, and known by the name of the Cow Pox.* London: Sampson Low; 'The Three Original Publications on Vaccination Against Smallpox.' *Harvard Classics 1909–14*, Vol. **38**, Part 4.

2. **Negri, A.** (1906). 'Über Filtration des Vaccine virus.' *Hyg. InfektKrankh.*, **54**: 327–46.

3. **Jenner, E.** (1809). 'Two cases of small-pox infection communicated to the fœtus in utero under peculiar circumstances, with additional remarks.' *Med Chir Trans.*, **1**: 271–7.

4. **Locke, J.** (1689). *Essay Concerning Human Understanding*, Book II, Ch. 1, sec. 19.

5. **Koch, R.** (1881). 'Zur Ätiologie des Milzbrandes.' *Gesammelte Werke*, **1**: 174–206.

6. **Bassi, A.** (1835) and (1836). *Del Mal del Segno Calcinaccio o Moscardino: Parte Prima: Teoria* (1835) and *Parte Seconda: Practica* (1836).

7. **Porter, R. J.** (1973). 'Agostino Bassi bicentennial (1773–1973).' *Bacteriological Reviews*, **37**: 284–8.

8. **Vallery-Radot, R.** (2009). *La Vie de Pasteur.* France: L'Harmattan, p. 372.

9. **Rayer, P. F. O** (1850). *Comptes Rendus des séances et memoires de la Société de Biologies*, **2**: 141–4.

10. **Davaine, C.** (1863). 'Recherches sur les infusoires du sang dans la maladie connue sous le nom de sang de rate.' *Acad. Sci.*, **57**: 220, 351, 386; Théodoridès, J. (1966). 'Casimir Davaine (1812–1882): a precursor of Pasteur.' *Med Hist.*, **10**(2): 155–65.

11. **Codell Carter, K.** (1988), 'The Koch–Pasteur Dispute on Establishing the Cause of Anthrax.' *Bull. Hist. Med.*, **62**: 42–57.

12. **Brauell, F. A.** (1866). 'Zur Milzbrand-Frage.' *Virchous Archiv.*, **36**: 292–7.

13. **Koch, R.** (1912). 'Untersuchungen uber die Aetiologie der Wundinfektionskrankheiten', in J. Schwalbe (editor), *Gesammelte Werke von Robert Koch*, Vol. 1, pp. 61–108. Leipzig: Georg Thieme.

14. **Codell Carter, K.** (1985). 'Koch's postulates in relation to the work of Jacob Henle and Edwin Klebs.' *Med Hist.*, **29**: 353–74.

15. **Anonymous** (1839). 'Das enträthselte Geheimniss der geistigen Gährung.' *Ann Pharm*, **29**: 100–4; Barnett, J. A. (2003). 'Beginnings of microbiology and biochemistry: the contribution of yeast research.'*Microbiology*, **149**: 557–67.

16. **Koch, R.** (1912). 'Zur Ätiologie des Milzbrandes', reprinted in J. Schwalbe (editor), *Gesammelte Werke von Robert Koch*, Vol. 1, pp. 174–206. Leipzig: Georg Thieme.

17. **Bert, P.** (1877). 'Du virus charbonneux.' *C. R. Mém. Sté Biologie*, séance 20 janvier, p. 70, analysé dans *Gazette des hôpitaux, civils et militaires*, 23 janvier 1877.

18. **Pasteur, L.** (1877). 'Etude sur la maladie Charbonneuse.' *Comptes Rendus de l'Académie des Sciences*; reprinted in R. Vallery-Radot, *Œuvres*, **6**: 164–71.

19. **Pasteur, L.**, Joubert, L., and Chamberland, C. E. (1878). 'La théorie des germes et ses applications à la medicine et à la chirurgie.' *Comptes Rendus de l'Académie des Sciences*, **86**: 1037–43.

20. **Bert, P.** (1877). 'Sur le sang dont la virulence résiste à l'action de l'oxygène comprimé et à celle de l'alcool.' Présenté par Claude Bernard, *Comptes Rendus de l'Académie des Sciences*, **85**: 293.

21. **Pasteur, L.** (1870). *Etudes sur la maladie des vers à soie: moyen pratique assure de la combattre et d'en prévenir le retour.* Paris: Gauthier-Villars; Valléry-Radot, R. (1926). *Oeuvres de Pasteur*, Vol. 4, pp. 153–4; 231–2.

22. **Koch, R.** (1876). 'Die Ätiologie des Milzbrandkrankheit, begründet auf die Entwicklungsgeschichte des Bacillis Anthracis.' Reprinted in J. Schwalbe (editor), *Gesammelte Werke von Robert Koch*, Vol. 1, pp. 5–26.. Leipzig: George Thieme.

23. **Koch, R.** (1876). 'Die Ätiologie des Milzbrandkrankheit, begründet auf die Entwicklungsgeschichte des Bacillis Anthracis.' Reprinted in J. Schwalbe (editor), *Gesammelte Werke von Robert Koch*. Leipzig: George Thieme, p. 185.

24. **Pasteur, L.** (1880). 'De l'attenuation du virus du choléra des poules.' *Comptes Rendus de l'Académie des Sciences*, **91**: 673–80.

25. **Pasteur, L.** (1881). 'De l'attenuation des virus et de leur retour à la virulence.' *Comptes Rendus de l'Académie des Sciences*, **92**; 429–35.

26. **Pasteur, L.** (1881). Comment to the French Academy on the topic 'Sur la cause de l'immunité des adultes de l'espèce bovine contre le charbon symptomatique ou bactérien, dans les localités où cette maladie est fréquente.' *Comptes Rendus de l'Académie des Sciences*, **93**: 608–9.

27. **Geison, G. L.** (1995). *The Private Science of Louis Pasteur*. Princeton, NJ: Princeton University Press, p. 162–3.

28. **Pasteur, L.** (1881). 'Compte rendu sommaire des expériences faites à Pouilly-Le-Fort, près de Meun, sur la vaccination charbonneuse (avec la collaboration de MM. Chamberland et Roux).' *Comptes Rendus de l'Académie des Sciences* **92**: 1378–83.

29. **Pasteur, L.** (2002) (with the collaboration of Mr. Chamberland and Mr. Roux). 'Summary report of the experiments conducted at Pouilly-le-Fort, near Melun, on the anthrax vaccination.'*Yale Journal of Biology & Medicine*, **75**: 59–62. Originally published in *Comptes Rendus de l'Academie des Science*, **92**: 1378–83. Translated by Tina Dasgupta.

30. **Geison, G. L.** (1995). *The Private Science of Louis Pasteur*. Princeton, NJ: Princeton University Press, pp. 151–9.

31. **Cassier, M.** (2005). 'Appropriation and commercialization of the Pasteur anthrax vaccine.' *Stud. Hist. Phil. Biol. & Biomed. Sci.*, **36**: 722–42.

32. **Geison, G. L.** (1995). *The Private Science of Louis Pasteur.* Princeton, NJ: Princeton University Press, p. 171.

33. **Koch, R.** (1884). 'Experimentale Studien über die künstliche Abschwächung der Milzbrandbazillen und Milzbrandinfektion durch Fütterung. Mitteilungen aus dem Kaiserlichen Gesundbeiramte. ' Reprinted in J. Schwalbe (editor), *Gesammelte Werke*, **1**: 232–70.

34. **Pasteur, L.** (1885). 'Méthode pour prévenir la rage après morsure.' *Comptes Rendus de l'Académie des Science*, séance du 26 octobre 1885, CI, p. 765–773 and p. 774.

35. **Hankins, D. G., and Rosekrans, J. A.** (2004). 'Overview, prevention, and treatment of rabies.' *Mayo Clin Proc.*, **79**: 671–6.

Chapter 2

Pre-molecular immunology: The dawn of mechanism

The cellular intrusion

The enormous success of vaccination approaches to disease prevention and cure, enabled through the frontier-pushing work of Jenner, Koch, Pasteur, and others was to have a major impact on mortality in both the domestic animal and more importantly the human population, particularly the fighting soldier, in the early twentieth century. As Fitzgerald observed in 1923, mortality due to typhoid and paratyphoid among members of the Canadian Expeditionary Force in the South African War of 1899–1901 was at a level of almost 20 per 1000. By contrast, after typhoid vaccination, the mortality in the 1914–18 war had dropped to 0.003 per 1000.[1] As Fitzgerald observed, between September 1917–May 1919, and with an average strength of more than two million soldiers in the American Expeditionary Force:

> … there were 213 deaths from typhoid fever. Had the Spanish–American War rate obtained there would have been 68,164 deaths instead of 213. Specific prevention through the use of typhoid vaccine more than any other factor was responsible for this splendid achievement.[1]

No-one doubts the enormous steps made in the late-nineteenth century in the discovery of how to achieve infectious disease control by attenuation of the infective agent and subsequent innoculation of animals or humans. What was lacking was an 'understanding' of just how these attenuated microorganisms induced the protective effect against the virulent form of the infective agent. It was over the turn of the nineteenth century that mechanistic insights began to emerge.

In the Straights of Messina, a Russian zoologist and prodigy, Elie Metchnikoff, was on course to take the scientific establishment into yet more controversy. It was while in his marine laboratory that he began the work that would seek to question current thinking on the role of phagocytic cells in the blood. One of his target organisms was the water flea Daphnia, a small and more or less transparent crustacean. Metchnikoff observed over many hours at a time the course of infection of Daphnia by a fungus he named *Monospora bicuspidata* (he was unsure if it was a yeast or a fungus going through a yeast-like stage). The extraordinary events that Metchnikoff recorded in his paper of 1884[2] were a paradigm of observational science. During the infection of Daphnia by the fungus, he observed attachment of phagocytic 'blood corpuscles' around the spores.

As the spores were taken into the cells, changes in spore morphology were observed that suggested degradation of the spores, or as Metchnikoff expressed it:

> … probably through some sort of secretion—are killed and destroyed. In other words, the blood corpuscles have the role of protecting the organism from infectious materials.[2]

In areas of the body cavity where many cells surrounded the spores (see Fig. 2.1), Metchnikoff described the milieu as:

> … highly inflamed, so much as one can speak of inflammation in a vessel-less animal.[2]

Metchnikoff's observations, while interesting, are less revealing than the language he uses in interpreting these observations. His use of the terms 'killed', 'inflammation', 'destroyed', and his reference to Daphnia's blood corpuscles as '… the bearers of nature's healing power …' were in reality the language of an iconoclast. The scientific icon under attack was the cellular model of Robert Koch in his observations of septicaemia in mice, that the white blood cells 'protected' the bacteria and allowed them to reproduce. Metchnikoff's view of Koch's observations was that the bacteria were '… eaten by the blood cells …'.

Here was a potential mechanism for protection, or perhaps more correctly, resistance, against bacterial infection. Furthermore, the pathological role of inflammation, hitherto considered harmful to the organism, was being proposed as a resistance mechanism. The controversy surrounding Metchnikoff's phagocytic theory and its ramifications has been beautifully explored by Silverstein[3] and others and no more will be said here except to add that one of its strongest opponents, Emil von Behring, was soon to publish results that would shift the balance of scientific opinion towards the humoral explanation of protection and away from cellular mechanisms. Ironically, Metchnikoff and von Behring would both receive the Nobel Prize, but Metchnikoff would have to wait seven years longer and share it with Paul Ehrlich, in what Silverstein suggests may have been an award of 'immunological reconciliation'.[4]

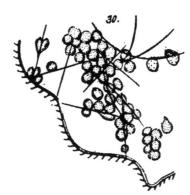

Fig. 2.1 Area of abdomen of another daphnia with intense accumulation of phagocytes around the spores.

von Behring and Kitasato—the humoral *putsch*

Emil von Behring (see Fig. 2.2) studied medicine at the Army Medical College in Berlin. His early research focused on gaining an understanding of the action of a number of widely used wound disinfectants, in particular iodoform (triiodomethane and a source of iodine), in arresting 'putrefaction'. This interest in the iodoform mechanism of action led him through various military appointments, including a period in the Institute of Pharmacology in Bonn under Carl Binz where he broadened his knowledge into bacteriology, and then on to Koch's institute in Berlin in 1889. His assumption that *cadaverine* was a product of the bacteria and toxic to the host led him to propose that such toxins could be responsible for diseases such as cholera,[5] and that the action of iodoform was to chemically neutralize the toxins. While his assumption about *cadaverine* was incorrect (rather than being a toxic product of the bacteria, it is produced during tissue degradation; specifically it is derived from decarboxylation of lysine during protein degradation)—the line of reasoning was to lead von Behring to a more important set of experiments two years later, the conclusions from which would get much closer to releasing the mechanistic genie.

In a critical collaboration, von Behring (now in Berlin) and Shibashaburo Kitasato, who was visiting Koch's laboratory in Berlin, pre-treated tetanus bacilli with iodoform and then injected rabbits with the 'disinfected' preparation. The cell-free blood, or serum, from these animals, when injected into mice, provided complete protection against the virulent form of tetanus.[6] Furthermore, when serum from immunized animals was mixed with the tetanus culture and allowed to incubate for 24 hours prior to administration of the culture, all animals receiving the preparation were protected. No protection was afforded by non-immune serum. This was a profound observation that gave von Behring the ammunition he needed to return to his own studies on diphtheria.

Later in 1890, von Behring reported follow-up experiments in which the tetanus detoxification protocols were tested using diphtheria. Although von Behring's work on using the blood of naturally immune animals (rats and mice) to protect sensitive animals (e.g. guinea pigs) from diphtheria challenge was referred to in the 1890 paper with Kitasato, no experimental evidence was produced. In this second paper[7] von Behring (as single author) describes use of the iodoform pre-treatment approach with diphtheria bacilli with outstanding results. His description of the injection of hydrogen peroxide some days before infection with the diphtheria culture as an alternative means of producing 'immunity' was a clear indication that the serum from exposed animals was believed by von Behring to operate as a chemical disinfectant in these animals, and that such serum contained a 'collection' of disinfectants.

This position was still taken by von Behring in a paper he published a year later:

> Thus, with respect to the therapeutic action of blood taken from other immunized animals, it is of little importance whether it has a direct influence on the bacteria or disables the pathogenic power of the bacterial metabolic product. I believe that I have the right to call both of these alternatives 'disinfection' of the living organism.[8]

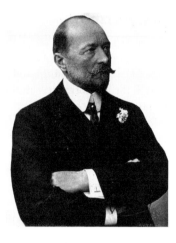

Fig. 2.2 Emil von Behring.
Reproduced courtesy of the Wellcome Library, London.

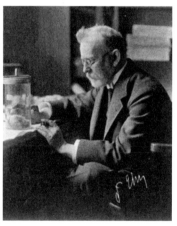

Fig. 2.3 Paul Ehrlich.
Reproduced courtesy of the Wellcome Library, London.

Despite that, what is clear is that the 'preferred' method of inducing immunity by pre-treatment of diphtheria cultures with iodoform was an undoubted success.

The key advance on the work of Pasteur was the observation that donor sera from animals receiving such cultures were able to pass on immunity to recipients. This was a true breakthrough and was to cement von Behring's position as the 'father of serum therapy'. In his Nobel Prize lecture in 1901, von Behring encapsulated his discovery in just a few words:

> If we now introduce the diphtheria serum as an antitoxin into the blood by injecting it under the skin, this antitoxin will reach all parts of the body to which the blood has access... We speak then of immunization or of preventative or prophylactic serum therapy.[9]

These extraordinary results would nurture the next developments in which his colleague Paul Ehrlich, also at the Koch Institute, would play a vital part.

Paul Ehrlich (see Fig. 2.3) was born in Strehlen, Upper Silesia. He studied medicine and during his doctorate in Leipzig in 1878 discovered, amongst other things, mast cells during experiments on histological colouring, the nature of which he postulated must involve chemical interaction between the 'cell' and the dye substance.[10] Shortly afterwards he contracted tuberculosis, and after a convalescence period in Egypt returned to Berlin in 1890, to a small laboratory financed by his father-in-law (who owned a thriving liqueur factory), receiving the appointment of *Professor extraordinarius* (more a personal Chair and typical in medicine) at the University of Berlin. During the next five years Ehrlich was to begin his collaboration with von Behring and breech the mechanism barrier that would set the humoral theory of immunity on an irrevocable course in which the antibody would become the principal runner.

Chemistry, interactions, and specificity

Ehrlich's studies on dyes and their selective staining of tissues and organs provided the blank manuscript on which he would draft small compositions, eventually leading to the great symphonic work describing specific toxin-antitoxin recognition and complement-mediated cell lysis. His preoccupation with redox dyes and their use in measuring the physiological status of specific biological 'targets' was a key platform for the later discoveries. In the early 1980s his focus was clinical diagnostics (under Frerich at the Charité hospital in Berlin), illustrated by development of the *bilirubin diazo* urine test, where sulfodiazobenzene added to urine triggered a colour change on reaction with bilirubin and/or its various forms (e.g. urobilinogen).[11] This test, involving a specific interaction of the dye with the tetrapyrrole moieties in bilirubin, turned out to be a good prognostic indicator for pneumonia and pleurisy.

It was during Ehrlich's *habilitation* (requirement to become a teaching professor) thesis in 1885 that his chemical intuition led to the proposal of a 'side-chain' theory to explain the binding of oxygen in the cytoplasm (protoplasm) of cells. By exposing animals to dyes (by infusion) and then performing time-dependent tissue analysis he could determine the oxygen 'affinity' of the various tissues via the dye uptake. However, it would be some 12 years before his side-chain notion was revisited in the context of toxin neutralization.

After his illness (tuberculosis) and convalescence in Egypt, Ehrlich was appointed as clinical supervisor in 1890 at the Hospital Berlin-Moabit by Robert Koch. It was here that the interaction with von Behring and Wassermann revitalized his interest in questions of theoretical immunology and their application in the clinical arena. While there he was asked to look at a critical issue of standardizing the dose of the diphtheria vaccine (antitoxin) developed by von Behring and being produced by the Hoechst Company. One of the issues was the variation in serum strengths prepared using diphtheria toxin as immunogen. Highlighting the magnitude of these discrepancies, *The Lancet* published its tests on nine different 'antitoxin' preparations from Germany, Britain, France, Belgium, and Switzerland, and the unacceptable variations therein.[12]

Ehrlich's contribution to the standardization of antitoxin units was ground-breaking. First, he observed that different cultures of *Corynebacterium diphtheria* produced different levels of toxin. Clearly the standardization of neutralization units could differ radically depending on the strain used, the age of the preparation, and the storage conditions. For example, if 50% of an antitoxin unit was added to the L_0 dose of toxin, the toxicity was not necessarily reduced by 50%, but could vary between 25% and 75%. Ehrlich developed procedures in which toxin and antitoxin preparations were dried and preserved as powders under vacuum, at low temperature and protected from light. Standard dilutions could then be repeatedly made at intervals, potentially without loss of activity of either component but where the activity of the serum was used as the standard since it was more stable than the toxin under storage. In this procedure two units of activity were proposed by Ehrlich. The first, L_0, was the amount of toxin which is completely neutralized by one unit of antitoxin in a guinea pig model (i.e. no death observed). The quantity L_+ represented the excess toxin required to exceed the neutralization dose such that a guinea pig (250g) exposed to this dose died by the fourth day.[13]

In parallel, similar methods had been designed by Emil Roux at the Pasteur Institute and were adopted in France. Roux's procedure—1mL of horse serum able to neutralize 20mL of a toxin solution, 0.1mL of which was able to kill a 500g guinea pig in 48h—differed from Ehrlich's standard procedure, although the neutralization units of the two approaches could be rationalized by a simple proportionality factor.

The observations that the toxicity and neutralization doses did not always correlate were critical observations in Ehrlich's attempts to understand the phenomena underlying diphtheria toxin-antitoxin interactions. The *loss* of *in vivo* toxicity on storage with *retention* of antitoxin binding units required explanation. How could toxicity decrease while 'binding' of the toxin by antitoxin remained? Ehrlich's insight led him to propose that there were different toxin components present, with differing 'affinities' for the antitoxin. The *toxophore Gruppe* was responsible for the *in vivo* toxicity and a secondary *haptophore Gruppe* present in the same toxin molecule mediated the antitoxin binding. Toxins which lacked or had lost the ability to kill but which retained antitoxin binding were called *toxoides*. These 'feeble' toxins had varying affinities for antitoxin—Ehrlich classified them as proto-, deutero-, and tritotoxins which subsequently degraded into proto-, deutero-, and tritotoxoids. These various toxoid species present generated a *Giftspektrum* in which the toxoid elements of differing affinities were consecutively neutralized.[14] Ehrlich's graphical explanation of this (see Fig. 2.4) revealed his prejudice for a chemical bonding model of toxin-antitoxin interaction, essentially requiring an irreversible (chemical) union.

In reality the multiple species present should have been a continuous curve but Ehrlich chose to represent it as a series of step neutralizations. This stepwise picture would only be seen if the highest affinity toxoid were to bind irreversibly until it was almost completely sequestered, followed by the next highest affinity and so on. This would occur of course if toxoid/toxin-antitoxin reactions formed covalent bonds on binding.

Immunology meets physical chemistry

It was in the interpretation of the solution behaviour of these mixtures that Ehrlich came firmly up against the Swedish physical chemist Svante Arrhenius and his Danish physician and bacteriologist colleague Thorvald Madsen. Arrhenius and Madsen accepted that different diphtheria toxoid species would be present but disagreed with

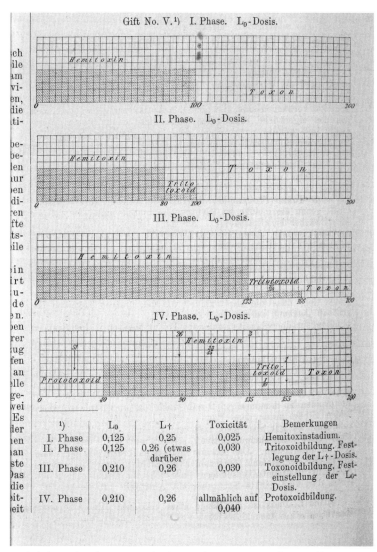

Fig. 2.4 Ehrlich's *Giftspektrum*[13] in which toxoid species with differing affinities are successively neutralized in a stepwise fashion (Phase I = > II = > III = > IV), as measured by remaining toxicity of diphtheria toxin, measured *in vivo*, as a function of added antitoxin.

Reproduced from Ehrlich, P, 'Die Wertbemessung des Diptherieheilserums und deren theoretische Grundlagen', KlinischeJahrbuch, Issue 6, pp. 299–326, 1897–8.

Ehrlich that the toxoid-antitoxin interaction was essentially 'irreversible', as suggested in Ehrlich's side-chain theory. Arrhenius took the view that such interactions were essentially driven by mass action, analogous to the manner in which a weak acid (e.g. boracic acid) would be neutralized by a weak base (e.g. ammonia). Thus, rather than the highest affinity toxoid being completely neutralized first, followed by the second highest affinity and so on as proposed by Ehrlich, the antitoxin interaction with all species would be driven by the laws of mass action as developed by the Norwegians, Guldberg and Waage.[15,16,17]

In their 1864 and 1867 papers Guldberg and Waage proposed that for the simple reaction

$$A + B = A' + B'$$

where A and B were typically simple ionic salts such a mixture of barium and potassium sulphates and carbonates, there would be an equilibrium driven by 'chemical forces' between molecules (their interatomic 'affinity') and that the rates of forward and backward reactions would depend on the strength of the chemical forces for the different species and by the relative concentrations of reactants. The key statement was that at a certain limiting situation *all four* substances would be present at the same time in equilibrium where forward and backward reactions were occurring simultaneously. This clearly would not be the case for an irreversible reaction between A and B where if A is a toxoid and B is an anti-toxin, and A and B have the same molar concentration, the reaction would proceed to form AB until no A or B remains, assuming a one-to-one stoichiometry.

The picture was further complicated by the fact that Ehrlich's toxin mixture contained multiple A species (toxoid, toxons etc.) at different concentrations, each with a different affinity for the anti-toxin. Adopting the reversible equilibrium approach in an extensive analysis of tetanus toxin, reported in 1902 on the occasion of the inauguration of the Danish Serum Institute in Copenhagen, Arrhenius and Madsen painted a radically different picture to that of Ehrlich and his 'step diagram'. Their study looked at the haemolytic activity of tetanus toxin (called tetanolysin) when titrated with anti-toxin. Their results are shown in Fig. 2.5 where the toxic quantity remaining, x obs (x observed), was plotted against the amount of anti-toxin added (n). The broken line (right-hand y-axis) shows the corrected toxicity (G) as a function of anti-toxin added. The conclusions from Arrhenius and Madsen were demonstrably at odds with those of Ehrlich:

> It appears that the values of x obs increase continuously and gradually with n. In consequence the G obs continuously decrease with increasing n. There is therefore no reason for drawing the G curve (the previously so-called 'toxinspectrum') as a line, formed like stairs, this would also be very improbable...[18]

Arrhenius would continue to plough the 'partial dissociation' furrow, maintaining his view that toxin-antitoxin neutralization could be explained by simple reversible equilibria.[19] Despite this scientific attack on his interpretation, Ehrlich stubbornly defended his assertion that toxoid and antitoxin formed a 'chemical' bond. Even as late as 1908, during his Nobel lecture, when considering the origin of the specificity of tetanus toxin for its antitoxin and diphtheria toxin for its 'antipode', he stated:

> ... the antipodes enter into a chemical bond which in view of its strict specificity is most easily explained by the existence of groups... which according to the comparison made by Emil Fischer fit each other by 'lock and key'. Considering the stability of the bond on

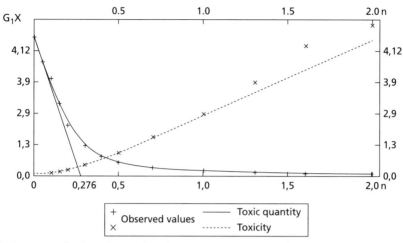

Fig. 2.5 Neutralization of tetanolysin by antitoxin. Reproduced from reference 18 with permission.

Reproduced from Arrhenius, S. and Madsen, T, 'Physical Chemistry applied to toxins and antitoxins' in *Festskrift ved indvielsen af Statens Seruminstitut 1902: Contributions from the University Laboratory for Medical Bacteriology to Celebrate the Inauguration of the State Serum Institute*, (Copenhagen: Olsen, 1902), III, pp. 58–59, with permission from the Statens Serum Institut.

> the one hand and the fact on the other that neutralization occurs even in very great dilu-
> tions... it must be assumed that this process... represents an analogue to actual chemical
> synthesis.[20]

This position would continue to be a cause for disagreement between Arrhenius and Ehrlich, although even contemporary physical chemistry 'giants' such as van't Hoff, Ostwald, and Nernst remained baffled by the apparent bonding contradictions. These scientific disagreements were not totally objective. When Arrhenius was appointed as a member of the Swedish Academy of Science in 1901 and sat on the Nobel Prize chemistry committee, views were expressed that Arrhenius' friends, van't Hoff, Ostwald, and others were likely to receive preference over his 'enemies', Ehrlich and Nernst. After Arrhenius' presentation of his 1904 paper, Nernst was critical of his interpretation if somewhat restrained in his language:

> If one assumes Arrhenius' idea of equilibrium, I cannot understand how to explain immu-
> nization. The bonding is supposed to be loose. But, in general, it is assumed that the free
> toxin is anchored by the tissues.[21]

And further:

> ... the concept of a reversible process collides with the facts...[21]

In this period of extraordinary discovery, the influence of Leibig's chemistry 'school' and the notion that specificity was linked to chemical 'bonding' continued to dominate the interpretive predispositions of even those scientists at the frontiers of the new immunology. This would slowly change.

Theoretical models and immunological reality

In his Croonian Lecture to the Royal Society of London in 1900 Ehrlich, then director of the Royal Prussian Institute of Experimental Therapeutics in Frankfurt, recapitulated his side-chain theory of 1897, with some considerable embellishment. In building the case he drew attention to a number of key observations, both by himself and others who observed that the toxicity of tetanus toxin post-injection could be reversed by antitoxin injection only for a limited period after dosing. This was explained as a time-dependent process of redistribution of toxin from the blood to the tissues. As the interval was extended the antidote effect could continue to be reversed by over-dosing of antitoxin until a time limit was reached, after which the toxin effect became irreversible. In interpreting this irreversible stage Ehrlich drew on his great love for dye chemistry:

> ...one was obliged to come to the conclusion that the union between toxine and the tissues, which could only be overcome by means of a specific chemically-related antagonizing agent, must itself depend on a chemical combination.[22]

Despite this chemical bond preoccupation, Ehrlich displayed outstanding insight as he developed his arguments. The tissue receptors to which the toxin molecules bind served normal functions in the animal and

> only incidentally and by pure chance possess the capacity to anchor themselves to this or that toxine.[22]

Here then was the concept of 'cross-reactivity' at the molecular level. But what were the 'receptors' to which toxin was bound fortuitously? Ehrlich supposed they were normal 'nutrient' receptors:

> We are obliged to adopt the view that the protoplasm is equipped with certain atomic groups, whose function especially consist in fixing to themselves certain food-stuffs, of importance to the cell life.[22]

As toxin levels began to saturate these food receptors, a regeneration process would be triggered resulting in an over-production and release into the blood of soluble receptors, viz antitoxin molecules. This was in accord with the stress-induced hyper-regeneration postulate of the pathologist Karl Weigert (who was also his cousin and from whom he learnt about aniline dyes in tissue staining[23]).

Quite extraordinarily, Ehrlich used language that immunologists would return to much later:

> In the course of the progress of typical systematic immunization, as this is practiced in the case of diphtheria and tetanus toxine especially, the cells become, so to say, educated or trained to reproduce the necessary side-chains in ever-increasing quantity.[22]

Ehrlich illustrated this nutrient receptor behaviour in his famous diagram (see Fig.2.6) from the Croonian Lecture, illustrating the following stages:

- challenge with toxin;
- cross-reactive recognition by particular nutrient receptors on cells from relevant tissues;
- over-production and secretion of soluble receptors (antikörper = antibodies).

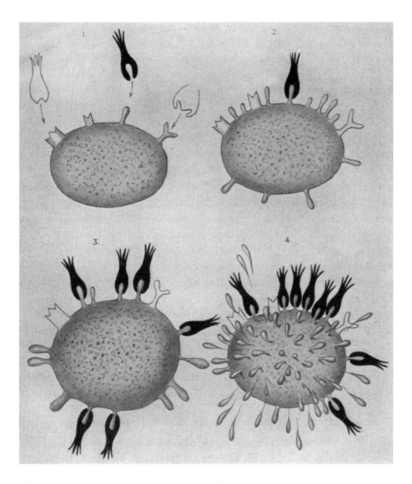

Fig. 2.6 Ehrlich's representation of the union of 'toxine' molecules with side-chains of the 'cell protoplasm' by means of their 'haptophore groups' as the first step in a toxic action.

Reproduced from Plate 6, Ehrlich, P., 'On Immunity with Special Reference to Cell Life', Royal Society Croonian Lecture 1900, in *Roy.Soc.Proc.* 1900, 66, pp. 424–448, Copyright © The Royal Society, with permission from the Royal Society, London, UK.

So, a mechanism for antitoxin production *in vivo* was proposed. However, scientific life is never that straightforward. An apparently simple model would need revision if several other biological effects were to be reconciled, effects that would yet again position Ehrlich against contemporaries such as Bordet and the developing Viennese 'unitarians' Buchner, von Gruber, and later Karl Landsteiner.

Antitoxins, agglutination, and cell lysis

In 1899 Ehrlich and his colleague Julius Morgenroth published the first of their papers[24] spanning six years of work on the action of anti-red blood cell antibodies (now referred to as 'immunkörper' or immune-body) raised by cross-species immunization. There followed five more papers between 1899 and 1901.[25] The antisera caused agglutination and red blood cell lysis or 'haemolysis' as Ehrlich called it. In 1895 Jules Bordet, the Belgian immunologist, published similar agglutination results for bacteria and in 1899 published his own hypothesis of the 'haemolysis' phenomenon,[26] mediated by the lytic substance 'alexine'. Their views on the mechanism of agglutination and cell lysis were diametrically opposed.

Ehrlich and his supporters favoured an expanded side-chain model in which the duality of antigen (bacteria or red blood cell) and alexine (or 'complement' as Ehrlich preferred to call the substance) recognition resided within the same 'amboreceptor' (an immune-body containing two haptophore groups).[27] Since each amboreceptor was specific for each antigen it met, Ehrlich was required to postulate a different complement substance for each lytic ensemble. This dual recognition process was illustrated in the second of his diagrams presented during the Croonian Lecture and shown in Fig. 2.7 (the amboreceptor is shown in the lower left as a dual specificity 'bridging' antibody in light grey, with recognition of both the cell and the complement molecule in black).

In contrast, Bordet proposed that the lysis (of bacteria) was due to an initial sensitization of the bacteria to alexine by the antibodies present in the serum after which the alexine would then exert its destructive effect. Explicit in Bordet's model was the absence of any direct interaction of antibody and alexine. Further, he proposed that in any serum there was a single, temperature-sensitive alexine substance that participated in all 'lytic' actions mediated by an immune serum. Bordet's mechanistic position was also taken by the Vienna group, exemplified by Buchner's argument[28] that the idea that two pre-existing substances, alexine (which Buchner himself had discovered) and amboreceptor should be required to interact prior to their action on the target cell was a contradiction to the notion of 'economy of thinking' (see Pauline Mazumdar's translation of Buchner's 1900 paper[29]).

Ehrlich himself was faced with several consequences of his model that required either explanation or dismissal. The first, which he dismissed as unlikely, was the possibility that immune-bodies, or antibodies, against self-molecules could lead to autoimmune disease. In describing this phenomenon as a *'horror autotoxicus'*[30] Ehrlich recognized the consequences if such autoimmune events were triggered. His presumption that physiological mechanisms existed to prevent such triggering (based on his own experimental attempts to induce such autoimmunity) would eventually be shown to be correct, but the seriousness with which the immunological community adopted this 'unlikely' view of autoimmunity would, as Arthur Silverstein notes, hamper research in the area for half a century.[31]

A further obstacle Ehrlich encountered was the *ad ridiculum* corollary that for every antigen there was a specific nutrient receptor, or antibody (antitoxin), and for each cellular lytic event there was a different immune-body (amboreceptor) with its own specific complement molecule. This proliferative model understandably received considerable scepticism. What evolutionary pressure would there have been for an organism to orchestrate a complete spectrum of nutrient receptors specific for all known antigens? The ridicule was particularly strong from the Vienna group of Buchner and von Gruber, the latter of whom criticized Ehrlich for 'too much fantasy and too little criticism'.[32]

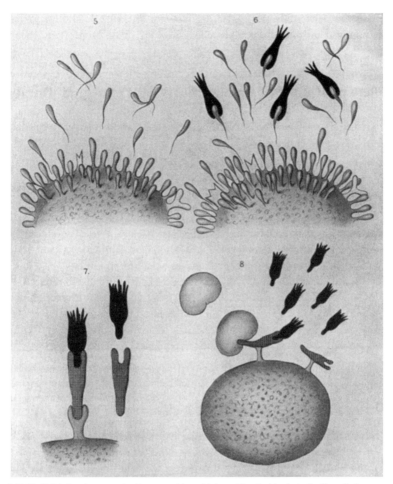

Fig. 2.7 Ehrlich's 'amboreceptor' concept in which antitoxin binds to both cellular side-chains and an 'alexine' molecule.

Reproduced from Plate 7, Ehrlich, P., 'On Immunity with Special Reference to Cell Life', Royal Society Croonian Lecture 1900, in Roy.Soc.Proc. 1900, 66, pp. 424–448, Copyright © The Royal Society, with permission from the Royal Society, London, UK.

In 1901, at the Institut Pasteur, the Polish bacteriologist Jean Danysz described a phenomenon with ricin which added further complexity to the toxin-antitoxin 'proportionality' debate and fuelled yet more exchanges between the Ehrlich and Bordet camps. When equivalent toxin and antitoxin amounts were added in one step, Danysz confirmed Ehrlich's result that neutralization was observed. However, when the same quantity of toxin was split into fractions and added over time to antitoxin, the neutralization was only partial. In other words, delaying the addition of toxin somehow either caused a change in the toxin so as to make it less avid for the antitoxin while retaining its toxicity, or the antitoxin was altered by its encounter with toxin. This behaviour (known as the Danysz effect) was clearly a blow for Ehrlich, and also for Arrhenius. Bordet pounced on this observation to question the 'fixed proportions' theory by stating:

> The point of importance is that these reactions differ from those of ordinary chemistry in that they are not expressed by equations: the proportions in which the substances unite vary according to the conditions of the experiment.[33]

In fact, it would be some considerable time before the Danysz effect was explained. As late as 1942 Pappenheimer stated:[34]

> Any theory of the toxin-antitoxin reaction should include an explanation of the following familiar phenomena:
> 1) The Danysz effect
> 2) The discrepancy between Ehrlich's L_0 and L_+ doses of toxin...[34]

Pappenheimer's explanation was based on the existence of a series of equilibria involving soluble and insoluble complexes. If toxin (T) and antitoxin (A) are added at their equivalent proportions, soluble complexes would form of the type TA and TA_2. However, if a smaller amount of T is added, higher-order complexes of high A, low T stoichiometry would form (e.g. TA_3 and TA_4). With subsequent further addition of T, the depleted A molecules would give an equilibrium mixture with an excess of free T. Some 15 years later Cinader used an enzymatic toxin model (based on the lecithinase from *Cl. welchii*) to confirm the aggregation hypothesis, concluding:

> The Danysz effect is shown to depend not only on the combination of antigen and antibody in multiple proportions but also on... restricted combination of compounds containing antibody with further antigen. This second reaction can be accounted for as the aggregation of the initial compound of antigen and antibody.[35]

The detailed molecular explanation would have to wait a further 20 years. The instability of diphtheria toxin due to proteolytic 'nicking' during preparation and storage (something Ehrlich would have been unaware of when he developed his method for preparation of stable toxin preparations), the cross-reactivity of toxin and nicked toxoid molecules with antitoxin antibodies, and the multi-epitope collection of antibodies raised during an immunization would eventually provide the key to the Danysz effect more than 70 years after its observation.[36]

A side-chain epilogue

It may be that Ehrlich was his own worst enemy in these often unpleasant debates, in which he appeared to draw regularly on diagrams and pictures to prove his point.[37] He seemed fully aware of and perhaps sensitized to the limitations of such 'immunological imagery', as he indicated in his Croonian Lecture:

> I have deemed it advisable to represent by means of some purely arbitrary diagrams (Plates 6 and 7) the views I have expressed regarding the relations of the cell considered in the manner I have been describing. Needless to say, these diagrams must be regarded quite apart from all morphological considerations, and as being merely a pictorial method of

presenting my views on cellular metabolism, and the method of toxine action and antitoxine formation during the process of immunisation.[38]

During their numerous exchanges, Jules Bordet referred to Ehrlich's graphical representations in his 1920 treatise on immunological infections as 'puerile' and suggested that their superficiality concealed the true inner meaning of what they were attempting to represent.

There is still a long-standing debate about the ability of visual imagery in communication to persuade the viewer or reader of the correctness of the scientific facts that models portray. As Kaplan observes:

> The danger is that the model limits our awareness of unexplored possibilities of conceptualization. We tinker with the model when we might be better occupied with the subject matter itself… incorporating it [our knowledge] in a model does not automatically give such knowledge scientific status.[39]

Not that such apparently *faux* imagery was restricted to Ehrlich. We have previously seen its power in the destructive criticism of Schwann by Leibig.[40] von Gruber himself used it to good effect when attempting to discredit Ehrlich's 'lysis' mechanism via a scurrilous letter from a 'Dr Phantasus', addressed to von Gruber, proposing that since water was able to lyse red blood cells, it must *strictu sensu* possess a multitude of water-toxins and toxoids (the Ehrlich–von Gruber exchanges are vividly reproduced by Pauline Mazumdar[41]).

In attempting to explain the various phenomena associated with toxin-antibody interactions or neutralization, observed both *in vitro* and *in vivo*, Ehrlich's contemporaries began to be drawn towards a different physical explanation. The rising scientific star whose studies would take an understanding of antibody mechanism one step further was a chemist turned immunologist, Karl Landsteiner.

References

1. Fitzgerald, J. G. (1923). 'Louis Pasteur—His contribution to the anthrax vaccination and the evolution of a principle of active immunization.' *California State Journal of Medicine*, **21**(3): 101–3.

2. Metchnikoff, E. (1884). 'Ueber eine Sprosspilzkrankheit der Daphnien. Beitrag zur Lehre über den Kampf der Phagocyten gegen Krankheitserreger.' *Archiv für Pathologische Anatomie und Physiologie und für Klinische Medecin*, **96**: 177–95. English version courtesy of the American Association of Microbiology archives.

3. Silverstein, A. M. (2009). *A History of Immunology* 2e. New York: Academic Press, pp. 25–35.

4. Silverstein, A. M. (2009). *A History of Immunology* 2e. New York: Academic Press, p. 37.

5. von Behring, E. A. (1888). 'Zur Kenntnis der physiologischen un der (cholerähnlichen) toxischen Wirkungen des Pentamethylendiamins (Cadaverin L. Brieger).' *Deutsche Med. Wochenschr.*, **14**(6), Nr. 24, 477–8.

6. **von Behring, E. A., and Kitasato, S.** (1890). 'Ueber das Zustandekommen der Diphtherie-Immunitat and der Tetanus-Immunitat bei Thieren.' *Deutsch Med. Wochenschr.*, **4**(12), Nr. 49, 1113–14.

7. **von Behring E. A.** (1890). 'Untersuchungen uber das Zustandekommen der Diphtherie-Immunitat and der Tetanus-Immunitat bei Thieren.' *Deutsch Med. Wochenschr.*, **11**(12), Nr. 50, 1145–8.

8. **von Behring, E. A.** (1891). 'Ueber Desinfection am lebenden Organismus.' *Deutsch Med. Wochenschr.*, **24**(12), Nr. 52, 1393–7.

9. **von Behring, E. A.** (1967). 'Serum therapy in immunity and medical science. Nobel Lecture, 1901.' *Nobel Lectures, Physiology or Medicine 1901–1921.* Amsterdam: Elsevier.

10. **Ehrlich, P.** (1878). 'Beiträge zur Theorie and Praxis der Histologischen Färbung.' Thesis, Leipzig University.

11. **Ehrlich, P.** (1883). 'Sulfodiazobenzol, ein Reagenz auf Bilirubin.' *Zentraalblatt für kilinische medizin*, **4**: 721–3.

12. **Report of The Lancet Special Commission** (1896) on the 'Relative serum strengths of diphtheria antitoxic serums.' *The Lancet*, **148**: 182–95.

13. **Ehrlich, P.** (1897–8). 'Die Wertbemessung des Diptherieheilserums und deren theoretische Grundlagen.' *KlinischeJahrbuch*, **6**: 299–326.

14. **Ehrlich, P.** (1898). 'Ü.d. Constitution des Diphtheriegiftes.' *Deutsche Med. Wochenschr.*, **24**(38): 597–600.

15. **Guldberg, C. M., and Waage, P.** (1864). 'Avhandl. Nomke Videnskws-Akademi Oslo' *Mat. Natorv. Kl.*, **35**.

16. **Guldberg, C. M., and Waage, P.** (1864). 'Etude sur les affinités.' *Les Mondes*, **12**: 107–13.

17. **Guldberg, C. M., and Waage, P.** (1867). 'Etudes sur les affinités chimique.' Christiania, 1867; Ostwald's Klassiker, 104.

18. **Arrhenius, S., and Madsen, T.** (1902). 'Physical chemistry applied to toxins and antitoxins' in *Festskrift ved indvielsen af Statens Seruminstitut 1902: Contributions from the University Laboratory for Medical Bacteriology to Celebrate the Inauguration of the State Serum Institute* III, pp. 58–9. Copenhagen: Olsen.

19. **Arrhenius, S.** (1904). 'Die Serumtherapie vom physikalisch-chemischen Gesichtspunkte.' *Z. f. Elektrochem.*, **10**: 661–8.

20. **Ehrlich, P.** (1908). 'Partial cell functions. Nobel Lecture, 11 December, 1908', in *Chemistry 1901–1921.* Amsterdam: Elsevier.

21. **Nernst, W.** (1904). 'Diskussion zu den Vortrage von Arrhenius über Serumtherapie.' *Z. f. Elektrochem.*, **10**: 668–79.

22. **Ehrlich, P.** (1900). 'On Immunity with Special Reference to Cell Life.' Royal Society Croonian Lecture 1900, in *Roy. Soc. Proc.*, **66**: 424–48.

23. **Rubin, L. P.** (1980). 'Styles in Scientific Explanation: Paul Ehrlich and Svante Arrhenius on Immunochemistry.' *Hist. Med. Allied Sci.*, **35**: 397–425.

24. **Ehrlich, P., and Morgenroth, J.** (1899). 'Zur Theorie der Lysinwirkung.' *Berl. Klin. Wochenschr.*, **36**: 6–9.

25. **Mazumdar, P. M. H.** (1995). *Species and Specificity.* Cambridge: Cambridge University Press, pp. 119–20.

26. **Bordet, J.** (1899). 'Agglutination et dissolution des globules rouges par le serum: deuxieme mémoire.' *Annales de l'Institute Pasteur*, **13**: 273–97.

27. **Ehrlich, P., and Morgenroth, C.** (1901). 'Über Hämolysine: sechste Mittheilung.' *Berl. Klin. Wochenschr.*, **38**: 569–74 and 598–604.

28. **Buchner, H.** (1900). 'Zur Kenntniss der Alexine, sowie deren specifisch-bactericiden und specifisch-haemolytischen Wirkung.' *Münch. Med. Wochenschr.*, **47**: 277–83.

29. **Mazumdar, P. M. H.** (1995). *Species and Specificity.* Cambridge: Cambridge University Press, pp. 121–2.

30. **Ehrlich, P., and Morgenroth, C.** (1901). 'Über Hämolysine: funfte Mittheilung.' *Berl. Klin. Wochenschr.*, **38**: 251–7.

31. **Silverstein, A. M.** (2009). *A History of Immunology* 2e. New York: Academic Press, pp. 154–64.

32. **von Gruber, M.** (1903). 'Toxin und antitoxin. Eine Replik auf Herrn Ehrlichs Entgegnung.' *Münchener Med. Wochenscr.*, **50**: 1825–8.

33. **Bordet, J.** (1903). 'Sur le mode d'action des antitoxines sur les toxines.' *Ann. L'Institut Pasteur.*, **17**: 161–86.

34. **Pappenheimer Jr., A. M.** (1942). 'Studies on diphtheria toxin and its reaction with antitoxin.' *J Bacteriology*, **43**: 273–89.

35. **Cinader, B.** (1957). 'The Danysz effect: an investigation of the reaction between an enzyme and its antibody.' *Br. J. Exp. Pathol.*, **38**: 362–76.

36. **Collier, R. J.** (1975). 'Diphtheria Toxin: Mode of Action and Structure.' *Bacteriol. Rev.*, **39**: 54–85.

37. **Marquart, M.** (1949). *Paul Ehrlich.* London: Heinemann.

38. **Ehrlich. P.** (1900). 'On Immunity with Special Reference to Cell Life.' Royal Society Croonian Lecture, in *Roy. Soc. Proc.*, **66**: 437.

39. **Kaplan, A.** (1964). *The Conduct of Enquiry: Methodology for Behavioural Science.* San Franciso: Chandler, p. 279.

40. **Anonymous** (1839). 'Das enträthselte Geheimniss der geistigen Gährung.' *Ann Pharm*, **29**: 100–104; Barnett, J. A. (2003). 'Beginnings of microbiology and biochemistry: the contribution of yeast research.'*Microbiology*, **149**: 557–67.

41. **Mazumdar, P. M. H.** (1995). *Species and Specificity.* Cambridge: Cambridge University Press, pp. 123–35.

Chapter 3

Structural chemistry: Locks, keys, and colloids

Landsteiner and post-Ehrlich developments

The breakthroughs of the Koch, von Behring, Pasteur, and Ehrlich era, though dramatic in relation to the *status quo* of contemporary chemistry and biology, were yet to explain the molecular basis of antibody action on toxins and viruses. While immunology made giant strides with its vaccine and immune serum advances, structural chemistry was uncertain about the exact nature of the large molecules that mediated those immunological effects. This was due in no small part to the confused perception of proteins, substances that were still somewhat 'mysterious' bodies. A number of proteins, well known to contain amino acids, had been crystallized,[1] although no structural methods (e.g. x-ray crystallography) were yet available to characterize such crystals. The structure of proteins as linear amino acid chains had been proposed by Emil Fischer, based on synthesis experiments, but analytical methods were too primitive to provide convincing evidence to gain widespread support for the idea that a protein with a molecular weight of 2000–6000 (proposed for albumin) could consist of a single linear chain of amino acids. While amino acids were known to be the products of protein hydrolysis, their large variety provided a conceptual challenge in contemplating the actual size of proteins, as Fischer commented in 1906:

> If they [the amino acids] were really components of the same molecule, this must be a frighteningly large complex... moreover, I believe that they are mixtures of substances whose composition is in fact much simpler than has been inferred hitherto from the results of elementary analysis and hydrolysis.[2]

In drawing conclusions about the nature of proteins, Fischer further commented in a Faraday Lecture before the Fellows of the Chemical Society in the theatre of the Royal Institution on Friday, 18 October, 1907, referring to his synthetic peptide work:

> ... the preparation of an octadecapeptide derived from fifteen molecules of glycine and three molecules of L-leucine, a substance which in its external properties closely resembles many natural proteins... Probably, too, the unpleasant discovery will be made that the natural proteins as we know them today are only to be obtained by mixing the homogeneous artificial [synthetic peptide] products.[3]

In the same year, in an experimental paper describing his further peptide synthesis results and commenting on the molecular weights of proteins and their possible composition, Fischer wrote:

> For…proteins the estimates are much higher, up to 12000 to 15000 but in my opinion these numbers are based on very insecure assumptions, since we do not have the slightest guarantee that the natural proteins are homogeneous substances.[4]

One reason for this notion that proteins were actually conglomerates of smaller molecules, explained by Edsall in his excellent retrospective,[5] was that protein purification and molecular weight determinations at the turn of the twentieth century were crude at best. None of the standard methods for measuring 'colligative properties' (e.g. melting point, vapour pressure depression, osmotic pressure, or conductivity) were appropriate for such large molecules, or where they were used, anomalous data resulted. The contemporary view of these large molecular weight systems fell back to the analogy of 'colloids'. Edsall makes further observations in explaining the preoccupation of chemists with colloidal science at this time:

> … objects of study were generally inorganic colloids—gold sols, mercury sols, sulfur sols. The particles in such preparations were always heterogeneous—their sizes had to be characterized by a distribution function, although the preparations could be made more uniform by careful fractionation. Inevitably investigators, whose first experience of colloids came through the study of such systems, thought about proteins in similar terms.[6]

The theories of *Haupt-* and *Nebenvalenzen* (primary and secondary valency) proposed by Werner in 1902 to explain the structures of inorganic coordination complexes (primary covalently-bonded moieties containing lower affinity secondary bonding potential) and polymers (small complexes held together by primary atom bonding and aggregated via secondary bonding) added weight to the notion that proteins were heterogeneous aggregates of smaller species. Werner's high reputation within the chemistry community (he was awarded the Nobel Prize in 1913 for his work on coordination chemistry[7]) would have been widely acknowledged and his theories would have readily fuelled arguments from the colloid mechanists. Within the physical chemistry community, the development of the equations of Brownian motion by Einstein and Smoluchowski (1905–6) and their experimental verification by Svedberg and Perrin would have sat comfortably with the colloid chemists who had long observed the molecular motion of colloidal substances in solution.

Against this chemistry backdrop, the key open question in immunology was still how antitoxin and toxin molecules interacted. It was now generally accepted that the bonding was not covalent, as implicit in Ehrlich's side-chain theory. In Vienna, Karl Landsteiner (see Fig. 3.1), a disciple of von Gruber, would seek to understand this question by initially taking a route along the colloid path, but would find mechanistic answers in another direction.

Karl Landsteiner's career began with medical training in Vienna followed by five years of structural chemistry in the laboratories of Emil Fischer in Würzburg, Arthur Hantzsch in Zurich, and Hamberger in Munich. This combination, not unusual among medics of the nineteenth century, honed his understanding of molecular interactions

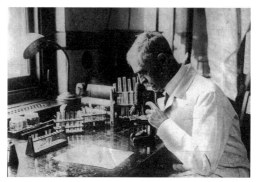

Fig. 3.1 Karl Landsteiner.
Reproduced with permission from Suddeutsche Zeitung and IBL Bildbyrå, Sweden.

and provided the foundation for his later discoveries. As early as 1903 he had already entered the 'reversible or irreversible' antibody-antigen debate by placing a stake in the ground in favour of a *form of irreversibility*, best explained by the same 'adsorption' forces at work in colloids and not necessarily conforming to the equilibrium hypothesis of Arrhenius.[8] This did not mean that he supported Ehrlich's 'covalent' side-chain position, since he also pointed out that the work of Eisenberg and Volk had clearly established that the 'law of fixed proportions', a corollary of Ehrlich's model, did not hold for typhoid serum and typhoid toxin agglutination, and that those interactions *ipso facto* could not be the result of 'chemical compound' formation.[7] His interpretation took its lead from the prevailing view[9] of the colloid chemistry school, championed in no small measure by another chemistry-practicing physician from the Vienna school, Wolfgang Pauli.

In the second of seven 'addresses', given between 1899 and 1906,[10] Pauli sets out his position by distinguishing proteins (colloids) and other high molecular weight substances from small hydrophilic molecules (crystalloids):

> All living matter is made up of colloidal and crystalloidal material … The colloids have for the most part a high molecular weight … a scarcely measurable osmotic pressure … do not conduct the electric current, yet they move, for the most part, in an electric current.[10]

In describing colloids further Pauli distinguishes the soluble protein state (sols) from the solid protein state which may be dry (coagulated by e.g. heat) or hydrated gels as a result of precipitation (by salts, urea etc.). In reflecting the primitiveness of the prevailing biochemical understanding of proteins, he poses the question on whether colloids of living matter exist in either the sol or the gel state. It may seem naïve to suggest that proteins might exist *in vivo* in a 'precipitated (gel) state'. However, the well-established experimental evidence on the avidity with which salts (charged or neutral) interacted with colloids, generating either soluble or gel states, provided a veil of uncertainty that would only be lifted some decades later.

In applying his scientific interpretation to 'that difficult and much-argued relation between toxin and antitoxin', Pauli laid out in his sixth address a quite detailed set of arguments on the similarity in behaviour of various inorganic colloids and toxin-antitoxin precipitation or agglutination reactions:

These precipitations are only possible in the presence of salts. If the protein or the bacteria under investigation are mixed with the specific substances in a salt free condition, no reaction occurs. These specific substances may, therefore, be looked upon as giving the colloidal proteins the properties of sensitive colloids, that of being precipitated through small amounts of salt ions…. Apparently all 'sensitizing' reactions encountered in the realm of the immune-body reactions are explainable in a similar way.[10]

This 'electrochemical' theory of immune reactions was adopted by Landsteiner and separated the 'sharp specificity, or receptor' school (Ehrlich and others) from the 'smooth, weak affinity interaction' school of Landsteiner, Pauli, Arrhenius, and even Bordet with his dye adsorption model.

The key breakthrough would require abandoning the colloid analogy in favour of a model where receptors, toxins, antitoxins, amboreceptors, haptophores, toxophores, complement, toxoids, and the like would all fall into a unified molecular explanation. Landsteiner would play a vital role in facilitating this important transition, but not before he had abandoned the physico-chemical colloid school of thought.

In 1903 he and Nikolaus von Jagić took the view that the specificity of toxin-antitoxin recognition could be regarded as the sum of a series of non-specific (and therefore, weak) interactions. The nature of these interactions was explained in a paper one year later as analogous to the charge-charge interactions of acids and bases (crystalloids). He concluded:

> … there is no sharp boundary separating the reactions of the immune bodies from chemical processes between crystalloids… The nearer the colloid particle approximates to that of the normal electrolyte, the nearer its compounds must obviously come to conforming to… simple chemical compounds.[11]

Landsteiner went on to compare his own ideas with those of Arrhenius and concluded that changes in acidity and basicity should be just as important in immune body interactions and protein interactions in general as in the interaction of dyes and other chemicals with tissues.

The foregoing should not be taken as an illustration of the negative influence organic and physical chemistry in the early 1900s may have had on biochemical and immunological development. Giants of chemistry such as Ostwald, Nernst, van't Hoff, Arrhenius, Fischer, and others created the chemical framework to which physiology and biology reached out for explanations of medically important observations. Clearly, charge-charge interactions are important in protein-protein interactions but as we now know are alone rarely capable of mediating the required specificity. Without a sustainable theory of protein structure and alongside it the nature of the spatio-chemical interface between interacting proteins, a viable theory of specificity would remain out of reach. It would be 20 years or so before that absence would be rectified.

As with the great nationalistic debate between Pasteur and Koch in the late 1800s, so the influence of the Great War on Teutonic models of immunology (in particular Ehrlich) and the corresponding effect on genuine mechanistic advances in immunology should not be understated. In the immediate post-war period the prevailing view in some quarters became more strongly wedded to the colloid science explanation for agglutination of bacteria by immune serum. As the retiring president of the Society of American Bacteriologists observed in an address delivered in December 1918:

> For many years the terminology, and conceptions of Ehrlich as they related to the phenomenon of agglutination have held sway in our texts and have in general proved fairly adequate for an introductory or rather casual explanation of this phase of immunology. They have served as guides in our discussions of the differentiation and recognition of bacteria by specific sera, and of the diagnosis of disease by use of specific bacteria. In some quarters, perhaps as a natural result of our anti-Teutonic bent in the Great War, there are signs of revolt against the dominance of such expressions.[12]

He concluded:

> There is ample justification for the conclusion that bacterial agglutination is a colloidal phenomenon that can best be studied in the light of the modern work on colloidal and physical chemistry.[12]

Exposure of the implausibility of the electrochemical theory of toxin-antitoxin interactions would actually come from another Teutonic quarter. Pauli and Landsteiner attempted to demonstrate the complementary charge model of protein interaction in apparatus that were essentially crude moving boundary electrophoresis devices. The mobilities observed of each of the supposedly oppositely charged species towards their respective electrodes were not as theory expected and led to the somewhat compromised proposal that specificity in agglutination reactions relied on weak charge-charge interactions and, with a somewhat stretched scientific proposition, that these weak interactions gave greater 'specificity'. In attempting to reconcile this modest behaviour of their experimental system with their interaction model, Pauli and Landsteiner ran into the opposing force of the Berlin physical chemist Leonor Michaelis (of Michaelis-Menten fame). In his *Handbook of Physical Chemistry and Medicine* Michaelis questioned the entire electrochemical explanation of toxin-antitoxin interactions:

> Everything we know points to the conclusion that specific affinity is chemical affinity in the purest sense, and is quite independent of electrical affinity, as Ehrlich has maintained from the beginning in spite of all the criticism...[13]

While Michaelis may have had a soft spot for the 'side-chain' theory, having been a private assistant of Ehrlich in the late 1890s, his powerful scientific influence would have caused many others to question the Pauli–Landsteiner model and look elsewhere for explanations of specificity.

Haptens and the continuing specificity debate

The concept of cross-species immunization had already been well studied before the turn of the century. A rabbit immunized with horse serum would generate rabbit anti-horse serum antibodies that would not react with serum from other species or be 'self-reactive', and so on. Immune specificity was thought to be a function of differences in the chemical groups present in various antigens (c.f. Ehrlich's 'haptophores'). However, what if the immunizing serum was chemically modified and then introduced into a host species? In 1906 Friedrich Obermayer and Ernst Peter Pick published the results of just such a set of experiments. Bovine serum albumin was chemically treated by iodine, nitric, or nitrous acids to form iodo-albumin, nitro-albumin, and diazo-albumin respectively. It was known that albumin is the most abundant serum protein and was therefore a reasonable surrogate for whole serum. An analysis by Mellanby in 1907 showed that three main components were present in (horse) serum with albumin (α) comprising the largest proportion (85%), followed by albumin (β) (12%), and globulin only representing 3%.[14]

On immunization of rabbits with the modified bovine albumins, the rabbit anti-serum reacted only with the chemically modified albumin and not with native albumin. More dramatically, the rabbit anti-sera were able to recognize the chemically modified albumins from *different* species. Furthermore, rabbits immunized with rabbit albumin modified by the same chemical treatments generated a rabbit anti-rabbit serum which only recognized the chemically altered rabbit albumin, in what Obermayer and Pick referred to as the *experimentum cruces*.[15] Knowing the typical chemistry of these particular reagents they suggested that their modifications had targeted aromatic groups and that these were responsible for the immune reactivity, although other changes from such strongly oxidising agents would certainly have occurred.

What Obermayer and Pick had done was to introduce side-chain modifications into albumin creating 'pseudo-haptens', whose ubiquity would have dominated the immune response. In fact their conditions were so harsh (heat under acidic (or basic) conditions with iodine and similar hot acidic denaturing conditions for nitration and diazotization), it is more than likely the albumin was totally denatured by the chemical derivatization, thus destroying the native epitopes.[16] Any remaining *native* linear epitopes after the chemical treatment that could have generated an antibody response would have been buried when they tested the native albumin cross-reactivity, leading them to the erroneous but understandable conclusion that specificity for the native protein had been completely lost.

Constructing a logical connection between these experimental results and a more profound model for protein structure would elude Obermayer, Pick, and many of their contemporaries due to the still primitive understanding of the nature of proteins. In 1908 Pick continued to assert the colloidal nature of proteins (as antigens in this instance):

> The only thing we know about the physico-chemical nature of antigens that is accepted by almost everyone, with few exceptions, is that they are colloids… nothing prevents us regarding the production of antibodies by antigens as the result of the formation of adsorption complexes between certain colloids and the toxins.[17]

Despite the experimental limitations, this was the first demonstration that antigenic or species specificity could be 'redirected' towards the modifications introduced into proteins by chemical reagents (notwithstanding the earlier work of Pasteur and others on attenuated vaccines). While the detailed interpretation of Obermayer and Pick was overly simplistic, the experimental model had set a tantalizing precedent which others such as Landsteiner would take one step further.

The stimulus for Landsteiner to enter the antigen arena may have been the publication of a review on antigens by Pick that appeared in 1912 in Kolle and von Wasserman's *Handbuch der pathogenen Mikroorganismen*, as suggested by Pauline Mazumdar.[18] Landsteiner's interest in the area was sufficiently strong that he repeated most of Pick's experiments with his co-worker Emil Prasek, although he came to somewhat different conclusions.

The question addressed by Landsteiner was whether the specificity change was due to antibody reactivity towards the chemical agent used in the modification or towards an altered protein moiety. His studies, spanning a decade or more, were brilliantly conceived and expertly executed. They addressed the unanswered question, if proteins were the *sine qua non* for an immunological response, how could this role be usurped by simple chemical structures? Chemical changes were not alone in this ability to divert or remove species specificity since exposure of protein antigens to enzymes (proteases) or alkaline treatment were known to have the same effect.

The relationship between 'haptenylated' proteins and their native protein progenitors was teased out by Landsteiner over a period of years.[19] His experimental plans had the objective of avoiding the unpredictable side effects of drastic modification by harsh chemicals in favour of gentle modification by reagents such as anhydrides to prepare acylated proteins and more importantly, with diazonium compounds to generate azo-proteins. In 1918 Landsteiner published the results of an exhaustive investigation of more than 20 haptens introduced via the azo reaction and the specificity of antisera generated therefrom.[20] These methods for generation of anti-hapten responses and the propensity of different haptens to give more or less strong responses, with some modifications, were used for more than 50 years after these series of studies. An example of the recognition capabilities of antibodies when the position in space of functional groups on small haptens was moved around is illustrated in some of his results on benzene sulphonic acids[21] (see Fig. 3.2).

What Landsteiner's results showed (he referred to them as 'striking') was that the position on the benzene ring was of greater influence on antibody recognition than the nature of the substituent (sulphonic acid) itself so that an antibody directed to a para-substituent regardless of its nature would react less well with a meta-substituent and poorly with an ortho-substituent.

The messages from Landsteiner's hapten studies were a blow for Ehrlich's 'selection theory'. Most of the chemical structures generated by Landsteiner would never have been seen by a living animal so how could preformed antibodies already be present that would recognize such structures? Adding insult to injury, although incorrectly assuming that anti-protein antibodies do not normally exist in non-immune serum, he noted:

… the hypothesis is untenable on account of the unlimited number of physiological substances which it would presuppose.[22]

Text extract reproduced from Landsteiner, K., *The Specificity of Serological Reactions*, Revised Edition, p.169, Dover Publications, New York, USA, Copyright ©1962, by permission of Dover Books Inc.

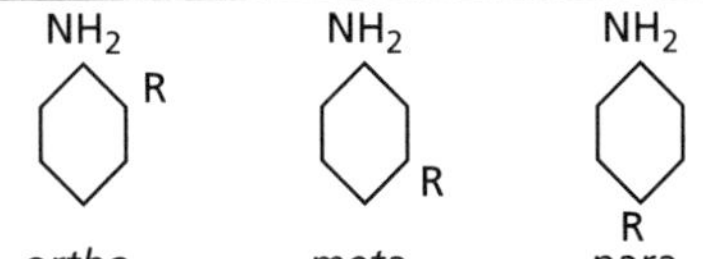

Antigens	NH$_2$ R ortho-	NH$_2$ R meta-	NH$_2$ R para-
Aminobenzene sulfonic acid..................	+ ±	+ + ±	±
Aminobenzene arsenic acid...................	o	+	o
Aminobenzoic acid	o	±	o

R designates the acid groups (COOH or SO$_3$H or AsO$_3$H$_2$).

Fig. 3.2 Antigens tested with immune serum for meta-aminobenzoic acid.

Reproduced from Landsteiner, K., *The Specificity of Serological Reactions*, Revised Edition, p.169, Dover Publications, New York, USA, Copyright ©1962, by permission of Dover Books Inc.

The advances of Landsteiner and the frustration he and others[16] experienced in trying to understand the phenomena they were generating is *de rigeu*r for precocious research. Parallel fields of study are not always at equal stages of advancement. The structural nature of proteins was not fully understood and when others showed that non-protein antigens (e.g. Oswald Avery using a protein-free capsular polysaccharide of pneumococcus) could also act as antigens, further confusion arose.

Using the anaphylaxis technique in the guinea pig—sensitizing the animals with pure vegetable proteins and challenging them with the same or related proteins—Harry Gideon Wells (a different H. G. Wells!) established the dependence of specificity on the chemical nature of proteins rather than their biologic origin. This was an important step but, equally frustrated by the 'antibody structure' lacunae, Wells further observed in 1928:

> ... we do not know whether they [*antibodies*] actually are proteins with a special molecular structure or with some special radical attached.... we do not know whether the immune bodies [*antibodies*] are serum proteins modified by the process of immunization, or specific proteins formed and secreted by cells to unite with the antigen, or specific chemical radicals either attached to or forming part of the protein molecule.[23]

Antibodies, agglutination, and blood groups

Despite the prevailing ignorance of protein structure, the phenomenon of intra-species versus inter-species specificity of antibody responses was moved forward by the elegant work of Landsteiner. In these studies spanning several decades Landsteiner expanded the earlier erythrocyte agglutination work of Ehrlich, Bordet, and others and defined the basic structure of the blood group system. Blood cells from closely allied species had been previously shown by Ehrlich and Morgenroth to be distinguished by either the agglutinin titre or by absorption experiments.[24] However, what Landsteiner explored was whether the agglutination behaviour of blood cells of individuals *within* the same species showed differences. As early as 1901 he demonstrated that:

> ... normal sera may agglutinate or hemolize the erythrocytes of other individuals of the same species and that on injection of red blood cells antibodies may be formed which by agglutination or hemolysis differentiate the blood corpuscles of various individuals in a species.[25,26]

Figure 3.3 shows Landsteiner's early results and the designation of the O, A, B, and AB sub-groups based on these agglutination experiments.

As Landsteiner further observes, the blood groups are 'sharply differentiated'. This conclusion has some significance since its recognition would later bring him back to the Ehrlich notion of 'sharp specificity' in antibody-antigen interactions. The further extensive work on blood group antigens is beyond the scope of this book, but the reader is directed to the excellent review of this important area by Landsteiner himself.[27]

A key breakthrough by Landsteiner, Avery, Heidelberger, and others was to provide convincing evidence that blood group and other antigens were antigenically dissociable from the proteins they accompanied. In studies of Pneumococci I, Avery and Heidelberger demonstrated that antibodies were able to agglutinate intact cells but that antibodies were also present that could precipitate the polysaccharides present in the S form of the bacteria (S = smooth and characterized by a polysaccharide capsular layer around the cell).[28] As with Landsteiner's blood group antigen experiments, reactions of immune sera raised against complete antigen were strong and specific when measured against the separated carbohydrate component. However, neither group was able to generate specific immune responses using the carbohydrate alone but only when it was in combination with the original protein or complete cellular matrix. In summary, using this antigen 'reconstruction', antibodies could be identified against both the carrier protein and the carbohydrate component.[29] This was important for two reasons. First, it clarified the earlier results of Bang and Forssman who in 1906 suggested that alcohol extracts of red blood cells were able to induce haemolytic antibodies[30] (the so-called Forssman antigen) but whose results were likely to have been the result of the presence of small amounts of protein in the immunizing material. Second, it discredited the notion that antibody responses were always directed towards proteins and that other chemical substances possessed antigenic potential if presented in combination with protein. This phenomenon would be elegantly exploited in Landsteiner's hapten-protein experiments, but would have to wait for a full mechanistic explanation until the role of major histocompatibility complex (MHC) proteins in antigen processing was discovered.

Groups	Agglutinins in the serum	Red blood corpuscles of groups			
		O	A	B	AB
O	α and β	o	+	+	+
A	β	o	o	+	+
B	α	o	+	o	+
AB	..	o	o	o	o

Fig. 3.3 Landsteiner's early results and the designation of the O, A, B, and AB sub-groups based on this agglutination experiment.

On the detailed chemistry underlying antigen-antibody interactions, an acceptable mechanism proved as elusive as ever. As Landsteiner observes as late as 1936, the mechanisms of Ehrlich (now largely abandoned according to Landsteiner), Bordet, and Arrhenius and Madsen were apropos at their time but contained irreconcilable components that did not satisfy a single theory:[31]

> ...no finished theory of antibody reactions has yet been attained that is comparable to those that cover and make it possible to formulate the reactions of organic chemistry. This is not too surprising in view of the fact that... the chemical structures responsible for the specificity of one of the reactants—the antibodies—are still unknown.[32]

> Text extract reproduced from Landsteiner, K., *The Specificity of Serological Reactions*, Revised Edition, p. 169, Dover Publications, New York, USA, Copyright ©1962, by permission of Dover Books Inc.

The open question about proteins and their exact chemical composition still remained, despite significant advances being made by physical chemists such as Gilbert Adair, who made much more accurate measurement of protein molecular weights by using low temperatures (to improve protein stability) in his osmotic pressure measurements. On the basis of this work he proposed that the molecular weight of haemoglobin was not ~16,700 as suggested from earlier measurements of the iron content, but four times that at 66,800.[33] His measurement of the molecular weight in both buffer solutions and water dispelled the notion that aggregation (leading to higher molecular weight estimates) was induced by salts. Adair's results were confirmed by Svedberg (Uppsala), who demonstrated that by observing sedimentation rates using his recently invented ultracentrifuge technique, molecular weights could be derived with high accuracy and also purity, and eventually shapes of the proteins could be determined (see Fig. 3.4) below on Svedberg's measurements for haemoglobin, published in 1927).[34]

Armed with this information, it may seem surprising that the peer scientific community was not more aligned with the notion that proteins and hence antibody molecules were homogeneous chemical 'chains' whose length and arrangement in space gave rise to the large molecular weights observed. But this is to deny the stranglehold conventional scientific wisdom had over all who ventured into this divisive space. This was a period when Fischer's chain hypothesis was still 'out of the question', when even Svedberg himself as late as 1937 proposed that all proteins were composed of a few 'definite units' where only a limited number of masses are possible[35] (even though Svedberg's units were much larger than Fischer's artificial peptides), and when the chemistry of those fundamental units remained uncertain, with propositions that either dipeptides or diketopiperazines (the latter were routinely seen after protein hydrolysis) were the protein building blocks held together in non-covalent strings.

Even with the advent of x-ray diffraction, the prevailing chemical dogma influenced interpretation. In diffraction studies of silk fibroin, Brill and his colleagues concluded that they were unable to distinguish between a polymer containing repeating glycyl and alanyl units (a polypeptide model) and a non-covalent aggregate of diketopiperazine units.[36] Similar conclusions were reached by Polyani using diffraction studies on cellulose where the small aggregating unit in this instance was the disaccharide anhydride.[37] It would not be long however before physical chemistry would again provide the tools

Interval (hours)	Δx per (1/2 hour)	x-med. (cm)	Speed (r.p.m.)	dx/dt: ω²x (cm/sec)	M
0.5–1	0.074	4.525	39,300	5.36×10^{-13}	67,770
1–1.5	0.078	4.601	39,400	5.44×10^{-13}	68,720
1.5–2	0.078	4.679	39,300	5.47×10^{-13}	69,090
2–2.5	0.077	4.757	39,300	5.34×10^{-13}	67,450
2.5–3	0.080	4.840	39,200	5.44×10^{-13}	68,720
					Mean: 68,350

Fig. 3.4 Svedberg's results for ultracentrifugation of haemoglobin.

Reproduced with permission from *Theodor (The) Svedberg's Nobel Lecture in Chemistry 1926*, Table 1, p. 79, Copyright © The Nobel Foundation (1908).

and spawn a new generation of scientific endeavour that would lead to a new molecular description of the antibody molecule. This chemistry would come at the hands of such scientific greats as Astbury, Pauling, Tiselius, Kabat, and others.

Acknowledgements

Text extracts reproduced from Edsall, J.T., The Development of the Physical Chemistry of Proteins, 1898–1940, *Annals of the New York Academy of Sciences*, Volume 325, p.53–76, Copyright © 1979, with permission from John Wiley and Sons.

References

1. **Chulz, F. N.** (1901). *Die Krystallisation von Eiweisstoffen und ihre Bedeutung fur die Eiweisschemie*. Jena: Gustav Fischer.
2. **Fischer, E.** (1906). 'Untersuchungen über Aminosäuren, Polypeptide und Proteine.' *Ber. Chem. Ges.*, **39**: 530–610.
3. **Fischer, E.** (1907). 'Synthetical chemistry in its relation to biology.' *J. Chem. Soc. Transac.*, **91**: 1741–65.
4. **Fischer, E.** (1907). 'Synthesen von polypeptiden.' *Ber. Chem. Ges.*, **40**: 1754–67.
5. **Edsall, J. T.** (1979). 'The Development of the Physical Chemistry of Proteins, 1898–1940.' *Ann. N.Y. Acad. Sci.*, **325**: 53–73.
6. **Edsall, J. T.** (1979). The Development of the Physical Chemistry of Proteins, 1898–1940.' *Ann. N.Y. Acad. Sci.*, **325**: 59.
7. **Werner, A.** (1913). 'On the constitution and configuration of higher-order compounds.' *Nobel Lectures, 1913, Chemistry 1901–1921*. Amsterdam: Elsevier.
8. **Landsteiner, K. and von Jagić, N.** (1903). 'Über die verbindungenen und die enstehung von immunokörpern.' *Münch.Med.Wochenschr.*, **50**: 764–8.
9. **Craw, J. A.** (1905). 'On the Mechanism of Agglutination.' *J. Hyg. (Lond)*, **5**(1): 113–28.
10. **Pauli, W.** (1907). *Physical Chemistry in the Service of Medicine*. 6th Address. Translated by Martin H. Fischer. New York: John Wiley & Sons.

11. **Landsteiner, K., and von Jagić, N.** (1904). 'Über analogiern der wirkung koloidaler kieselsäure mit der reaktionen der immunokörper und verwandte stoffe.' *Münch. Med. Wochenschr.*, **5**: 1185–9. English translation taken from P. M. H. Mazumdar (1995), *Species and Specificity*. Cambridge: Cambridge University Press, p. 225.

12. **Buchanan, R. E.** (1919). 'Agglutination.' *J. Bacteriol.* **4**(2): 73.

13. **Michaelis, L.** (1908). *Physikalische Chemie und Medizin: ein Handbuch*. Leipzig:Thieme. English translation taken from P. M. H. Mazumdar (1995), *Species and Specificity*. Cambridge: Cambridge University Press, p. 236.

14. **Mellanby, J.** (1907). 'The precipitation of the proteins of horse serum.' *J. Physiol.*, **36**(4–5): 288–333.

15. **Obermayer, F. and Pick, E. P.** (1906). 'Über die chemischen Grundlagen der Arteigen schaften der Eiweisskörper. Bildung von Immonoräzipitin durch chemisch veränderte Eiweisskörper.' *Wiener Klin. Wochenschr.*, **19**: 327–33.

16. **Wormall, A.** (1930). 'The immunological specificity of chemically altered proteins.' *J. Exp. Med.*, **51**: 295–317.

17. **Pick, E. P.** (1908). 'Darstellung der Antigene mit chemischen und physikalischen methoden', in Rudolf Krause and Constantin Levaditi (eds), *Hanbuch der Technik und Methodik der Immunitätsforschung*, V1: Antigene, p. 332. Jena: Fischer. English translation taken from P. M. H. Mazumdar (1995), *Species and Specificity*. Cambridge: Cambridge University Press, p. 241.

18. **Mazumdar, P. M. H.** (1995). *Species and Specificity*. Cambridge: Cambridge University Press, p. 242–3.

19. **Landsteiner, K.** (1962). *The Specificity of Serological Reactions*, revised edition. New York: Dover Publications, pp. 164–5.

20. **Landsteiner, K., and Lampl, H.** (1918). 'Über die Abhängigheit der serologischen Spezificität von der chemischen Struktur.' *Biochem. Ztschr.*, **86**: 343.

21. **Landsteiner, K.** (1962). *The Specificity of Serological Reactions*, revised edition. New York: Dover Publications, p. 169.

22. **Landsteiner, K.** (1962). *The Specificity of Serological Reactions*, revised edition. New York: Dover Publications, p. 148.

23. **Wells, H. G.** (1928). 'Immunity: The chemical warfare of existence.' In J. Stieglitz (ed.), *Chemistry in Medicine*. New York: Chemical Foundation, pp. 559–77.

24. **Ehrlich, P., and Morgenroth, C.** (1899). 'Über Hämolysine: zweite mittheilung.'*Berliner Klin. Wochschr.*, **36**: 481–6; (1900) 'Über Hämolysine: dritte mittheilung.' *Berliner Klin. Wochschr.*, **37**: 453–8; (1900) 'Über Hämolysine: vierte mittheilung.' *Berliner Klin. Wochschr.*, **37**: 681–7; (1901) 'Über Hämolysine: fünfte mittheilung.' *Berliner Klin. Wochschr.*, **38**: 251–7; and 'Über Hämolysine: sechste mittheilung.' *Berliner Klin. Wochschr.*, **38**: 569–74, 598–604.

25. **Landsteiner, K.** (1900). 'Zur kenntniss der antifermentiven, lytischen und agglutineier-enden wirkung des blutserums und der lymphe.' *Centralblätt für Bakt.*, **27**: 357–62.

26. **Landsteiner, K.** (1962). *The Specificity of Serological Reactions*, revised edition. New York: Dover Publications, p. 84.

27. **Landsteiner, K.** (1962). *The Specificity of Serological Reactions*, revised edition. New York: Dover Publications, pp. 75–126.

28. **Avery, O. T. and Landsteiner, M.** (1925). 'Immunological relationships of cell constituents of Pneumococcus.' *J. Exp. Med.*, **42**: 367–76.

29. **Landsteiner, K.** (1921). 'Ober heterogenetische Antigen und I-Iapten XV: Mitteilung über Antigene.' *Biochem. Ztschr.*, **119**: 294–306.

30. **Bang, I., and Forssman, J.** (1906). 'Untersuchungen über die Hämolysinbildung.' *Beitr. z. chem. Physiol. und Path.*, **8**: 238–75.

31. **Landsteiner, K.** (1962). *The Specificity of Serological Reactions*, revised edition. New York: Dover Publications, pp. 240–1.

32. **Landsteiner, K.** (1962). *The Specificity of Serological Reactions*, revised edition. New York: Dover Publications, p. 260.

33. **Adair, G. S.** (1925). 'The osmotic pressure of haemoglobin in the absence of salts.' *Proc. Roy. Soc. A.*, **109**: 292–300.

34. **Svedberg, T.** (1926). *The Nobel Lecture*, 19 May, 1927, Table 1, p. 79. Stockholm: The Nobel Foundation.

35. **Svedberg, T.** (1937). 'The ultra-centrifuge and the study of high-molecular compounds.' *Nature*, **139**: 1051–62.

36. **Brill, R.** (1926). 'Bemerkung zu meiner Arbeit Über Seidenfibroin.' *Annal. Chem.*, **446**: 307–8.

37. **Polyani, M.** (1921). 'Die Chemische Konstitution der Zellulose.' *Naturwiss.*, **9**: 288.

Chapter 4

The foundations of antibody-antigen recognition emerge

Protein chemistry breaks its organic chemistry reins

Our current understanding of antibody structure emerged through systematic chemical and physical studies spanning many decades. Through scientific endeavour in the 1930s, chemists and immunologists began to define the globular nature of antibodies, their continuous polypeptide chain nature, bi- and multi-specificity within the same molecule, and early notions of how antigen binding occurred. These were real breakthrough years, even though cellular mechanisms leading to antibody induction and production were to prove less tractable.

Numerous studies on proteins had established that they could be denatured by salts (including urea), pH changes, heat, and addition of organic solvents, and that denaturation also revealed previously buried SH groups. What was lacking was an understanding of what was occurring during this denaturation which was always accompanied by inactivation of the protein: loss of catalytic activity if an enzyme and loss of antigen binding if an antibody. Further, experimental observations of denaturation sought to distinguish loss of activity per se from coagulation, a 'change of state' invariably accompanied by an irreversible flocculation state. This was an active period in which information was widely disseminated through scientific journals. What it required was a change of direction, a unification of the multitude of observations by organic chemists, physical chemists, and the fledgling protein chemists and biochemists. Such unification came from an unlikely geographical source, unlikely that is for a Europe that considered itself to be the stronghold of the 'chemistry of life'.

Hsien Wu was educated at MIT and Harvard and then took up his position as head of biochemistry at Peiping (Beijing) Union Medical College in 1924. Five years later he presented the core arguments of a protein denaturation theory to the American Physiological Society. It is worth reproducing the abstract:

> The protein molecule is not to be regarded as a long straight chain but rather as a compact structure. Besides the peptide linkage by which the amino acids are joined 'end to end' there are other kinds of linkages which unite different portions of the chain laterally. These lateral linkages are very labile. The chain may be conceived to fold repeatedly at short intervals forming a three-dimensional network somewhat resembling a crystal lattice in which the atoms are replaced by molecules of amino acids. Denaturation is the breaking

up of these labile linkages. Instead of being compact the protein molecule now becomes a 'diffuse' structure. The surface is altered and the interior of the molecule is exposed. This explains the decrease in solubility, increase in acid and base binding power, and the change in immunological specificity which are known to accompany denaturation.[1]

Two years later he published in the *Chinese Journal of Physiology* what was undoubtedly the seminal paper on denaturation theory at that time.[2] The paper was republished in English in 1996.[3] Wu collected all the observations on denaturation, examined the results against a backdrop of chemical logic, and drew some incisive, though still at the time controversial conclusions, summarized below:

1. Denaturation and coagulation are essentially part of the same process;

2. 'If a chain is very long, it should be able by molecular attraction to fold upon itself repeatedly';[3]

3. Despite current uncertainties on the peptide chain structure 'the peptide linkage remains the best supported theory regarding the constitution of the protein';[3]

4. 'Denaturation per se involves no change of molecular weight';[3]

5. Denaturation changes antigen properties;

6. Denaturation is accompanied by an increase in viscosity (shown both by Wu & Yen[4] and Mirsky & Anson[5]);

7. Long chain or linear structures for native proteins are incompatible with observed molecular weights and the associated molecular dimensions of an extended structure. The probability of random linear chains being able to crystallize in regular arrays is '… so small as to be negligible';[3]

8. Protein molecules are not open chain, flexible molecules but have a compact structure.

It would be five years after Wu's paper before Mirsky and Pauling would publish their famous paper 'On the structure of native, denatured, and coagulated proteins'[6] although puzzlingly at this stage without any reference to the work of Wu (this would be corrected in the Pauling and Niemann paper published in 1939—see reference 18). The content of the Mirsky and Pauling paper superficially had startling resemblances to that of Wu's paper, but in describing the hydrogen bond as the non-covalent 'glue' that holds folded chains together, Mirsky and Pauling presented a thermodynamically more rigorous treatment of what Wu describes as 'labile linkages'. In defining their model for protein structure, Mirsky and Pauling assert:

Our conception of a native protein molecule (showing specific properties) is… one polypeptide chain… folded into a uniquely defined configuration, in which it is held by hydrogen bonds.[6]

By considering the magnitude of the entropy change during denaturation, Mirsky and Pauling proposed that the denatured form is a more flexible form of the native state with many conformations (they use 'configurations') available to it, hence the positive entropy change. While their assumption that the hydrogen bonding holding the native state together is between side-chain carboxyl groups and amino groups was not entirely correct (a conclusion that might be considered a little curious given Wu's assertion that the interior of the native protein is less soluble in water after denaturation, which is why aggregation occurs), the energetic description was essentially correct, if lacking the detail that would shortly arrive.

It could be said that the 1930s was the defining decade in protein science. From this time forward protein chemists would shed their colloidal skins and adopt the language of biophysics. In spite of lingering nostalgia for the 'old chemistry' from Linderström-Lang, Haldane, Astbury, Wrinch, Langmuir, and others (Wrinch proposed the 'cyclol' theory of protein structure that was espoused by Langmuir—cyclols were structural units formed by ring formation between the NH of one amino acid and the CO group of another, forming six membered rings that *en masse* would form a three-dimensional honeycomb structure)[7], the polypeptide theory would displace the *status quo*. In immunology, the convergence of physical chemistry and protein chemistry lifted the study of plasma proteins out of the domain of organic chemistry, and in doing so consolidated a language and nomenclature for immunoglobulins that was to give a true identity to molecular immunology.

Ultracentrifugation and electrophoresis—a revolutionary immunological toolbox

Contemporaneous with the work of Mirsky and Pauling at Caltech, two peculiarly Swedish developments would take the field one step further forward. In a study using Svedberg's recently developed technique of ultracentrifugation, Heidelberger and Pedersen, working in Uppsala, described the results of 29 experiments on normal and immune rabbit and horse serum (immunized against pneumococcus antigens) samples.[8] In their conclusions they state:

> It appears, therefore, that the molecular weight, at least of the two classes of rabbit antibodies included in this study, is very close to that of normal serum globulin, about 150,000.[8]

They continue further in the same article:

> On the basis of the observed sedimentation constant it would appear that antibody in the rabbit is formed either from the principal globulin component of the serum or possibly by the cells or tissues responsible for the building up of the principal component of normal serum globulin.

Text extracts © 1937 Rockefeller University Press. Originally published in *The Journal of Experimental Medicine*, Volume 65: pp. 393–414.

Studies on horse anti-pneumococcus serum in the same project produced different molecular weight estimates but these were open to some uncertainty due to the lower stability of the horse sera preparations. Despite this the authors suggested a larger molecular weight (three to four times the 150 000 size) for the horse anti-pneumococcus fraction. This must have been the first sighting of IgM, size discrepancy notwithstanding!

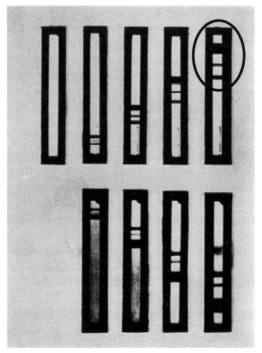

Fig. 4.1 Tiselius' analysis of blood serum by electrophoresis.

From Tiselius, A., A new apparatus for electrophoretic analysis of colloidal mixtures, *Journal of the Chemical Society, Faraday Transactions*, Issue 33, pp. 524–531, Copyright © 1937. Reproduced by permission of The Royal Society of Chemistry, http://dx.doi.org/10.1039/TF9373300524

Plasma samples were also being studied by Tiselius using his recently developed moving boundary electrophoresis apparatus. This work was published in the same year as Heidelberger and Pedersen's work (1937) and since both groups were working in the department of The Svedberg in Uppsala their studies would likely have been well known to each other. In his 'apparatus' paper[9] Tiselius's brief electrophoresis results on plasma protein separation (the title betrays perhaps his scientific prejudice on the nature of proteins) are reproduced in Fig. 4.1.

The circled region (author's addition) shows serum albumin as the topmost dense band and two globulin fractions. However, no reliable molecular weight information would be derived from Tiselius' studies since both mass and charge (at pH 8.06 in this experiment) would have been co-determinants of the mobilities observed. In the same year Tiselius followed up this initial observation with a more detailed study[10] in which, explaining the results (see Fig. 4.2) from horse serum electrophoresis, he comments:

> The fastest of these components could be identified with serum albumin. The other three are found in varying amounts in all serum globulin preparations investigated, and are more or less completely precipitated by half saturation with ammonium sulphate. They will therefore be named α, β, and γ serum globulin.[10]

On a technical note, Tiselius' development of the boundary electrophoresis method was based on the earlier work of Pauli, Landsteiner, and others.[11] For visualizing the protein bands the Topler *schlieren* method was used in which the light intensity passing through the glass tubes containing the moving plasma components would be altered as a result of protein effects on the refractive index. Against a grey background any large refractive index changes from high protein concentration would be indicated by darkened bands. Also, Tiselius' naming of the globulin bands bears no direct relationship to modern immunoglobulin nomenclature but was merely the classical way of naming different experimentally observed species.

But which of these fractions was associated with antibodies appearing after immunization with a specific antigen? The results were striking and unexpected. Working together in Uppsala, Tiselius and Elvin Kabat (an ex-student of Heidelberger and on a Rockefeller Foundation Fellowship during 1937–8) examined the electrophoretic behaviour of rabbit and horse serum fractions before and after absorption of specific anti-pneumococcus antibody. The preliminary report of this work[12] and the more extensive later paper[13] explained the ultracentrifugation results of Heidelberger and Pedersen and demonstrated that the γ band was increased in immune sera compared to normal sera but was significantly reduced in intensity after absorption with antigen, while in the horse serum samples a new band between the β and γ bands was present in immune sera but disappeared completely after antigen absorption. In studies of these fractions using the ultracentrifuge, Kabat determined the molecular weights of the normal gamma band and the 'heavy band' fractions to be around 160 000 for the gamma band and 900 000 for the heavy band. What is more, similar data were obtained for sera from different species, although the antibody size profiles were divided into two distinct species classes: pig, cow, and horse responses produced the 900 000 molecule as the predominant species while human, rabbit, and monkey gave the more commonly observed gamma globulin response at 160 000 with a small but definite 900 000 fraction in the monkey sera. Furthermore, both antibody size fractions bound pneumococcus

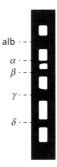

Fig. 4.2 Photograph of the migrating boundaries of horse serum after 80 min. at 7–25 V. per cm.

Reproduced with permission from Tiselius, A. CLXXXII. Electrophoresis of serum globulin. II. Electrophoretic analysis of normal and immune sera, *Biochemical Journal*, Volume 31, Part 9, pp. 1464–1477, Copyright © 1937, The Biochemical Society.

and caused agglutination but only the gamma fractions were found to fix complement, in accord with observations made by Goodner and Horsfall some years earlier.[14]

Here then was a milestone in the path to understanding Ehrlich's 'immunotoxins' and Buchner and Bordet's 'alexin'. Distinct globulin fractions with specific antigen agglutination ability were now assigned molecular weights, had known electrophoretic behaviour, appeared after an immune challenge with protein and non-protein (e.g. carbohydrate) antigens and disappeared from the serum fraction after absorption with the antigen, had similar sizes by ultracentrifugation and mobilities by electrophoresis in a number of animal species, and had been scored for their ability to fix complement. Despite this, doubt still remained about whether immune globulin differed structurally from normal globulin in some way. As Marrack observed in 1938:

> The power to act as an antibody must depend on some difference from normal globulin...[15]

Was this an immunological 'tipping point'? It was certainly an exciting time for new ideas although as we shall see, the protein science prejudices of the key scientific opinion makers would continue to walk the immunology corridors until the protein structure question was resolved.

Protein structure and theories of antibody formation

The principal protein structure virtuosi of the 1930s offered a series of incompatible theories on protein structure and antibody formation. The structural principle of Max Bergmann and Carl Niemann was based on an interpretation of both x-ray crystallographic data on fibrous proteins and amino acid compositions of these and other proteins. The total number of amino acids in the proteins haemoglobin, albumin, fibrin, silk fibroin, and gelatin, whose compositions had been analysed, appeared to fall into a series of multiples of 288, or $(2^n \times 3^m)$. Thus fibrin had 576 amino acids $(2^6 \times 3^2)$ and a molecular weight of 69 000, while silk fibroin had 2592 amino acids $(2^5 \times 3^4)$ and a molecular weight of 217 000. The reliance on fibrous protein structural data to derive a general model led Bergmann and Niemann to propose a 'law' for all protein structures and to include in that law a requirement that certain amino acids are repeated at regular intervals along the protein chain.[16] This $2^n \times 3^m$ notion was consistent with Frank and Wrinch's cyclol theory of protein structure by a mathematical coincidence. Svedberg has suggested a modular unit for proteins of 35 000 on the basis of his ultracentrifugation studies, which would correspond to a structural unit of about 288 amino acids, a unit size also proposed by Bergmann and Niemann.

Both models were unceremoniously 'dumped' by Pauling and Niemann (now having joined the group of Pauling at Caltech) in their 1939 critical analysis, based on symmetry and other chemical illogicality arguments. A particular feature of the cyclol model was its heavy configurational (we would now use 'conformational') restrictions for proteins and, in particular, antibodies, arising directly from the symmetry imposed by its hexagonal cage form.

In March of 1939 Pauling wrote to a colleague in Wisconsin:

> … Niemann and I have just finished preparing a criticism of the cyclol theory, and we hope the J.A.C.S. will publish it. The x-ray results aren't any good, and we have examined all of the other arguments and decided that no proteins have a cyclol structure…[17] [J.A.C.S = Journal of the American Chemical Society]

The paper appeared later in 1939 in which he and Niemann commented on the implications of considering antibody structure in terms of a cyclol model:

> … the restriction of a molecule to one of a few configurations… seems to us unsatisfactory rather than desirable. The great versatility of antibodies in complementing antigens of the most varied nature must be the reflection of a correspondingly wide choice of configuration by the antibody precursor.[18]

As a result of this damning publication and subsequent vigorous exchanges between Pauling and Wrinch, the cyclol theory entered its demise and the polypeptide theory of protein structure emerged as the accepted model, although not without some lingering uncertainties about the periodicity with which certain amino acids (e.g. glycine) along the chain might need to be represented to generate the large numbers of possible configurations required.

The preoccupation of so many great scientists with protein theoretical models is not so surprising given that this was a period when proteins were considered as the most likely chromosomal elements responsible for replication. The geneticist Goldschmidt actually proposed that the protein structural principle of Bergmann and Niemann might be the mathematical link between proteins and Mendel's laws.[19] In developing his famous theory on the structure of antibodies, published in 1940, even Pauling presumed of a sort of protein-templated biosynthesis:

> … postulated process of formation of a normal globulin molecule… the polypeptide chain has been synthesized, the amino acid residues have been marshaled into the proper order, presumably with the aid of polypeptidases and protein templates…[20]

Despite these predispositions, Pauling's 'theory' was a remarkable step forward in attempting to explain the origin of antibody structural diversity and the manner in which this might generate a multitude of antigen specificities.

In passing it should be noted that nucleic acids were of course not unknown. The chemistry of the mononucleotides, generated by enzymatic hydrolysis of yeast or animal thymus extracts, had been worked out by Levine and others, although the exact phosphodiester linkage eluded conclusive specification. Levine supposed that the nucleic acids were composed of four nucleotide units, forming tetranucleotide molecules.[21] Where higher molecular weight species were observed, the preferred view was that these were aggregates of these smaller units rather than covalently linked macromolecular chains, reflecting the still prevalent 'colloid' thinking. Until the seminal papers of Avery et al[22] in 1944 on the 'transforming principle' of the pneumococcus bacterium (for which mysteriously he did not receive the Nobel prize) and the base ratio analyses by Chargaff in 1950,[23] nucleic acids were considered somewhat dull, mere chemical curiosities with no clearly defined role. Even after the publications from the

Avery Laboratory (Rockefeller Hospital) the role of DNA as a ubiquitous transforming substance was not widely appreciated, even by Chargaff himself. This was partly because bacterial nucleic acid was considered somewhat irrelevant to the study of animal and plant nucleic acids, which themselves were considered different, but largely because the polymeric nature of DNA and RNA had not yet been unequivocally established, let alone the notion of one type of polymer being a template for synthesis of another. For a tantalizing discussion of this exciting era of nucleic acid discovery see Maclyn McCarty's excellent retrospective.[24]

Pauling and Heidelberger: the 'structure and formation of antibodies'

Even great scientists make wrong predictions. Pauling was no exception. His friend and colleague Neils Bohr allegedly observed that 'predictions are difficult, especially about the future'. In 1939 Pauling wrote:

> It has not yet been possible to make a complete determination with X-rays of the positions of the atoms in any protein crystal; and the great complexity of proteins makes it unlikely that a complete structure determination for a protein will ever be made by X-ray methods alone.[25]

Perhaps it was this conviction, the plethora of immunological data from Landsteiner (now working in New York), Tiselius, Kabat, Svedberg, Heidelberger, Haurowitz, and others, and his insatiable appetite for mechanistic explanations of molecular events that led Pauling to his 'Theory of the structure and process of formation of antibodies'. It was a theory that was accepted by many immunologists and was to sway scientific opinion on the origin of antibody diversity for some considerable time.

Pauling's assumptions were based on the following known facts, or his interpretation of those facts:

- Antibodies have complementarity to the antigen, the two being held together by 'strong' forces;
- Antibodies have a molecular weight of ~160 000 and probably arise from the γ fraction of serum;
- They are multivalent (required to get a 'framework' construction in the precipitin reaction);
- Antibodies are identical in amino acid composition;

In considering these and other facts Pauling drew the startling conclusion:

> The effect of an antigen in determining the structure of an antibody molecule might involve the ordering of the amino-acid residues in the polypeptide chains in a way different from that in the normal globulin, as suggested by Breinl and Haurowitz and Mudd. I assume, however, that this is not so, but that all antibody molecules contain the same polypeptide chains as normal globulin, and differ from normal globulin only in the configuration of the chain; that is, in the way that the chain is coiled in the molecule.[20]

The earlier models of Breinl and Haurowitz,[26] Alexander,[27] and later Mudd[28] that Pauling refers to presumed that the antibody receives its specificity by synthesis

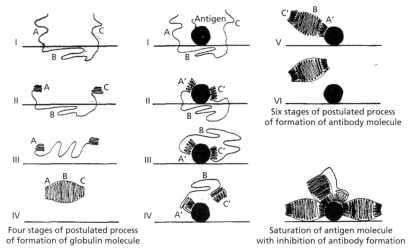

Fig. 4.3 Diagrams representing four stages in the process of formation of a molecule of normal serum globulin (left side of figure) and six stages in the process of formation of an antibody molecule as the result of interaction of the globulin polypeptide chain with an antigen molecule. There is also shown (lower right) an antigen molecule surrounded by attached antibody molecules or parts of molecules and thus inhibited from further antibody formation.

Reproduced with permission from Pauling, L. J., A theory of the structure and process of formation of antibodies, *Journal of the American Chemical Society*, Volume 62, Issue 10, pp. 2643–2657, Copyright © 1940 American Chemical Society.

'on the antigen surface' from peptide units ('building-stones' as Mudd calls them), adapted to the spatial and stereochemical features of the antigen. In short, the antigen directs the synthesis of the antibody in a one-to-one *pas de deux*. Pauling had no real evidence against this synthesis model but considered his 'one chain, different configurations' model more plausible and what is more, 'simple and reasonable', a mantra essential perhaps for someone constantly seeking to apply Occam's razor.

Pauling's model had two parts. The first required the synthesis of a generic globulin molecule containing a central, structurally non-changeable region (B in Fig. 4.3) and two terminal regions (A and C in Fig. 4.3), each with an 'unstable, extended configuration'. In the presence of an antigen the extended regions would then be 'instructed' to form a configuration complementary to the antigen.

When completed, the antigen could dissociate and act as a template for another antibody to form, and so on. The evidence Pauling called on to support the theory came from influential immunologists such as Landsteiner, Heidelberger, and others. Essentially, the facts were: globulin fractions were heterogeneous; antibodies had been shown to be multivalent; antibody responses to various well-studied antigenic systems such as the azo-proteins carrying various haptens (studied by Landsteiner and van der Scheer) and quantitative precipitin studies by Heidelberger and Kendall, demonstrated

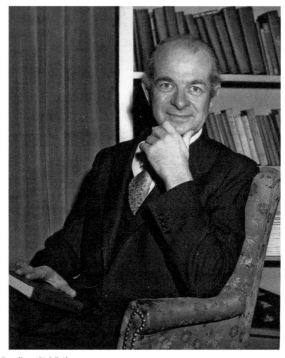

Fig. 4.4 Linus Pauling (1954).

Reproduced with permission from Pauling, L. J., A theory of the structure and process of formation of antibodies, *Journal of the American Chemical Society*, Volume 62, Issue 10, pp.2643–2657, Copyright © 1940 American Chemical Society.

the existence of heterogeneous antibody populations. Based on this evidence, Pauling could offer persuasive arguments in favour of the new theory (see Fig. 4.4).

Prior to Pauling's 1940 model, the question of antibody valency was still considered open. Heidelberger had published numerous papers on precipitation and/or agglutination reactions using both large antigens (e.g. pneumococcus) and hapten-protein conjugates such as azoproteins to examine antibodies to 'small antigens'. In a paper presented at a symposium on the physical chemistry of proteins in the American Chemical Society meeting in Milwaukee, Wisconsin, he draws together several strands of activity on antibody-antigen interactions based not just on his own work with collaborators such as Kabat and Kendall but also published work of Marrack, Avery, Felton, Tiselius, and many others.[29] A number of interesting conclusions from his review are worth considering (summarized below), a few of which represent something of an *umschwung* from his earlier position:

1. Using methods developed by Felton, analytically pure antibody from horse sera showing 100% reactivity with antigen could be prepared;

2. Antibody is 'protein';

3. Based on extensive experimental data, quantitative mathematical models could be drawn up to describe the process of antibody-antigen complexes in regions of antigen excess, equivalence, and antibody excess;

4. Antibodies are assumed (although not established with any certainty) to be 'multi-valent'—with a valency of two or more; '. . . if the conception of precipitate formation by the union of multivalent antigen with multivalent antibody is correct. . .'[29]

5. The composition of precipitates 'depends not upon the antibody concentration at equilibrium but on the proportions in which the components are mixed".[29] This con-clusion 'prevents a simple treatment of the precipitin reaction according to the law of mass action' (Arrhenius' position), 'but also blasts the hopes of the colloid enthu-siasts' (Buchner, Bordet, and others) 'who have endeavored to characterize this and other immune reactions by adsorption isotherms, for adsorption isotherms, too, contain a concentration term.'[29]

6. 'The process of aggregation, as well as the initial hapten-antibody combination, is considered to be a chemical reaction between definite molecular groupings.'[29] This comment was clearly a return to Ehrlich's position and something of a 'blast' for Bordet's colloidal model, at least in respect of how antigens and antibodies interact.

7. Ionic interactions are still considered important to drive the antigen-antibody inter-action, a view that would be put on a more detailed physicochemical framework by Pauling.

The alternative and typically parsimonius interpretation of the multivalency assump-tion of Heidelberger came via a particularly clever analysis by Pauling, from which a somewhat simpler model for antigen-antibody precipitation was derived. Pauling com-bined the antibody valency factor, which he proposed is 'at the most, bivalent' and the theoretical antigen-antibody packing possibilities required for the formation of pre-cipitin networks. Using spherical packing analogies from crystal structures, Pauling proposed that with a valency of two for the antibody and various sizes of antigen, the observed excess of antibody in precipitates could be explained by a simple ratio:

$$R = N_{eff}(antigen) / N_{eff}(antibody) \tag{1}$$

Where N_{eff} (antigen) and N_{eff} (antibody) are the average effective valences of antigen and antibody molecules respectively.[20]

By assuming that antibody valency had a maximum of two the formula simplified to:

$$R = N_{eff}(antigen) / 2 \tag{2}$$

Did this adequately explain the data from Heidelberger, Marrack, and Kendall, who had first propounded the network idea of antibody-antigen precipitation with antibodies having an undefined multivalency? Pauling calculated antibody-antigen ratios based on his spherical packing calculations and obtained the following results (see Table 4.1).

In this calculation, Pauling assumed that for an antibody and antigen of equal size (line one of Table 4.1) an N value of 12 (maximum number of antibodies able to pack around an antigen of the same size) would be possible, whence from equation (2) above, R would equal 6, and so on for antigens of decreasing size. Pauling was quite clear about the significance of the numbers given in Table 4.1 and that they should not

Table 4.1 Coordination of spherical antibody molecules about spherical antigen molecules

No. Ab mols around Ag	Min ratio of Ab radius to Ab radius	Min MW of Ag (Ab 160k)	Max molecular ratio of Ab to Ag in precipitate	Max mass ratio Ab/Ag
12	1.000	160 000	6	6
8	0.732	63 000	4	10
6	0.414	11 000	3	44
4	0.225	1 800	2	178

Reproduced with permission from Pauling, L. J., A theory of the structure and process of formation of antibodies, *Journal of the American Chemical Society*, Volume 62, Issue 10, pp. 2643–2657, Copyright © 1940 American Chemical Society.

have 'rigorous quantitative significance'.[20] A particularly clever conclusion was that 'in many sera the antibodies might be complementary in the main only to certain surface regions of the antigen, the number of these determining the valence of the antigen',[20] a piece of sagacity that Pauling may have 'borrowed' from Marrack who had observed two years earlier:

> … it appears probable that the immunological character of natural proteins is determined by the arrangement of amino-acids on the surface of the molecule. It may be either that individual acids act as 'determinant groups', in which case the character would depend on their distribution on the surface, or that several may together form an 'active patch' with a characteristic distribution of inter-molecular forces. Such a patch may be more or less completely altered by the molecular arrangements taking place on denaturation.[30]

These were the first real statements invoking the notion of a restricted number of antigenic determinants on a protein surface, although without the language of later immunology.

Heidelberger's experimental R values for antigens between 4000 and 700 000 molecular weight lay in the range 2.5 for the smaller antigens to 15 for the larger antigens. While the experimental R values were smaller than the calculated values, Pauling surmised that not all surface regions of an antigen are effectively antigenic leading to correspondingly lower than predicted values. Despite these discrepancies, Pauling was able to demonstrate that the observed precipitation framework stoichiometry could be generated by antibodies having a valency of two and no more.

A structural coda

A consequence of Pauling's 'wrap-around assembly' hypothesis was that each bivalent antibody molecule would carry two different specificities within the same molecule (see Fig. 4.3). Some of the evidence Pauling cited supported the theory (e.g. Haurowitz and co-workers[31]). Pauling's argument was simple but convincing:

- A bivalent antibody should form A-A, B-B, and A-B bivalent species in antigen excess with an antigen to which the two different haptenic groups A and B had been attached.

- The statistics predicted that the ratio of A-A, A-B, and B-B antibodies produced would be 1:2:1. This arises because when single hapten binding has occurred with either A or B, the probability of A-B pair formation is twice that of either A-A or B-B formation (A- and -B can both form A-B pairs).

Haurowitz's experiments seemed to support this, while Landsteiner and van der Scheer's experiments suggested otherwise. When these latter authors took immune sera raised against azoproteins containing two different haptenic groups and absorbed out the single hapten reacting antibodies, they found little evidence for heterobifunctional antibodies in the remaining serum. They concluded:

> Azoproteins have been prepared with azocomponents possessing two serologically active groups. On immunization with such antigens, immune sera were obtained containing two separate, unrelated antibodies, each specific for one of the two groups and separable by absorption. In other cases one of the two structures was dominant, in that antibodies were formed only towards this and not towards the other grouping.[32]

Text extracts © 1938 Rockefeller University Press. Originally published in *The Journal of Experimental Medicine*, Volume 67: pp. 709–723.

Clearly this was not compatible with Pauling's statistics. In commenting on this Pauling observed:

> It seems possible that the conclusion is not justified by the data, and, with the kind cooperation of Dr Landsteiner, we are continuing this investigation.[33]

A further problem with Pauling's model of the antibody flexible regions arose while considering the likely conformational preferences of globular proteins. Pauling's hydrogen bonding model for 'layers' (what we now call beta sheets) in proteins was an extraordinary *tour de force* although it was actually an extrapolation from the keratin structures that had been observed in Astbury's x-ray studies. Pauling lent on the fibrous protein structure analogy and by clever integration of amino acids such as proline and hydroxyproline (found in abundance in keratin) at particular intervals in his hydrogen-bonded 'layers' to facilitate turns, he suggested that a globular structure for the antibody could be built up like a 'stack of pancakes'. His 40Å cubed module example would contain four such anti-parallel layers each with eight strings (beta strands) and 12 residues in each string (see Fig. 4.5).

While beautiful in conception, the adoption of this structure by an entire antibody would present problems. How could a structure so stable and rigid be consistent with Pauling's flexible terminal regions? As with all beautiful theories, adulteration with unsightly elements is sometimes necessary to retain viability. Pauling's compromise was the addition of non-hydrogen bonding (and hence string breaking) proline and hydroxyproline residues, postulated to be at least one-third and maybe one-half of the total residues present in the terminal flexible regions. This would have introduced into these regions a limitation on recognition diversity—such a large proportion of essentially

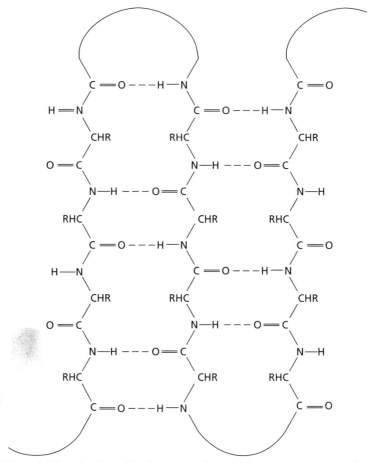

Fig. 4.5 The folding of polypeptide chains into a layer held together by imino-carbonyl hydrogen bonds.

Reproduced with permission from Pauling, L. J., A theory of the structure and process of formation of antibodies, *Journal of the American Chemical Society*, Volume 62, Issue 10, pp. 2643–2657, Copyright © 1940 American Chemical Society.

weakly functional amino acids with little or no hydrogen-bonding capability (a form of interaction highly espoused by Pauling) and no charge properties would have severely limited their capability to form specific binding sites for the myriad of antigens out there. But this was Linus Pauling, and as with the great organic chemists of the nineteenth and early-twentieth century, scientific giants create scientific dogma, 'warts an' all'.

A potentially exciting spin-off from Pauling's instructive theory was that it should be possible to form antigen-specific antibodies *in vitro* by mixing the non-immune globulin fraction with antigen under specified conditions. In a short piece published in *Science* in April 1942, he and Dan Campbell declared, in what might be considered a sort of 'press release':

> By following the general procedure proposed in connection with a theory of serological phenomena, we have succeeded in making antibodies in the laboratory. The procedure

consists in subjecting normal globulin or other protein to the action of denaturing reagents or conditions in the presence of an antigen. The protein molecule unfolds, and then refolds in such a way as to assume a configuration complementary to that of the antigen, thus acquiring the properties of a specific homologous antibody.[34]

Text extract reproduced with permission from Pauling, L. and Campbell, D.H., *The manufacture of antibodies in vitro*, *Science*, Volume 95, Issue 2498, pp. 440–441, Copyright ©1942

Although further work was published on this 'in vitro instruction', others could not reproduce it and the phenomenon passed quietly into obscurity.

Chemistry gives way to biology

Given the knowledge of antibodies and their interactions with antigens at the time, the instructive theory of Pauling had enormous merits. It explained how diversity to the enormous variety of antigens could be generated when the antigen came into contact with cellular sites that produced the antibodies. It explained the phenomenon of precipitation and agglutination based on Heidelberger's data and Pauling's simple quantitative model. It defined the nature of the bonding between antibody and antigen and proposed a structure for antibodies compatible with the 'instruction' believed to be occurring.

But, it could not explain the phenomenon of antibody persistence in the serum even after disappearance of antigen, nor affinity improvement (maturation), occurring after multiple immunizations. Once the antibody with its limited if any sequence diversity had met its antigen and folded itself around the antigenic site, the chemistry of bonding would be fixed for all time. As Marrack observed:

A difficulty that arises with all theories of antibody production is the prolonged formation of antibodies after the injection of antigen and particularly the phenomenon of 'anamnesis'—the stimulation of a fresh production to one antigen, when a new antigen is injected. It seems necessary to suppose that immunization has some permanent effect on the organism...[35]

Marrack, in concluding his extensive review of 'Antigens and Antibodies', nails his colours to the Ehrlich mast, a move reflecting perhaps the veil of mechanistic uncertainty still pervading the views of the principal antibody players:

... insofar as he considered that specific combination depends on specific configurations of atoms representable by chemical formulae, the developments of immunology appear to have confirmed Ehrlich's views.[36]

The landscape was about to change, however. Physical and organic chemistry would make way for a cell biology 'Restoration' and the rise of protein chemistry with its new power techniques. In concluding her paper on antibody formation in 1939, Florence Sabin (a pioneer of women in science; she was the first woman to be elected to the US National Academy of Sciences), working at the Rockefeller Institute, observed:

1. The use of an antigen which can be seen within cells demonstrates that one may stimulate the phagocytic cells either of the liver and spleen or of the tissues and lymph nodes to produce antibodies.

2. The appearance of antibodies in the serum correlates with the time when the dye-protein is no longer visible within the cells and with the phenomenon of a partial shedding of their surface films.

3. It is thus inferred that the cells of the reticulo-endothelial system normally produce globulin and that antibody globulin represents the synthesis of a new kind of protein under the influence of an antigen.

4. An antigen is a substance which can specifically modify the synthesis of the cytoplasm of the cells of the reticulo-endothelial system.[37]

Text extract © 1939 Rockefeller University Press. Originally published in *The Journal of Experimental Medicine*, Volume 70: pp. 67–83.

While Sabin's conclusion that Kuppfer cells, macrophages, and monocytes appeared to be the target cells for antigen processing and hence antibody production were not correct, they shifted the bias away from chemistry towards cellular biology, notwithstanding the earlier proposals of Ehrlich and others on the cellular origin of antitoxins. As we shall see, this shift allowed dramatic progress during the following decade or so.

Meanwhile, in a quiet laboratory in Melbourne, a microbiologist was about to begin rewriting immunology, although it would take time and journeys down many mechanistic *culs de sacs* before the true picture of antibody formation would emerge. Frank Macfarlane Burnet had studied animal viruses and bacteriophages with a particular interest in influenza virus, its genetics, propagation in chick embryos, and methods for its use in vaccination. As a physician and microbiologist his familiarity with antibody serology was extensive. He routinely used antisera in characterization of bacteriophages, but studies of antibody responses to staphylococcus toxins seem to have triggered a much more significant surge in his activity in this area. In 1941 he assembled a number of ideas in a monograph that captured his thinking about the antibody formation process (see Fig. 4.6).

Burnet was obviously familiar with the current 'instructive theories' of antibody formation. His issue was not with the notion of instruction itself but rather in the mechanism by which antibodies became instructed. How could a conformational mechanism (of Pauling) that required antigen to be present to generate each antibody explain both antibody increase with declining antigen and the large increase in antibody production and improved affinity on secondary antigen challenge? Burnet posed the problem in his 1941 monograph. Essentially the 'antigen as a template' synthesis model of Haurowitz–Mudd should give a regular antibody output resulting in a linear titre increase. In fact, many antigens (e.g. staphylococcal toxoid) show a logarithmic increase in titre after secondary challenge. Burnet's explanation was that the logarithmic rise was '... because the entities ... are ... multiplying or are being produced by multiplying agents'. His conclusion was that 'contact of the antigen with a cell which has previously encountered the same antigen, results in a proliferation of the antibody-producing mechanism...' and that it is 'immaterial whether the proliferating units are the cells themselves or some sub-cellular units...'.[38]

During the 1940s Burnet and others would attempt to identify the antibody-producing cells and the mechanism by which antibody persistence

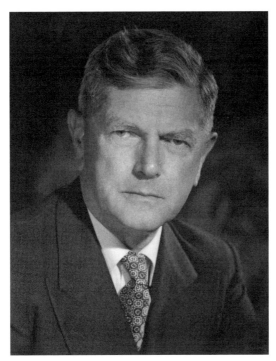

Fig. 4.6 Frank Marfarlane Burnet.

Reproduced from the Royal Society of London, *Biographical Memoirs of Fellows of the Royal Society*, Volume 33 (Dec., 1987), pp. 100–162, Image IM/GA/WRS/5496, Copyright © 1987 Godfrey Argent Studio, with permission from the Royal Society, London, UK.

occurred. In his 1941 monograph Burnet was still ambivalent about the exact cellular sites involved, citing many published experimental attempts to tie antibody production to the spleen, lymph nodes, and other tissues of the reticulo-endothelial system, including Kupffer cells and bone marrow cells. Burnet's own experiments pointed to spleen and lymph nodes as the most likely sites for antibody production. In one of his own experiments he reports a clear mediastinal lymph-node response in mice challenged with influenza virus intranasally. From the fifth day onwards after injection, more antibody was detected in the node than in the serum, and none in the lung. Burnet observed that proof of the antibody being produced in the lymph node was '... almost conclusive'.[39] However discrepancies between the response of lymphatic tissues to antigens of different types presented some challenges. Particulate antigens (bacteria, viruses) seemed to obey Burnet's hypothesis while soluble antigens (toxoids etc.) did not, leading him to speculate that such antigens pass into the blood and that responses to these antigens in the form of anti-toxins are exclusively associated with the reticulo-endothelial system.

On the question of antibody production in the absence of antigen, the picture painted by Burnet in 1941 was less convincing. The difficulty was not in conceiving of the right experiment but rather how to follow disappearance of any injected antigen(s) and then to correlate this with antibody production. For example, as Burnet suggested, the ideal experimental system would involve linking a chemical determinant such as the arsenilic acid radical to a carrier and then following its disappearance from spleen, liver, and bone marrow while measuring antibody production. Indirect support for the loss of antigen long before the cell loses its capacity to produce antigen had been produced by Haurowitz and Kraus but 'direct evidence' for complete antigen loss from all tissues was more difficult to come by.

The question of lifetime antibody immunity (e.g. against certain viruses) was more perplexing to Burnet. Data from measles and yellow fever epidemiology provided convincing evidence that circulating antibody persisted long after the antigen would be expected to have disappeared, in the measles case for up to 75 years! As Burnet noted:

> It is quite impossible to think of reticulo-endothelial cells maintaining individual existences for 75 years, or of fragments of virus being retained as antigenic pattern for so long.[40]

At this time Burnet's conclusion was that the time period of protection was likely to correlate with the concentration of antigen in the bloodstream at immunization. In developing further his views, Burnet favoured the model in which antibody synthesis was mediated by the 'proteinase unit' of Bergmann and Niemann. His rationalization of the 'no template, no antibody synthesis' issue was that after the initial specific template synthesis of antibodies by the protease unit, further antigen exposure to other antigens would generate sufficient cross-reactive determinants that a response to some of the determinants on the original antigen would be maintained. This 'adaptive response' of the protein synthesis machinery took its cue from the bacterial world in which enzymes were known to undergo adaptive changes in response to changes in food molecule sources.[41]

A further 'unsolved problem' for Burnet concerned the difference in globulin size generated by different species and the relation to antibody-producing cells. The antibody response in ungulates (e.g. horse) giving mainly high molecular weight globulin (the 'heavy fraction') while the rodent (e.g. rabbit) response generated mostly globulin in the gamma fraction posed a conundrum. His conclusion (really a speculation) was that in the different species, and even within a species showing different responses to large antigen and small toxoid molecules, different cells are responsible for the different antibodies generated. But the question remained which cells, and how did they direct the synthesis of specific antibodies?

After a further eight years of experimentation and theoretical analysis based on his own published work and that of others, Burnet recapitulated the issue of antibody production in an updated version of his 1941 monograph:

> Unless the antigen or its determinants can be so built into the cellular mechanism that it is capable of multiplication through successive cell generation there is no conceivable place in the body where it can be stored. Nor does this theory (*referring to Breinl and Haurowitz, Mudd, and Pauling*) provide any framework for an interpretation of the difference between primary and secondary types of response or the changing character of antibody in the course of repeated immunization.'[42]

Significantly, the possibility that heavy fraction globulin (mw 900 000) and gamma fraction (150–160 000) are produced by the same cells, reacting in different ways to different types of stimulus, was now entertained. Some contradictions were still outstanding, in particular with regard to the specificity of primary versus intermediate and late secondary responses. In some instances secondary response antibodies appeared to be less specific for the immunizing antigen than primary response antibody, though sometimes with a broadening of the specificity for related antigens. In other instances, cross-reacting antibodies diminished, giving a more specific response after repeated immunizations (e.g. in a study with Mavis Freeman on phage C16 responses[42]). The interpretation of the published experiments would have been complicated by the multitude of events occurring simultaneously. Heidelberger and Kendall's study on the response to crystalline (and hence pure) albumin in rabbits suggested that as the immunization course progressed, the antibody repertoire incorporated more and more chemically distinct groups on the albumin molecule. This could have given the impression of reducing the specificity, since as more and more determinants were included, the probability of them being represented in other antigens would be increased.

As far as identification of the cellular origin of antibodies, Burnet strongly subscribed to the emerging view that when particulate antigens are inoculated at peripheral sites, the major source of circulating antibody is the regional lymph nodes. However, it was less evident which cells within the lymph were responsible for production. When antigen is present in the blood, the spleen is the critical site for production, the most likely candidates being lymphocytes, plasma cells, and macrophages. As outlined by Burnet, the prevailing view was that 'macrophages are responsible for taking up the antigen molecules or particles and in them the initial stages of antibody production take place. The plasma cell is a cell in which rapid production of antibody... globulin is taking place'.[43] The transfer of this information to plasma cells is made possible either because plasma cells are descended directly from macrophages or from reticulum cells to which the antigen stimulus has somehow been transferred.

A great deal of data generated by Ehrich,[44] White and Dougherty,[45] and others suggested that antibody passes from the lymph to the circulation within the cytoplasm of lymphocytes and plasma cells in the efferent lymph stream. A further, more controversial proposal discussed and to some extent accepted by Burnet was that liberation of antibody occurs via cytoplasmic dissolution controlled by adreno-cortical hormones, a hypothesis strongly disputed by Robertson,[46] based on his own experiments carried out at the Dunn School of Pathology in Oxford and the published work of others.

Perhaps the most convincing evidence of the identity of antibody-producing cells came from the elegant work of Astrid Fagraeus, working at the Caroline Institute (now the Karolinska Institute) in Stockholm. Fagraeus' experiments were a model of clarity and experimental rigour. Fagraeus injected rabbits subcutaneously with live *Salmonella typhi* on day one and again 14–25 days later intravenously. She then followed the histology in the spleen and measured the levels of antibody produced by the spleen *in vitro* for a number of days after the second injection (she was interested in the secondary response) and in the serum. Her conclusions were clear-cut. Initially transitional cells were observed followed at a later time point by immature plasma cells culminating in mature plasma cells.

The appearance of antibody, both circulating and splenic, correlated with the growth in numbers of the immature plasma cells. Fagraeus' conclusions are worth stating in their original:

1. During secondary response, elicited in sensitized rabbits by means of intravenous injections of antigen, a great increase in the number of plasma cells (pl.c.) in the spleen was recorded simultaneously with the increase of circulating antibodies.

2. Pl.c. were confined almost exclusively to the red pulp, especially after the injection of living S. typhi. They originated apparently from reticulum cells, passing through a chain of development: transitional cell —+ immature pl.c. —~ mature pl.c.

3. Pieces of spleen were excised at different times during the period of antibody formation in rabbits, differential cell counts were made and the capacity of excised splenic tissue to form antibodies in vitro was investigated. The following observations were made:

   a. The amount of antibody liberated in plain tissue extracts, under conditions preventing growth or metabolism of cells, was very low, whereas significant yields were obtained in tissue cultures.

   b. The capacity of the red pulp abundant in pl.c. to produce antibodies in vitro was considerably superior to that of lymph follicles, rich in lymphocytes but devoid of pl.c.

   c. Antibody production was comparatively poor in tissue containing only transitional cells, reached a maximum when numerous immature pl.c. were present and receded when predominantly mature pl.c. were found.

4. After intravenous injections the antigen accumulated in those places where pl.c. subsequently developed. The conclusion is drawn that antibodies under the conditions of the experiments, are formed by cells of the R.E.S., passing through a chain of development, the final link of which is the mature pl.c.[47]

While Burnet was aware of Fagraeus' work and similar studies of others, he was not yet convinced the issue of antibody production had yet been resolved, drawing his own conclusions on the area 'with some diffidence'. What was clear to Burnet and others was that antigen-specific antibody production could continue long after the antigen had disappeared from the organism. This was perhaps the most difficult phenomenon to understand, particularly as the turnover of the candidate cells was believed to be from hours to days while specific antibody could be measured for very much longer, even years after inoculation. This required invoking a 'cell descendent' model in which the information present in an initially stimulated cell would be passed on to descendent cells, but by what mechanism?

The concept of the gene in 1949 was still firmly embedded in proteinology. As Burnet observes:

… (a) From the chemical point of view virtually nothing is known of the details of protein synthesis in vivo; (b) there is an increasing tendency for biologists to use explicitly or implicitly the conception that significant intracellular proteins, particularly enzymes, are synthesized by a process of replication (an essentially biological concept) not yet expressible in chemical terms.[48]

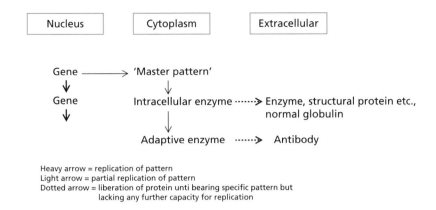

Fig. 4.7 Scheme of protein and antibody replication.

Reproduced with from Burnet F.M and Fenner F., *The Production of Antibodies*, Second Edition, p.94, Macmillan, Melbourne, Australia, Copyright © 1949, reproduced with permission of Macmillan Australia.

Monod, writing in 1947, stated that the formation of these highly complex and highly specific molecules (enzymes) must involve a sort of prototype mechanism involving a pre-existing 'master pattern', speculating that the pattern need only include a small element of the specific molecule.[49] Based on the available evidence Burnet proposed his own schema for protein and antibody synthesis (see Fig. 4.7).

There are several points to be made from this schema. First, the gene is as yet an undefined entity but thought to be a protein-like template. Second, the adaptive enzyme mechanism for protein replication, borrowed from bacteriology, is still the favored biosynthetic mechanism for specific antibody production. Third, the synthetic origin of normal globulins and antibodies differ in that antibodies require the specific action of the adaptive enzymes to impart the antigenic specificity. Finally, when cells carrying the particular adaptive enzyme multiply, their descendants maintain the new character.

The uncertainty of the nature of the 'gene' and its presumptive protein nature by Burnet may seem a little curious given the already-published work of Avery and Chargaff. The reluctance of the scientific community at this time to accept that DNA is the 'transforming material' is explored by McCarty at length in his book *The Transforming Principle*, in a sometimes melancholy final chapter,[50] attributing the low impact of the work of Avery and co-workers to a combination of poor scientific communication in the immediate post-war period, the perhaps obscure nature of the journals the Avery laboratory published in at this time, and the abiding view that bacteria were not like higher organisms, even though it seemed quite acceptable to borrow their adaptive enzymology! As Virgil aptly put it (*Aeneid* VI, 100), *obscuris vera involvens*.

The emergence of the 'self-marker' concept

By the time Burnet penned his 1949 monograph, recognition that the antibody 'machinery' is able to distinguish foreign from autologous antigens was well known, even if the mechanisms by which self-reacting antibody avoidance occurs were not understood (see Ehrlich[51] and the concept of *horror autotoxicus*). In exploring this concept Burnet and Fenner speculated that the avoidance mechanism originated with the ability of the 'adaptive enzymes' tuned to antibody production to adapt their antibody synthesis to recognize foreign antigens that were similar enough to self-antigens (or 'markers') to avoid 'large adaptations'. As Burnet stated:

> A very minor difference might not act as a stimulus to adaptation and too remote a resemblance might make adaptation impossible.[52]

Enzymes involved in cellular turnover are adapted to recognize a small number of markers in such cells (e.g. the ABO blood groups in erythrocytes) and such enzymes are:

> ... brought into being in the cells that destroy erythrocytes. This newly patterned enzyme becomes stabilized as part of the inheritable structure of these cells and is transmitted indefinitely to their descendants.[53]

Taking this concept further, Burnet also proposed that self-marker recognition must occur during the embryonic and post-embryonic stages of growth. A consequence of this hypothesis was that introduction of a foreign antigen into the foetal system (either experimentally or naturally via placental or yolk sac transmission) should render the animal immunologically tolerant on challenge with the same antigen in adult life. Some data from Traub[54] supported this concept but it was by no means fully proven.

In extending the self- versus non-self-argument, Burnet commented on the observations of Medawar[55] and others on graft-host responses, in particular the rejection of skin grafts. Neither Medawar nor Burnet had any explanation for the rejections observed and were somewhat perplexed by the absence of specific anti-graft tissue antibodies. Medawar's studies included grafts to the brain and the anterior chamber of the eye in which the presence (tissue rejection) or absence (no rejection) of vascularization suggested that the immune response was mediated by the blood stream but that rejection also required a working lymphatic drainage system, at least to create a state of immunity. Burnet's working hypothesis drew on his experience with known anti-tuberculin hypersensitivity reactions. On first exposure the foreign antigens are distributed throughout many host-cell types. On re-challenge a liberation may occur of 'the same pharmacologically active substances as are responsible for the necrosis of a fully developed tuberculin reaction'.[55] It would be some considerable time before the cellular basis of graft rejection would become known, but what a remarkable insight Burnet displayed as he unwittingly attempted to unlock the closely guarded secrets of cellular immunology.

Acknowledgements

Text extracts from Pauling, L. and Niemann, C., The structure of proteins, *Journal of the American Chemical Society*, Volume 61, Issue 7, pp.1860–1867, Copyright © 1939 American Chemical Society, reprinted with permission.

Text extracts from Pauling, L. J., A theory of the structure and process of formation of antibodies, *Journal of the American Chemical Society*, Volume 62, Issue 10, pp. 2643–2657, Copyright © 1940 American Chemical Society, reprinted with permission.

Text extracts from Marrack, J.R., Report No.230 of the Medical Research Council, HM Stationary Office, London, UK Copyright © 1938, reproduced with permission from the Medical Research Council.

Text extracts from Heidelberger, M and Pedersen, K. O., The molecular weight of antibodies, *The Journal of Experimental Medicine*, Volume 65, pp. 393–414, Copyright © 1937 American Chemical Society, reprinted with permission.

Text extracts from Burnet F.M, The Production of Antibodies, Macmillan, Melbourne, Australia, Copyright © 1941 reproduced with permission of Macmillan Australia.

Text extracts from Burnet F.M and Fenner F., *The Production of Antibodies*, Second Edition, Macmillan, Melbourne, Australia, Copyright © 1949 reproduced with permission of Macmillan Australia.

References

1. **Wu, H. A.** (1929). 'Theory of denaturation and coagulation of proteins.' *Amer. J. Physiol.*, **90**: 562–3.
2. **Wu, H. A.** (1931). 'Studies on Denaturation of Proteins. XIII. A Theory of Denaturation.'*Chinese Journal of Physiology*, **5**(4): 321–44.
3. **Wu, H. A.** (1995). 'Studies in denaturation of proteins. XIII. A theory of denaturation.' *Adv. Prot. Chem.*, **46**: 6–25. Reprinted in English from reference 2.
4. **Wu, H. A. and Yen, D.** (1924). 'Studies of denaturation of proteins: I. Some new observations concerning the effects of dilute acids and alkalies on proteins.' *J. Biochem.* (Jpn), **4**: 345–84.
5. **Mirsky, A. E., and Anson, M.** (1929). 'Protein coagulation and its reversal: the reversal of the coagulation of hemoglobin.' *J. Gen. Physiol.*, **13**: 133–43.
6. **Mirsky, A. E., and Pauling, L.** (1936). 'On the structure of native, denatured and coagulated proteins.' *Proc. Natl. Acad. Sci.*, **22**: 439–47.
7. **Fruton, J. S.** (1999). *Proteins, Enzymes, Genes.* Yale: Yale University Press, pp. 208–10.
8. **Heidelberger, M., and Pedersen, K. O.** (1937). 'The molecular weight of antibodies.' *J. Exp. Med.*, **65**: 393–414.
9. **Tiselius, A.** (1937). 'A new apparatus for electrophoretic analysis of colloidal mixtures.' *Transac. Faraday Soc.*, **33**: 524–31.
10. **Tiselius, A.** (1937). CLXXXII. 'Electrophoresis of serum globulin. II. Electrophoretic analysis of normal and immune sera.' *J. Biochem.*, **31**: 1464–77.
11. **Pauli, W., and Valkó, E.** (1933). *Kolloidchemie der Eiweisskörper* 2e (Chapter 10). Dresden: Steinkopff.
12. **Tiselius, A., and Kabat, E. A.** (1938). 'Electrophoresis of immune serum.' *Science*, **87**: 416–17.
13. **Tiselius, A., and Kabat, E. A.** (1939). 'An electrophoretic study of immune sera and purified antibody preparations.' *J. Exp. Med.*, **69**: 119–31.
14. **Goodner, K., and Horsfall, F. L. Jr.** (1936). 'Lipids and immunological reactions II. Further experiments on the relation of lipids to the type-specific reactions.' *J. Immunol.*, **31**: 135–40.
15. **Marrack, J. R.** (1938). *Report No. 230 of the Medical Research Council.* London: HM Stationary Office, p. 65.
16. **Bergmann, M.** (1938). 'The structure of proteins in relation to biological problems.' *Chem Revs.*, **22**: 423–35. The text of this paper was delivered by invitation at the seventh National

Organic Chemistry Symposium of the American Chemical Society, 29 December, 1937, Richmond, Virginia, USA.

17. **Pauling. L.** (1939). Letter to Thomas Anderson, Wisconsin, 17 March, 1939. Taken from Linus Pauling (2012), *Day by Day*, Special Collections, OSU Libraries, Oregon State University.

18. **Pauling, L., and Niemann, C.** (1939). 'The structure of proteins.' *J. Amer. Chem. Soc.*, **61**: 1860–7.

19. **Goldschmidt, R.** (1938). 'The theory of the gene.' *Sci. Mon.*, **46**: 268–73.

20. **Pauling, L. J.** (1940). 'A theory of the structure and process of formation of antibodies.' *J. Amer. Chem. Soc.*, **62**: 2643–57.

21. **Levene, P. A., and London, E. S.** (1929). 'The structure of thymonucleic acid.' *J. Biol. Chem.*, **83**: 793–802.

22. **Avery, O. T, MacLeod, C., and McCarty, C.** (1944). 'Studies on the chemical nature of the substance inducing transformation of pneumococcal types: Induction of transformation by a deoxyribonucleic acid fraction isolated from pneumococcus type III.' *J. Exp. Med.*, **79**: 137–58.

23. **Chargaff, E.** (1950). 'Chemical specificity of nucleic acids and mechanism of their enzymatic degradation.' *Experentia*, **6**: 201–9.

24. **McCarty, M.** (1985). *The Transforming Principle*. New York: W. W. Norton & Co.

25. **Pauling, L., and Niemann, C.** (1939). 'The structure of proteins.' *J. Amer. Chem. Soc.*, **61**: 1860–7.

26. **Breinl, F., and Haurowitz, F.** (1930). 'Untersuchung des Präzipitates aus Hämoglobin und anti-Hämoglobin serum und Bemerkungen über die Natur der Antikörper.' *Z. Physiol. Chem.*, **192**: 45–57.

27. **Alexander, J.** (1931). 'Some intercellular aspects of life and disease.' *Protoplasma*, **14**: 296.

28. **Mudd, S.** (1932). 'A hypothetical mechanism of antibody formation.' *J. Immunol.*, **23**: 423–27.

29. **Heidelberger, M.** (1939). 'Chemical aspects of the precipitin and agglutinin reactions.' *Chem. Rev.*, **24**: 323–42.

30. **Marrack, J. R.** (1938). *Report No. 230 of the Medical Research Council*. London: HM Stationary Office, p. 89.

31. **Haurowitz, F., Kraus, F., and Marx, F.** (1936). 'Über die Bindung zwischen Antigen und präzipitierendem Antikörper.' *Z. Physiol. Chem.*, **245**: 23.

32. **Landsteiner, M. D., and van der Scheer, J.** (1938). 'On cross reactions of immune sera to azoproteins. II. Antigens with azocomponents containing two determinant groups.' *J. Exp. Med.*, **67**: 709–23.

33. **Pauling, L.** (1940). 'A theory of the structure and process of formation of antibodies.' *J. Amer. Chem. Soc.*, **62**: 2654.

34. **Pauling, L., and Campbell, D. H.** (1942). 'The manufacture of antibodies in vitro.' *Science*, **95**: 440–1.

35. **Marrack, J. R.** (1938). *Report No. 230 of the Medical Research Council*. London: HM Stationary Office, p. 182.

36. **Marrack, J. R.** (1938). *Report No. 230 of the Medical Research Council*. London: HM Stationary Office, p. 188.

37. **Sabin, F. R.** (1939). 'Cellular reactions to a dye-protein with a concept of the mechanism of antibody formation.' *J. Exp. Med.*, **70**: 67–83.

38. **Burnet, F. M.** (1941). *The Production of Antibodies*. Melbourne: Macmillan, pp. 23–4.

39. **Burnet, F. M.** (1941). *The Production of Antibodies*. Melbourne: Macmillan, p. 37.

40. **Burnet, F. M.** (1941). *The Production of Antibodies*. Melbourne: Macmillan, pp. 42–3.

41. **Burnet, F. M.** (1941). *The Production of Antibodies*. Melbourne: Macmillan, pp. 62–4.

42. **Burnet, F. M., and Fenner, F.** (1949). *The Production of Antibodies* 2e. Melbourne: Macmillan, p. 2.

43. **Burnet, F. M., and Fenner, F.** (1949). *The Production of Antibodies* 2e. Melbourne: Macmillan, p. 97.

44. **Ehrich, W. E., and Harris, T. N.** (1942). 'The formation of antibodies in the popliteal lymph node in rabbits.' *J. Exp. Med.*, **76**: 335–47.

45. **White, A., and Dougherty, T. F.** (1945). 'Effect of prolonged stimulation of the adrenal cortex and of adrenalectomy on the numbers of circulating erythrocytes and lymphocytes.' *Endocrinol.*, **36**: 16.

46. **Robertson, J. S.** (1948). 'Failure of adrenal cortical extracts to cause lysis of living lympho-cytes in vitro.' *Nature*, **161**: 814.

47. **Fagraeus, A.** (1948). 'The plasma cellular reaction and its relation to the formation of anti-bodies in vitro.' *J. Immunology*, **58**: 1–13.

48. **Burnet, F. M., and Fenner, F.** (1949). *The Production of Antibodies* 2e. Melbourne: Macmillan, p. 92.

49. **Monod, J.** (1947). 'The phenomenon of enzymatic adaptation and its bearing on the prob-lems of genetics and differentiation.' *Growth Symp.*, **11**: 223–89.

50. **McCarty, M.** (1985). *The Transforming Principle*. New York: W. W. Norton & Co., pp. 213–35.

51. **Ehrlich, P., and Morgenroth, J.** (1901). 'Über Hämolysine: funfte Mittheilung.' *Berlin Klin. Wochenschr.*, **38**: 251–7.

52. **Burnet, F. M., and Fenner, F.** (1949). *The Production of Antibodies* 2e. Melbourne: Macmillan, pp. 100–2.

53. **Burnet, F. M., and Fenner, F.** (1949). *The Production of Antibodies* 2e. Melbourne: Macmillan, pp. 102–3.

54. **Traub, E.** (1939). 'Epidemiology of lymphocytic choriomeningitis in a mouse stock observed for four years.' *J. Exp. Med.*, **69**(6): 801–17.

55. **Medawar, P. B.** (1948). 'Immunity to homologous grafted skin. III. The fate of skin homo-grafts transplanted to the brain, to subcutaneous tissue and to the anterior chamber of the eye.' *Br. J. Exp. Pathol.*, **29**: 58–69.

Chapter 5

The cellular reformation

Immunology breaks its organic chemistry reins

By the early 1950s no definitive structural description of antibodies was known, no explanation of how the antibody response could be retained in the absence of antigen was
provided by 'instructional' theories, and the exact cellular origins of antibodies and the
mechanism by which antibody reproduction occurred with the required fidelity was not
yet firmly established. It can be argued that this was largely because an accepted body of
evidence defining protein structural principles was still absent and scientific models of
the gene remained hostage to chemical predispositions. If any decade can be described as
a 'decade of enlightenment', the post-war 1950s can lay claim *nonpareil*. From here on in,
cell biology and protein chemistry would become inextricably bound together.

Instruction gives way to natural selection

Driven by the shortcomings of the prevailing models of antibody induction and propagation, three different research groups in Copenhagen, Melbourne, and Chicago were
walking the same path but would come to slightly different conclusions that together
would form a realistic, collectively attractive theory of antibody production. The earlier
of the ideas, at least in terms of date of publication, came from the group of Niels Jerne,
based in Copenhagen but on a visiting fellowship to Caltech at the time of the publication. His seminal paper entitled 'The natural selection theory of antibody formation'
was a major departure from the earlier instructional theories and in some respects a
recapitulation of Ehrlich's side-chain theory with differences. Jerne's theory postulated
that the role of the antigen was to transport its cognate antibody to a cellular site for
reproduction of the antibody. On arrival at its cellular target and entry into the cell
by phagocytosis, the antigen would have served its purpose and would be eliminated
while the receiving cell would be triggered to reproduce the antibody delivered. In
describing this theoretical process Jerne proposed that:

> Among the population of circulating globulin molecules there will, spontaneously, be frac-
> tions possessing affinity toward any antigen to which the animal can respond. These are the
> so-called 'natural' antibodies.[1]

Jerne thus allowed for the presence of chance affinity between the natural antibody population and any antigen. Their pairing would require complementarity between antigen
and antibody and would be a prerequisite to the cellular targeting and reproduction.

To effect this Jerne proposed that antibody molecules would be selectively attached to the antigen surface.

A novel aspect of Jerne's theory was the proposed elimination of self-reactive antibodies during development (either early in life or continuously) leading to autoimmune avoidance. This was a subject Burnet had also addressed in his 1949 monograph (briefly discussed in Chapter 4) by suggesting that elimination occurred in the foetal stage of development via a sort of pre-exposure of self markers to the adaptive enzyme system resulting in tolerance to self. The same adaptive enzyme system would, he surmised, later introduce the specific elements that would endow antibodies with recognition features structurally complementary to their foreign cognate antigens.

On the question of how antibodies were reproduced, Jerne was still mechanistically wedded to the adaptive enzyme mechanism, noting that prior to induction a small amount of enzyme appears to be already present in the cells and speculating that induction of antibody synthesis would involve replication of the enzyme or its constituents (by some as yet unknown mechanism). He does comment on the possible role of RNA in directing the synthesis by acting as a template on which the amino acids are assembled. RNA would then direct the order of amino acids in the chain and potentially vice versa. In pursuing this line of reasoning some doubtful consequences had to be contemplated such as, if RNA is the protein assembly template, an antibody when introduced into a cell would either have to encounter a pre-existing RNA molecule or be capable of initiating synthesis of an RNA molecule specific to that antibody.

The pre-existing RNA model would require that in order for the cell to synthesize a variety of different antibodies, cells may:

> … already contain a large variety of RNA structures of various specificities…[2]

An alternative mechanism would require antibodies to impose their specificity on a small number of related RNA molecules.

While Jerne's natural selection theory showed gifted insight, his explanation of the mechanism by which specific antibody induction and synthesis occurred had not yet invoked the 'cell' as the responsible reproduction unit except as an enzymatic synthesis 'receptacle'. Like Ehrlich 40 years earlier, Jerne postulated a large pre-existing antibody population—although Ehrlich thought the antitoxin was actually a surface-located, naturally-occurring nutrient receptor (a model that Burnet would shortly return to) that adventitiously cross-reacted with a foreign antigen (toxin)—that was then reproduced by elements within the cell and released into the circulation in a sort of compensatory over-production. From Jerne's repertoire, the antigen would select a candidate pre-existing antibody on the basis of avidity and transport the assembly to an adaptive cell in which antibody production would occur, mediated by adaptive enzymes. Thus, Jerne's selection was at the level of the antibody-antigen complex, not the cell. Ehrlich's notion foundered on the rocks of hapten immunology, largely due as we have seen to Landsteiner's persuasive arguments on the impossibility of an organism retaining a repertoire large enough to recognize all known antigens. This limitation had to be addressed if new theories were to gain traction.

The continued place Jerne gave to adaptive enzyme synthesis of antibodies may seem at first sight to be rather surprising. The DNA double-helix revelation by Watson and Crick two years earlier and their subsequent mechanism paper one month later proposing that each of the two DNA chains could serve as a template for itself generating a new pair of exact copies, a requirement for replication of DNA, might have been expected to take the genomic 'material' debate by storm. These two *Nature* papers would have been well known to all scientists, since they clearly represented a revolution in biological mechanism, but their impact on immunologists and others looking to understand protein synthesis may not have been as obvious as hindsight would suggest. Despite the attractiveness of the double helix (putting to rest the triple helix proposal of Pauling and Cory, developed by the way without consideration of the important concept in Chargaff's base ratio analysis), there remained many unknowns that would have denied an obvious explanation for antibody and indeed any other protein synthesis. Watson and Crick still were not sure how DNA and protein interacted in the replicative mode, whether the genetic unit ('gene'—coined by Johanssen in 1909) was just DNA or a mixture of DNA and protein, and whether the replicative machinery (e.g. enzymatic activity) resided in a protein or indeed in the DNA itself. These facts and the embedded 'protein as gene' prejudices conspired to minimize the immediate impact. As Crick recollected 40 years later:

> How was the double helix received? There was rather little about it in the newspapers, if only because there was much less scientific journalism then. The reactions of the scientific community were mixed. The X-ray evidence supporting the double helix was, at that time, only suggestive. It was not enough to establish the structure beyond a reasonable doubt. To some, the whole idea seemed too simplistic. It certainly lacked biochemical support. In spite of this, most of the members of the phage group were enthusiastic about our ideas, especially as Max Delbruck liked both the structure and its implications. Others were not impressed. Some years later, Jean Brachet, the Belgian biochemist and embryologist, told me that when he read our papers, he thought ours was another silly theoretical idea, better ignored. Arthur Kornberg also thought nothing of it (perhaps because DNA did not appear to be an enzyme) and dismissed it as mere speculation. The reactions of many biochemists, such as Joseph Fruton, ranged from coolness to muted hostility. They had long considered the biochemistry of the gene to be based on proteins, not nucleic acids, and thought the problem far too difficult to tackle in the immediate future. It did not help that the structure had been put forward by two people who were obviously not card-carrying biochemists.[2]

Two years after Jerne's paper, David Talmage published his 'Allergy and Immunology' review article,[3] followed some eight months later by Burnet's[15] short paper proposing a clonal selection adaptation of Jerne's theory. Talmage had sent his manuscript to Burnet for pre-publication comments (probably late in 1956 since the review was published in February 1957), an event that has caused a great deal of debate among medical historians about the origin of the 'clonal selection' idea. Both Talmage and Burnet seemed to have realized the importance of nucleic acids, Talmage noting that the configuration of a protein molecule is contained in the nucleic acids as the hereditary units of the cell, although without any explanation of just how the cell got from one to the other. As we shall see, Burnet's thinking on the potential role of DNA was somewhat 'busier'.

In his review, which was actually about allergic responses, Talmage cites two pieces of evidence that support the proposition that the cell is the unit of antibody production, a proposition that was actually the core of Ehrlich's side-chain hypothesis and was the 'passive' production unit of Jerne's specific antibody populations. The first was a series of experiments by Roberts and Dixon, published in 1955, demonstrating that after transfer of cells from spleen or peritoneal exudates from immunized to non-immunized animals and subsequent challenge with the relevant antigen, a prompt anamnestic response occurred.[4] Talmage himself had also shown that transfer of serum under the same conditions caused suppression rather than accentuation of the antigenic response.[5] He dismisses Jerne's suggestion that these results could be explained by a foreign-antigen versus self-antigen recognition mechanism that operates even within animals of the same species, … *a feat that antibody-producing systems have never been shown to accomplish, and Jerne's explanation does not account for the successful transfer of sensitization with cells.*[4]

Talmage concludes the section in his review on 'Production of Antibodies' with a tantalizing proposition that contains the elements of a cellular model, while lacking perhaps some personal conviction and the specific language defining a genuine clonal selection hypothesis:

> As a working hypothesis **it is tempting to consider that one of the multiplying units in the antibody response is the cell itself**. According to this hypothesis, **only those cells are selected for multiplication whose synthesized product has affinity for the antigen injected.** This would have the disadvantage of requiring a **different species of cell for each species of protein produced**, but would not increase the total amount of configurational information required of the hereditary process. Three experimental observations may have bearing on this question. (a) The time required to sensitize an animal for a maximum anamnestic response is usually 30 days or more. This suggests that **multiplication of cells is required rather than multiplication of subcellular units**. The latter is a much more rapid process which may be important in the primary response. (b) Sensitization once established persists for a long time. This suggests the **persistence of an already differentiated cell type**. It might be expected that **a multipotential cell would revert to the presensitized state after a few cell divisions performed in the absence of antigen.** (c) **The protein produced by the rapidly reproducing myeloma cells is remarkably homogeneous**. Putnam suggests that in an individual case there is **massive production of one globulin randomly selected from the family of normal globulins**.[6]

Talmage subscribed to the notion that antigens select antibodies from a pre-formed population and having selected on the basis of affinity, some event occurs that triggers a cell-based proliferation. In fact, Talmage proposes that it is a multipotential cell that becomes sensitized by antigen, enters a pre-sensitized state, and after antigen disappearance reverts to its pre-sensitized state. The idea as presented lacked the element of perspicacious simplicity that would characterize Burnet's formulation.

About eight months after Talmage's review appeared, Burnet published a short communication in the little known *Australian Journal of Science*. There have been many opinions cast on the origin of Burnet's ideas in this second paper, his choice of journal giving as it did a rapid route to publication and his knowledge of Talmage's thinking in the area. Forsdyke goes further, implying that Burnet may have been heavily influenced by Talmage's idea and rapidly published to get 'into the game':

> Burnet's short paper (1), dated 21st October 1957, is described as a 'preliminary account' and cites Talmage's paper. It seems probable that the entire paper was drafted after the receipt of the Talmage manuscript.[7]

The University of Colorado's School of Medicine website goes perhaps one step beyond historical probity:

> It was David Talmage... who first put forward an explanation, now called the clonal selection theory. David suggested that each B cell might be able to make only one antibody sequence, and that each B cell synthesized its personal antibody.... David's clonal selection theory turned out to be correct...[8]

It would be disingenuous to suggest that this extract (written perhaps by enthusiastic supporters) is an example of 'creeping determinism' (something Jordan and Baxter comment on in another context[9]) since Talmage's contribution to immunology has been immense. Was Talmage the first to suggest the cell as the production 'unit' of antibodies? Certainly not, and neither was Burnet perhaps.

Ehrlich had invoked the cell as the site of antitoxin production and the role of lymph tissue in antibody production had been documented by McMaster and Kidd in 1937:

> ... An antiviral principle is elaborated within the regional lymph nodes draining skin into which vaccinia is injected. The immunity conferred by clinical Jennerian vaccination may be largely of lymph node origin.[10]

It was also documented by Sabin in 1939:

> It is thus inferred that the cells of the reticulo-endothelial system normally produce globulin and that antibody globulin represents the synthesis of a new kind of protein under the influence of an antigen.[11]

Astrid Fagraeus made more explicit mention of plasma cells in 1948:

> The conclusion is drawn that antibodies under the conditions of the experiments, are formed by cells of the R.E.S., passing through a chain of development, the final link of which is the mature pl.c.[12] [R.E.S = reticulo-endothelial system and pl.c = plasma cells]

Were Talmage and Burnet at equivalent points in their intellectual thinking about antibody production and clonal selection? Simultaneity in scientific discovery is a tricky phenomenon to quantitate and consequently difficult to accurately assign discovery 'rights'. How does one assess, for example, the originality of a slightly earlier but contemporaneous study by Askonas, Humphrey, and Porter reported in 1956 on the incorporation of radiolabelled amino acids into globulin fractions being synthesized by lymphatic tissues? During discussion of the observed synthesis activity in spleen, lymph nodes, and bone marrow *in vitro,* these authors concluded:

> As all the tissues examined synthesize all the fractions, though at different rates, the sim-
> plest explanation appears to be that individual cells are synthesizing characteristic types of
> γ-globulin, and that the distribution of these cells is different in the various organs.[13]

They made no reference to the work of Fagraeus or Roberts and Dixon since presumably they were unaware of either study and furthermore, gave no indication of
how the cell produced the correct antibody. Certainly no concept of clonal selection
was stated or even implied. Yet, their experimental track led them to the cell as the
antibody production unit, albeit allowing for multiple globulin types being produced
by individual cells, a possibility also entertained by Talmage as late as 1959 (see reference 18).

For Burnet, the timing of his papers is perhaps less relevant than the timing of
his ideas. In 1958 Burnet delivered a series of lectures at Vanderbilt University, the
Abraham Flexner lectures, and participated in an immunity and virus infection symposium. Those lectures were subsequently published by Vanderbilt University Press
in 1958 and republished in 1959[14] by Cambridge University Press, the latter being the
most frequently cited reference. In those lectures Burnet elaborated on his 1957 ideas,
and while further refinement would take place over the following decade, the essential
ingredients were fixed. Figure 5.1 shows Burnet's comparison of the prevailing theories
of antibody production at the time.

In Fig. 5.2 Burnet's clonal selection model is shown in more detail, clearly indicating
the selection of pre-existing lymphocytes by antigen, clonal expansion, and differentiation into antibody-secreting plasma cells.

Whatever the exact chain of events at the time, the massive contribution of Burnet
in the immunology area, particularly in virology, the antibody production ideas already
developed in Jerne's 1955 paper, and the elegant simplicity of Burnet's clonal model presented in 1957, suggested his engagement in a continuous process of intellectual thinking.

In comparing the Talmage paper to his own work, Burnet observes:

> Talmage (1957) has suggested that Jerne's view is basically an extension of Ehrlich's
> side chain theory of antitoxin production and that it would be more satisfactory if the
> replicating elements essential to any such theory were cellular in character ab initio
> rather than extracellular protein which can replicate only when taken into an appropri-
> ate cell. **Talmage does not elaborate this point of view but clearly accepts it as the
> best basis for the future development of antibody theory.** He stresses the multiplicity
> of the globulin types that can be present in the blood and is profoundly skeptical of
> any approach which attempts too 'unitarian' an interpretation of antibody. **In his view
> properdin has as much right to be called an antibody as any other globulin.**[15] (This
> author's bold emphasis.)

As an aside, the 'properdin' reference comes from a statement by Talmage in his 1957
review:

> The only properties common to all antibodies are (a) their protein nature, (b) an increased
> production following exposure to antigen, and (c) affinity for the antigen. In these respects,
> properdin is an antibody...[6]

Clonal selection theory

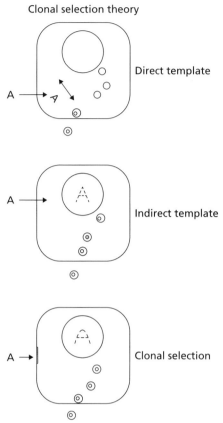

Direct template

Indirect template

Clonal selection

Fig. 5.1 The direct template model required the antigen to enter the cell and stamp a complementary pattern on the antibody molecule (Haurowitz, Pauling et al); in the indirect template model (Burnet & Fenner) the antibody synthesis is directed by cellular 'adaptive' enzymes in the presence of the antigen. Burnet's clonal selection theory required the antigen only to bind to the selected antibody displayed on the target cell surface after which its work was done.

Originally published in Burnet, F.M., *The Clonal Selection Theory of Acquired Immunity*, p.57, Cambridge University Press, Cambridge, UK, Copyright © 1959, with kind permission from Elizabeth Dexter and the University of Melbourne Archives.

Properdin was discovered in 1954 by Louis Pillemer and was later to become an important part of the alternative complement pathway. It is somewhat surprising that Talmage makes the statement he does about properdin when Pillemer himself stated:

> Properdin is a normal serum constituent and differs from antibody in many respects, particularly in its lack of specificity and in its exact requirements for its interactions.[16]

Text extract from Pillemer, L. et al., The properdin system and immunity. I. Demonstration and isolation of a new serum protein, properdin, and its role in immune phenomena, *Science*, Volume 120, Issue 3112, pp. 279–285, Copyright ©1954. Reprinted with permission from AAAS.

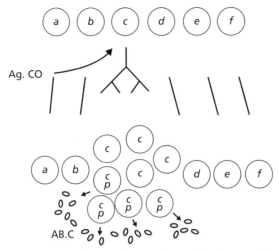

Fig. 5.2 To illustrate the clonal selection theory of immunity. Contact of the corresponding antigenic determinant *Ag. C* with cells of clone *c* stimulates proliferation to antibody-producing plasma cells *cp* and non-antibody producing types *c*.

Originally published in Burnet, F.M., *The Clonal Selection Theory of Acquired Immunity*, p. 59, Cambridge University Press, Cambridge, UK, Copyright © 1959, with kind permission from Elizabeth Dexter and the University of Melbourne Archives.

In addition, as the title of his paper suggests, Burnet attempted to reconcile those elements of Jerne's theory that Talmage (and others) were uncertain about. The kernel of Burnet's theory was that foreign antigen recognition is ascribed to clones of lymphocytic cells and not to circulating antibody. In elaborating this concept of antibodies containing 'patterns' of recognition for all possible foreign antigens, Burnet states:

> Each type of pattern is a specific product of a clone of mesenchymal cells and it is the essence of the hypothesis that **each cell automatically has available on its surface representative reactive sites equivalent to those of the globulin they produce.** For the sake of ease of exposition these cells will be referred to as lymphocytes, it being understood that other mesenchymal types may also be involved. Under appropriate conditions, **cells of most clones can either liberate soluble antibody or give rise to descendent cells which can.**[15] (This author's bold emphasis.)

So, it was actually Burnet who proposed that the interaction of antigen that leads to proliferation of antibody occurs at the cell surface with a 'natural antibody' (c.f. Ehrlich's nutrient receptor) after which the selected cell undergoes proliferation to produce a variety of descendants:

> In this way preferential proliferation will be initiated of all those clones whose reactive sites correspond to the antigenic determinants on the antigen used. The descendants will include plasmacytoid forms capable of active liberation of soluble antibody and lymphocytes which can fulfill the same functions as the parental forms.[15]

The essential elements of memory necessary for affective secondary responses were assumed to be due to the increase in circulating lymphocytes of the clones concerned. Burnet did not comment at this stage on how longevity of antigen responses can be sustained by cells known to have a relatively short lifetime.

A clonal selection coda

An important concept addressed by Burnet in a very preliminary way was the origin of antibody diversity. His notion was that during embryogenesis, the genomes of early mesenchymal cells would undergo '... randomization of the coding responsible for part of the specification of gamma globulin molecules.'[15] This would result in specifications in the genome of '... virtually every variant that can exist as a gamma globulin molecule' followed by some genomic stabilization and transfer to descendent cells.[15] Taking a cue from Jerne's current thinking, Burnet surmised that elimination of self-reactive clones would take place late in embryo development resulting in tolerance to those self-antigens.

Nowhere in the published 1957 paper does Burnet refer to nucleic acids in the context of his 'genome', although an early draft of the paper contained speculations on how certain regions of DNA could be randomized by somatic mutation during embryogenesis and then eventually 'fixed' in the genome for successive generations of each of the different antibody clones (see Fig. 5.3). His crude drawings clearly show a double-stranded nucleic acid as the target material in which somatic mutation would take place. Such somatic changes were even suggested to occur later in life, giving rise to autoimmune antibodies able to fix complement (the so-called AICF antibodies).

Some key elements of this short unpublished draft that would become important later are clearly already present in Burnet's thinking:

♦ The body must be able to generate a large enough antibody repertoire to accommodate all antigen species;

♦ To avoid self-recognition, the antibody-producing capacity of self-reactive clones must somehow be switched off *or* the clones must be eliminated;

♦ The lymphocyte surface after reaction with a specific antigen is primed to adopt a 'niche' role as a parent antibody-producing cell (thus giving a possible mechanism for Jerne's hypothesis);

♦ In early development lymphocyte 'molding' is occurring to induce tolerance to self-antigens;

♦ A globulin randomization mechanism must be present to generate the wide repertoire required, made possible by:
  • Restricted DNA segments of mesenchymal ancestor cells, randomized during embryonic life, and;
  • Stabilization of the random sequences subsequently occurs.

(a)

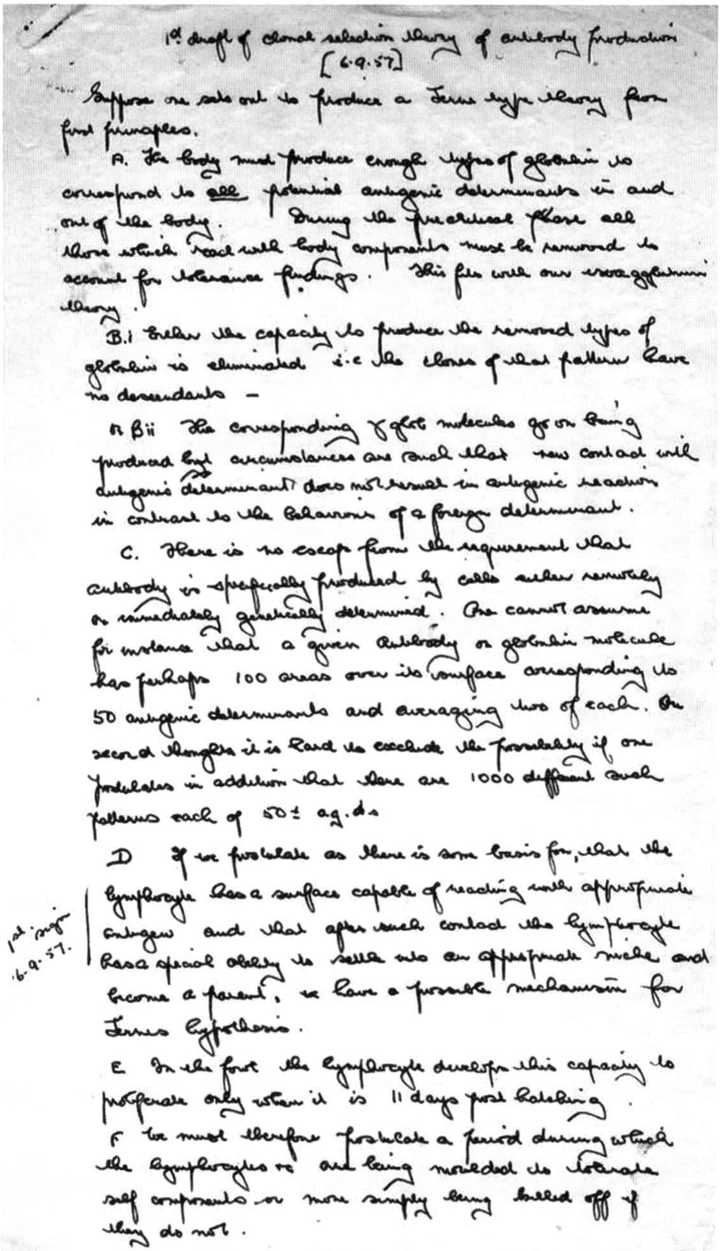

Fig. 5.3 Copy of an early draft of Burnet's 1957 paper.

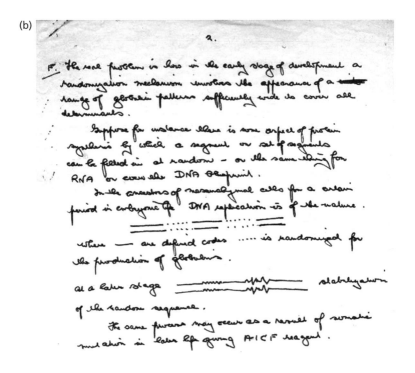

Fig. 5.3 (*Continued*).

The view that Burnet's 1957 'published' paper, which lacked some of the ideas in the draft version above for reasons best known to Burnet, contained clear and testable statements is not shared by all those who have followed the Talmage–Burnet interplay. Jordan and Baxter argue that Burnet's model was *qualitative* while Talmage presented a *quantitative* theory.[17] They argue that Burnet appeared incapable of devising an experiment to test his own clonal selection theory (citing Burnet's own PhD student Nossal who allegedly made such a comment) and that he acknowledged the priority of Talmage in formulating the cellular origin of antibodies. The courteous view, taken by both men themselves incidentally, would be that Talmage and Burnet had simultaneous thoughts on the importance of the cell as the 'reproduction unit' for antibodies *based on published work of others* while the degree of acuity with which those ideas were developed into a clonal model differed.

As late as 1959 Talmage himself expressed uncertainty about the 'clonality' of the cellular protein product, stating when considering the single cell studies of Nossal and Lederberg and the double immunization experiments of Coons:

> … impossible to conclude from both of these experiments that cells do not make more than one type of protein, but only that the number of types any cell can make is greatly

restricted compared with the capacity of the organism as a whole. In this sense they are highly specialized.[18]

In this statement Talmage seems to define 'specialization' in a qualitative way, allowing some restricted multiplicity of antibodies produced by individual cells, a conclusion resonating with the ideas of Askonas, Humphrey, and Porter published some years earlier.

What is clear from the way events played out is that Burnet's formulation of clonal selection intellectually was a more discrete set of ideas. The fact is it was Burnet's concepts that influenced the experimental path of cellular immunology for the next decade.

The negative connotation of 'qualitative' as applied to Burnet's clonal model and indeed his science as a whole is interesting. One is reminded of Einstein's 'qualitative' thought experiment, his 'glücklichste Gedanke' ('luckiest/happiest thought'),[19] in which he conceptualized the principle of general relativity by considering a man falling in free space who is unable to feel his own weight. It took him eight more years and the help of Marcel Grossman's mathematical expertise (the 'quantitative' contribution) to complete the generalization of his theory of special relativity. Although Poincaré and Lorentz were considered by some of Einstein's contemporaries to be at the same cusp of relativistic thinking, their attachment to current dogma (the 'ether' as a fixed frame of reference) acted as a heavy veil obscuring the real content of Einstein's model.[20] Often, 'thought' experiments can lead to scientific leaps as astounding as those arising from detailed experimental design and analysis. In the end it is the model that makes the most comprehensible conceptual leap, casts off the incompatible dogma, and amasses the largest portfolio of experimental proof that wins the prize.

The first actual experiments that would firmly establish the cell as the 'clonal' unit of antibody production, ironically, were carried out in Burnet's Institute (WEHI) by one of his PhD students, Gustav Nossal, working together with Joshua Lederberg on a Visiting Fulbright Fellowship from Wisconsin. The experimental system involved immunization of rabbits with two different *Salmonella* serotypes, followed by removal of lymph nodes and dispersion of lymphatic cells to obtain single cells in droplets (the expertise of Lederberg), some of which would be expected to be secreting specific antibody. On challenge with either bacterial cell a motility assay was used since it was known that anti-flagellar antibodies could inhibit bacterial motility. The results showed that single cells could only inhibit the flagella-dependent motility of one or other of the two serotypes injected but not both. As the authors observed, the results were consistent with the hypotheses of Talmage and Burnet:

> These results imply that when an animal is stimulated with two contrasting antigens individual cells tend to form one species of antibody… The experiments were provoked by current hypotheses on the role of clonal individuation in antibody formation.[21]

Thus, in what was essentially an extension of the work of Fagraeus, Nossal and Lederberg produced the first evidence for 'one cell, one antibody'. While clearly an exciting advance, it left open the question of exactly how the specificity of individual antibodies was translated from the genome into a plausible protein structure that differed in those parts responsible for antigen binding but was structurally homogeneous in non-antigen binding regions. The answer to that question would come from the developing arts of protein chemistry and molecular biology.

Acknowledgements

Text extracts from Talmage, D.W., Allergy and Immunology, *Annual Review of Medicine*®, Volume 8, pp. 239–245, Copyright © 1957, republished with permission of Annual Review of Medicine®, from permission covered through Copyright Clearance Center, Inc.

Text extracts from Burnet, F.M., A modification of Jerne's theory of antibody production using the concept of clonal selection, *The Australia Journal of Science*, Volume 20, pp. 67–69, Copyright © 1957, reproduced by permission of the Australian and New Zealand Association for the Advancement of Science.

Text extract reproduced from *Gene*, Volume 135, Issue 1–2, Crick, F.H.C., Looking backwards: a birthday card for the double helix, p.17, Copyright © 1993, with permission from Elsevier: http://www.sciencedirect.com/science/journal/03781119

References

1. **Jerne, N. K.** (1955). 'The natural selection theory of antibody formation.' *Proc. Natl. Acad. Sci.*, **41**: 849–57.
2. **Crick, F. H. C.** (1993). 'Looking backwards: a birthday card for the double helix.' *Gene*, **135**: 17.
3. **Talmage, D. W.** (1957). 'Allergy and Immunology.' *Ann. Rev. Med.*, **8**: 239–56.
4. **Roberts, J. C., and Dixon, F. J.** (1955). 'The transfer of lymph node cells in the study of the immune response to foreign proteins.' *J. Exp. Med.*, **102**: 379.
5. **Talmage, D. W., Freter, G. G., and Thomson, A.** (1956). 'The effect of whole body x-radiation on the specific anamnestic response in the rabbit.' *J. Infect. Diseases*, **99**: 246–52.
6. **Talmage, D. W.** (1957). 'Allergy and Immunology.' *Ann. Rev. Med.*, **8**: 239–56; Putnam, F. W., and Udin, B. (1953). 'Proteins in multiple myeloma. I. Physicochemical study of serum proteins.' *J. Biol. Chem.*, **202**: 727.
7. **Forsdyke, D. R.** (1995). 'The origins of the clonal selection theory of immunity as a case study for evaluation in science.' *FASEB J.*, **9**: 164–6.
8. **Integrated Department of Immunology, History of Immunology in Denver**, available from: http://www.ucdenver.edu/academics/colleges/medicalschool/departments/immunology/Pages/History.aspx
9. **Jordan, M. A., and Baxter, A. G.** (2008). 'Quantitative and qualitative approaches to GOD: the first 10 years of the clonal selection theory.' *Immunol. & Cell Biol.*, **86**: 72–9.
10. **McMaster, P. D., and Kidd, J. G.** (1937). 'Lymph nodes as a source of neutralizing principle for vaccinia.' *J. Exp. Med.*, **66**: 73–100.
11. **Sabin, F. R.** (1939). 'Cellular reactions to a dye-protein with a concept of the mechanism of antibody formation.' *J. Exp. Med.*, **70**: 67–82.

12. **Fagraeus, A.** (1948). 'The plasma cellular reaction and its relation to the formation of antibodies in vitro.' *J. Immunol.*, **58**: 1–13.

13. **Askonas, B. A., Humphrey, J. H.**, and Porter, R. R. (1956). 'On the origin of the multiple forms of rabbit gamma-globulin.' *Biochem. J.*, **63**: 412–19.

14. **Burnet, F. M.** (1959). *The Clonal Selection Theory of Acquired Immunity.* Cambridge: Cambridge University Press.

15. **Burnet, F. M.** (1957). 'A modification of Jerne's theory of antibody production using the concept of clonal selection.' *Aust. J. Science*, **20**: 67–9.

16. **Pillemer, L., Blum, L., Lepow, I. H., Ross, O. A., Todd, E.W.**, and **Wardlaw, A. C.** (1954). 'The properdin system and immunity. I. Demonstration and isolation of a new serum protein, properdin, and its role in immune phenomena.' *Science*, **120**: 279–85.

17. **Jordan, M. A.**, and **Baxter, A. G.** (2008). 'Quantitative and qualitative approaches to GOD: the first 10 years of the clonal selection theory.' *Immunol. & Cell Biol.*, **86**: 72–9.

18. **Talmage, D. W.** (1959). 'Immunological specificity.' *Science*, **129**: 1634–48.

19. **Isaacson, W.** (2007). *Einstein, His Life and Universe.* New York: Simon & Schuster, pp. 145–7.

20. **Isaacson, W.** (2007). *Einstein, His Life and Universe.* New York: Simon & Schuster, pp. 132–5.

21. **Nossal, G. J. V.**, and **Lederberg, J.** (1958). 'Antibody production by single cells.' *Nature*, **181**: 1419–20.

Chapter 6

The molecular path unfolds

An understanding of protein properties begins to emerge

As with the introduction of ultracentrifugation and electrophoresis in the 1920s and 1930s, techniques that allowed characterization of serum globulin fractions in some qualitative detail, so the development of chromatography and automated UV-visible spectrophotometry in the 1950s provided the essential tools for protein chemists to purify proteins, a prerequisite to unravelling their molecular structures. Chromatography of small molecules was well known using solid-phase supports and mixtures of various solvents and salts to allow differential elution of chemically different compounds. Proteins however were different. With organic solvents they would denature and with certain salts (e.g. urea) they would unfold or exhibit stability problems. Further, complex mixtures of proteins such as presented by normal serum—essentially 'polyelectrolytes'—would introduce new separation challenges. Given the continuing uncertainty about the chemical differences between normal and immune globulin, new approaches were required, approaches that only those knowledgeable in the fledgling field of protein chemistry would have the skills to develop.

Enzymes were proteins that had been extensively studied since they seemed to hold so many keys to biological processes. Their molecular characterization however was hampered by impure preparations. A critical breakthrough was made by Moses Kunitz, working at the Rockefeller Institute in Princeton, who developed preparations of both ribonuclease[1] in 1940, and ten years later 'crystalline deoxyribonuclease'.[2] In the Kunitz purification protocols, which relied heavily on crystallization, pure enzymes were produced that allowed both stability (thermodynamic) and kinetic characterizations. A further major step forward was the introduction of partition chromatography of proteins hitherto only used for small molecule separations.

In Cambridge, England, two new 'kids on the block' were also making significant headway in protein science. Rodney Porter was working with Fred Sanger (as his PhD student) on characterization of the terminal amino acids in various haemoglobins and the relationship between the inter-species (or intra- in the case of human adult versus foetal) N-terminal variation and the antibody responses thereof reported in published work of many other groups (see Fig. 6.1). What these studies had shown, subsequently reinforced by work on ribonuclease, was that proteins with identical activities (either O_2 binding or RNA hydrolysis) may have different terminal sequences, even if this difference is slight.[3] If this were also true of globulin and immune globulin protein, so that antibodies with different specificities may exhibit amino acid sequence diversity

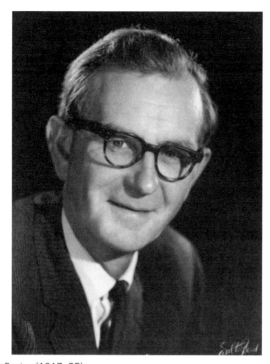

Fig. 6.1 Rodney Porter (1917–85).

without compromising their ability to act as antigen-binding proteins, it would place Pauling's 'configurational diversity' theory in jeopardy.

During a one-year post-doctoral period in Sanger's laboratory from 1948 to 1949 Porter began his immunological journey. The results of several Cambridge studies on rabbit globulin and specific anti-ovalbumin antibodies reflected Porter's experimental flair reinforced by skill sets developed with Sanger. His conclusions after purification of immune and non-immune rabbit serum gamma fractions and N-terminal sequence analysis were as follows:

1. There was no difference in the amino terminal residue in any of the immune or non-immune globulin fractions studied. A single N-terminal residue, alanine, was found.
2. All globulin fractions had the same N-terminal sequence Ala-Leu-Val-Asp-(Glu?).
3. Reduction of the disulphide bonds had no apparent effect on the antigen binding.
4. The flocculation (precipitation) time increased by five times.

While the science was impeccable, Porter's interpretation of the results led him to an unfortunate conclusion. He was unaware at that time that the heavy chains (not yet discovered!) of rabbit globulins are N-terminally blocked and that his uniform N-terminal alanine would have been from the light chains only. Knowing the molecular weight of

~150 000 for globulins in the gamma fraction, his understandable conclusion was that globulins must therefore be single chain molecules of around 1500 amino acids. This apparent chemical homogeneity of globulins led Porter to acknowledge that Pauling's structural diversity model was alive and kicking:

> The results described are in agreement with Pauling's theory of antibody formation in that no chemical distinction between the fractions could be found… it is clear that the chemical evidence described here, contrary to the physiological evidence discussed in the introduction [those of Haurowitz & Breinl, Mudd, and even Burnet], is in accordance with Pauling's theory.[4]

In a follow-up study while still in Cambridge, some preliminary results were obtained using enzymatic degradation of impure rabbit globulin. Porter's conclusion would hold the key for his later work on the chain structure of gamma fraction rabbit antibodies. By treatment of rabbit globulin with papain, Porter showed that a fragment was generated that was able to inhibit the precipitin reaction in a dose-dependent manner. Furthermore, when precipitating globulin was added, the fragment was carried down with the precipitate. In addressing the question of heterogeneous bivalency Porter noted:

> … hydrolysis would be expected to produce two inhibitors arising from two combining centres in different parts of the molecule… it appears that only one inhibitor, from the terminal quarter of the molecule, is produced by papain-HCN hydrolysis… possible that a second combining centre was destroyed during the hydrolysis.[5]

Porter's data should have told him the two combining sites were identical, thus explaining the single inhibition activity, but he was still influenced by the Landsteiner/Pauling school of thinking and would need to take a different path to shake free of this influence.

In 1949 Porter moved to the MRC National Institute of Medical Research (NIMR) in London. Having realized that chromatography was likely to be very important for further characterization of proteins, he took a position in the group of AJP Martin. During his first year at NIMR, working with Martin—Archer Martin would receive the Nobel Prize for Chemistry with Richard Synge in 1952 for the invention of partition chromatography—Porter focused on use of this new technique for protein purification.[6] This would eventually lead him to revise his initial view of antibody structure, although it would take more than ten painstaking years to fully understand the immunoglobulin chain structure.

Antibody chain structure revealed

In Cambridge, Sanger was making headway on methods for protein sequencing. His determination of the primary structure of insulin shattered all the early 'colloid-based' theories of protein structure, but not without niggling uncertainty along the way—he initially thought there were four chains of insulin joined by disulphide bonds due to an incorrect published molecular weight value of 12 000. His methods involved splitting the individual chains of insulin into peptide fragments, either chemically or by use of proteases, and then decoding their reconstruction into a linear sequence using overlapping peptides generated by the different methods of hydrolysis. Despite these significant advances Sanger was still not sure of the general nature of protein structure:

> It is impossible with the small amount of experimental evidence at present available to form any general theory of protein structure or to form any principles that govern the arrangement of amino acids in proteins…[7]

It was in this scientific climate that Porter returned to his antibody studies after several years working with protein chromatography in Martin's group. When applying his knowledge to the fractionation of immune rabbit globulin, the results were complex but at the same time ripe for speculation. His initial purifications showed chromatographic differences between immune and non-immune globulin with a series of overlapping fractions in the gammaglobulin region. All these fractions possessed antigen-specific antibody (against ovalbumin) but moved position on his chromatographic columns as the multiple immunizations moved the rabbit through primary and then secondary responses. Porter speculated that this could have been due to 1) the γ-globulin types varying during synthesis within the same or different antibody-producing cells; 2) environmental influences on the synthesis 'system' could result in small differences in the protein product, or 3) γ-globulins are labile and this instability might result in heterogeneous physical properties (in a reference back to the instructional theory of Pauling).[8]

A year later, working with John Humphrey, Porter demonstrated that this heterogeneous gamma-globulin behaviour was repeatable with totally different antigens (polysaccharide from pneumococcus type II killed bacteria and live influenza type A virus). In concluding their summary of these experiments Humphrey and Porter speculated:

> The findings suggest that different cells, capable of producing slightly different globulins, may predominate in antibody production according to the route of injection and duration of the antigenic stimulus.[9]

This was still one year before Burnet and Talmage would propose the cellular basis of antibody production, although without any explanation yet of the genetic origin of antibody heterogeneity.

In studies on bovine serum albumin published in 1957[10] Porter adopted a fragmentation approach to dissect this antigen in an attempt to define a smaller unit (referred to as 'inhibitor') that still retained the ability to unite with its antibody. This approach was a cue for the future methods Porter would apply to the antibody itself. The study was not remarkable but it did introduce for the first time in Porter's studies an important technique for measuring antibody-antigen interactions, the agar gel precipitation method of Ouchterlony[11] (see Fig. 6.2).

During 1958 Porter, working essentially alone, made a key breakthrough. By using a pure preparation of the proteolytic enzyme papain he reproduced and improved on his 1950 studies, generating three fragments of approximately equal size, two of which displayed antigen binding (fragments I and II), with a third fragment (III) having no antigen binding but with lower solubility and hence easily crystallizable. The separation of the two antigen-binding fragments into two chromatographically different fractions (if classical Fab fragments they should not have been separable) was probably due to

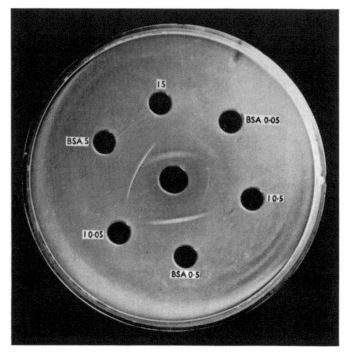

Fig. 6.2 Comparison of behaviour of bovine-serum albumin (BSA) and inhibitor (I) on diffusion into antiserum in agar gel by the method of Ouchterlony. Centre cup contains rabbit anti-bovine-serum albumin. This photograph was taken after the plate had been standing for five days at 20C.

Reproduced with permission from Porter, R.R., The Isolation and Properties of a Fragment of Bovine-Serum Albumin which Retains the Ability to Combine with Rabbit Antiserum, *Biochemical Journal*, Volume 66, Part 4, pp. 677–685, Copyright © 1957 the Biochemical Society.

differential glycosylation, noted by Porter after analysis of total hexose content and adding weight to the notion that the two antigen-binding arms were actually structurally different. His view of the antibody as a single linear chain remained an *idée fixe* and he was forced to propose a number of rather odd variations to explain the fragmentation, faced with the topological conundrum of how two fragments of equal size could display antigen-binding activity in a linear chain while attached to a non-antigen binding piece. Further, the intrinsic errors in amino acid analysis and N-terminal sequencing still allowed for the possibility that the two antigen-binding fragments were different in specificity, a conclusion that pushed Porter back into the comfort zone of Pauling's conformational instruction theory—two different antigen-binding fragments could be 'conformationally different' in the presence of a structurally stable core! Despite these exegetical difficulties his concluding statement was less dogmatic and even rather premonitory:

> I and II are extremely similar in chemical and biological properties, and III differs very widely in all respects. This has led to the suggestion that rabbit γ-globulin is formed of two pieces with very similar structure joined to a third piece of quite different character.[12]

Protein chemistry meets genetics

The 'embryonic antibody diversification' mechanism initiated by Burnet was renovated by Lederberg in 1959, invoking a continuous process of somatic mutation throughout lymphocyte proliferation. Lederberg provided his analysis in a set of analytical dissections of current thinking, his 'nine propositions', in what was essentially a *coup de grace* for much of the contemporary antibody mechanistic dogma. In this theoretical exposition[13] he buried instructive theories, laid the foundation for one antibody, one gene, proposed a mechanism for lifetime somatic mutation in the context of neo-Darwinian selection with hypermutation occurring via gene randomization (admitting this was the 'least defensible' proposition), and anticipated that antibody-producing cells spontaneously produce antibody prior to antigen exposure (no instruction here), aligned with the notion that exposure of immature antibody-producing cells induces tolerance to those (self-) antigens and that '… some role of cellular destruction of immature antibody-forming cells in the induction of tolerance' is plausible. He also accepted that maturation and differentiation into plasma cells marks the acceleration of protein synthesis and increased antibody production, and commented on the clone persistence issue required to explain life-long immunity:

> … a substantial reservoir of immunological memory should be inherent from one cycle of expansion of a given clone. Its ultimate decay might be mitigated either by continued selection (that is, persistence of the antigen) stabilization of genotypes, or dormancy (to cell division or remutation, or both) on the part of a fraction of the clone.[13]

> Text extract reproduced from Lederberg, L. Genes and Antibodies, *Science*, Volume 129, Issue 3364, pp. 1649–1653, Copyright ©1959. Reprinted with permission from AAAS.

By coincidence, in the same year (in fact the same month) Gerald Edelman, working at the Rockefeller Institute in New York, published a short but devastatingly simple observation that would completely change the direction of thinking about antibody structure. His results from use of reducing chemicals in the presence of protein-denaturing agents, along with sedimentation experiments, demonstrated that gamma globulin could be dissociated into smaller subunits simply by reduction of disulphide bonds. In an extension of these studies Edelman, now working with Poulik, proposed a multi-chain structure for gamma globulin (so-called 7S γ-globulin) that cast major doubt on the single chain model proposed by Porter arising from his N-terminal studies, despite the fact that the relation between Porter's papain fragments and Edelman's reduced and alkylated chains must *de facto* have been orthogonal, a distinction noted by Edelman:

> The fragments obtained by treatment with papain do not seem to be identifiable with the subunits described above.[14]

> Text extract © 1939 Rockefeller University Press. Originally published in *The Journal of Experimental Medicine,* Volume 113, pp. 861–884.

In their 'Discussion' Edelman and Poulik propose a model for gamma-globulin structure, also suggesting an explanation for the structural differences in myeloma (Bence-Jones) proteins:

A unifying hypothesis may be formulated for the structure of proteins in the γ-globulin family based on the findings presented above … 7S γ-globulin molecules appear to consist of several polypeptide chains linked by disulfide bonds. Bivalent antibodies may contain two chains that are similar or identical in structure…. A provisional explanation for the wide molecular weight range of antigenically related globulins from Bence-Jones proteins to macroglobulins is suggested by this model…. may arise from various combinations of different chains as well as from differences in the sequence of amino acids within each type of chain.[14]

In 1962 and now at the Department of Immunology, St Mary's Hospital Medical School in London, Porter presented his own model for immunoglobulin structure at a celebratory symposium at Columbia University[15] (commemorating the fiftieth anniversary of the Institute of Cancer Research, Columbia University, and the tenth anniversary of the Francis Delafield Hospital, 12–14 March, 1962), followed in 1963 by what could be described as the defining paper in the field, at the same time acknowledging the critical observations of Edelman and others. The title, 'The arrangement of the peptide chains in γ-globulin',[16] provided the evidence for Porter's symposium model, shown in Fig. 6.3. With this chain structure and the underlying experimental data five conclusions were drawn by Porter and colleagues:

1. The proposed structure, of four peptide chains with five interchain disulphide bonds, of γ-globulin has been tested by isolation and characterization of the constituent chains.
2. The amino acids, carbohydrate and N-terminal amino acids of rabbit γ-globulin have been accounted for in terms of the chains.
3. The papain digestion pieces have been correlated with peptide chains and they have themselves been dissociated into their respective chains. These have in turn been analysed and characterized.
4. The carbohydrate associated with papain digestion piece I has been shown to be due to non-covalently bound glycopeptide, and analysis suggested that the carbohydrate of rabbit γ-globulin is present on the molecule in two parts.
5. The antibody-combining site of horse antibody is associated with chain A.[16]

The amassed data that now began to emerge tempted both Edelman and Porter to play the chain topology game. How were the chains disposed one to another and which chains were involved in antigen binding? The question of the antigen-binding site location separated the two camps. Porter speculated that antigen interacted with the heavy chain only[16] while Edelman adduced evidence for both light- and heavy-chain roles. In doing so, Edelman constructed an interchain-interaction zone and an antigen-recognition zone (see Fig. 6.4). He also allowed for regions that could 'modulate' the binding site conformation and that any heavy chain could pair with any light chain. Interestingly, the perceived dominance of the heavy chain in antigen binding would continue to be a controversial topic right into the 1990s.

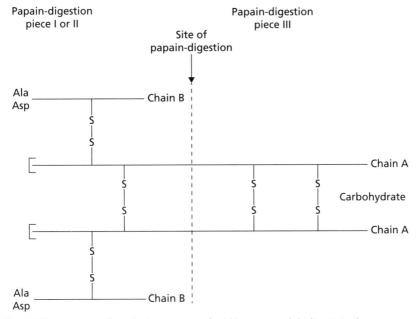

Fig. 6.3 The proposed four chain structure of rabbit gamma globulin. Note the now accepted blocked ([ ) N-terminus of the heavy chain.

Reproduced with permission from Fleischman, J.B., et al., The Arrangement of the Peptide Chains in γ-Globulin, *Biochemical Journal*, Volume 88, Part 2, pp. 220–228, Copyright © 1963 the Biochemical Society.

Edelman concluded that his rigid chain model:

> … meets the requirements for symmetry, arrangement in the known molecular shape and volume, chain interaction, site location and consistency with known degradative steps.[17]

Edelman further concluded:

> Changes of the amino acid residues in the site region can directly alter the specificity of the antibody, whereas changes in the modulating region alter the conformation of the binding site only indirectly.[17]

Topologically Edelman's model was correct but lacked the fact that heavy chains also interacted with each other—bending about the two-fold axis to allow the two heavy chain C-terminal regions to interact, forming the Fc region would in any event have been a quite extraordinary prediction had it occurred to him and for which there was no direct evidence anyway.

Progress on the question of the involvement of both antibody chains in antigen binding and *a priori* that a defined amino acid sequence must dictate the antibody specificity came from the independent studies of Edgar Haber at Harvard Medical School and Charles Tanford at Duke University. Haber prepared rabbit antibodies to the enzyme ribonuclease and enzymatically digested the IgG with papain, according to Porter's procedure, producing pure Fab fragments. Under fully denaturing

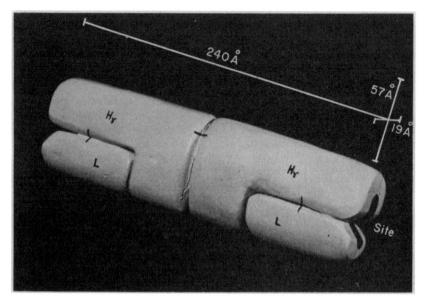

Fig. 6.4 Edelman and Gally's model of the 7S antibody molecule.

Reproduced with permission from Edelman, G.M and Gally, J.A., A model for the 7S antibody molecule, *Proceedings of the National Academy of Science (PNAS)*, Volume, 51, Number 5, pp. 846–853, Copyright © 1964, with permission from the author.

conditions including reducing the disulphide bonds to dissociate the chains, Haber showed that virtually no residual structure remained in the denatured molecule. Anti-ribonuclease binding activity was then regained by removal of the denaturant and reoxidation of the disulphide bridges.[18] This was important for two reasons. Haber was able to conclude that both the heavy chain and light chain were required for antigen binding, and more importantly that the information for antibody specificity resided solely within the antibody sequence itself, a serious blow for the conformational theory of antibody specificity. A year later, Charles Tanford produced identical results but this time with a rabbit antibody directed towards the much studied dinitrophenyl (DNP) hapten, attached in this instance to the amino acid lysine forming DNP-lysine.[19] Tanford's conclusions were even more important in some respects. The spontaneous regain of Tanford's folded conformation in the two-chain antibody fragment was exactly in line with Anfinson's hypothesis that protein folding was mediated solely by the amino acid sequence.[20] Furthermore, the regain of anti-hapten activity in the absence of hapten during the folding process was formal proof that antigen-directed antibody folding is unlikely. A further nail was driven into the conformational-theory coffin by Tanford when, after renaturation of non-specific Fab fragment chains in the presence of a 100-fold excess of DNP-lysine, no binding of hapten to this Fab could be seen. In the same year, the Tanford group made a remarkably premonitory proposal for the shape of the IgG molecule, based on solution sedimentation and viscosity data together with the results from different

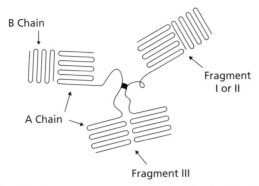

Fig. 6.5 Model of IgG chain arrangement, as predicted by Tanford in 1965. A chain = heavy chain, B chain = light chain.

spectroscopy techniques (see Fig. 6.5).[21] While the quaternary arrangement of the light and heavy chains was not correct in this cartoon—the light (B) chain was shown as a separate 'globule' from the heavy-chain component of fragment I or II (the Fab fragment)—the overall Y-shape was tantalizingly close to what would later be confirmed by electron microscopy experiments.

Despite the advancing understanding of gamma-globulin chain structure, the distinction between the so-called 7S (containing γ_1A and γ_2 fractions by immunoelectrophoresis) and 19S (γ_1M) globulin forms was still unclear. Porter and his colleague Cohen from the same department (St Mary's, London) who had looked at human 7S gamma globulin, while accepting that A-chains (H or heavy chains by the recent nomenclature of Edelman and Benaceraff) from the three distinct species were different structurally (they had different electrophoretic and chromatographic behaviour for example), believed that they were still 'gamma globulins' and that any differences were likely to be due to differential glycosylation. Edelman and Benaceraff, heavily influenced by their interest in Bence-Jones proteins, proposed that the heavy chains were less variable than light chains:

> The scheme would suggest that the genes controlling H chains would have undergone less variation than those containing the highly variable set of light chains.[22]

The implications of this proposal for the number of different light chains required to account for the breadth of antigen specificity received a mitigating option from Edelman that, in the event, would prove closer to the reality:

> It has the inherent disadvantage of requiring a rather large number of L chains of different amino acid composition and sequence. On the other hand, if the active site were determined by the interaction of more than one chain, a limited number of chains of different sequence might provide an adequate range of specificity and still be consistent with a selective mechanism.[22]

In the same year, Edelman and Gally presented the results of a pivotal study on Bence-Jones proteins and normal light chains, using various electrophoretic, chromatographic, amino acid composition, and spectroscopic methods, and concluded:

> The findings suggest that Bence-Jones proteins are composed of L chains of the type found in normal and pathological γ-globulins.[23]

Although in 1962 firm sequence information to fully confirm this proposition was lacking, this was remedied three years later by two of Edelman's colleagues at the same institute, Norbert Hilschman and Lyman Craig, who took the Bence-Jones proteins from several donors, generated partial sequences by peptide mapping (all of them kappa chains), and concluded when comparing two of the donor proteins (Roy and Cummings):

> It seems likely, therefore, that the entire sequence in Roy from 106 to 212 is also present in Cummings except for the single Val-Leu replacement at position 189.[24]

This was the first proof that the C-terminal portions of light chains were identical (aside from the allotypic differences). In comparing the N-terminal portions of the same donor chains, Hilschman and Craig found that they varied significantly in sequence, representing evidence of a variable plus constant region construction. In concluding their paper, Hilschman and Craig, who were aware of Smithies' theory of antibody variability generation by genetic inversion, did not believe they had provided sufficient evidence to support or refute this proposed mechanism for the observed variability in the N-terminal region, despite the fact that Smithies had suggested sequencing of Bence-Jones proteins as a way to test his theory.[25] Notwithstanding the exotic proposition from Smithies, the impact of Hilschman and Craig's findings would have provided the molecular trigger for more testable genetic models of antibody diversity that would explain how an antibody gene could exhibit diversity in one region while remaining constant in another and further, how Darwinian selection could operate on such a construction.

It would be just a few short months later that Edelman and Gally would make the first attempt to explain the observed sequence results (see Fig. 6.6). In their 1967 paper they state the problem:

1. The multiplicity of amino acid replacements in the variable half (V) and the relative invariance of sequence in the constant half (C).
2. The presence of a majority of amino acid interchanges consistent with single base replacements in the genetic code.
3. The similarity in lengths of the V and C regions (in the case of the light chains).
4. The occurrence of invariant segments within the V region as well as the finding that certain positions show interchanges among only a few amino acids (e.g., N-terminal glu or asp in K chains).
5. The failure to observe a high recombination frequency among allotypes.
6. The fact that a particular plasma cell tumor can produce a single well defined protein, the sequence of which does not change from generation to generation. This may be correlated with the finding that the majority of single plasma cells from animals immunized with two unrelated antigens produce antibodies either against one or the other antigen.[26]

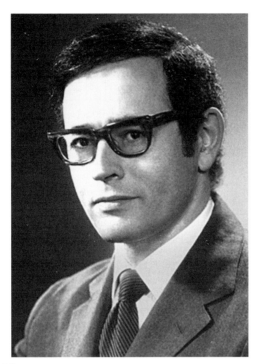

Fig. 6.6 Gerald Edelman.
Reproduced with kind permission from Gerald Edelman.

Their genetic model of the variable region genes invoked gene duplication followed by accumulation of random mutation in the tandem duplicate genes with somatic crossing-over during recombination generating the diversity. This was in contradistinction to the germ-line theory in which all antibody specificities must be encoded by separate genes. The enormously large number of genes required to explain the germ-line theory was well recognized and no method yet existed to 'count' the number of genes. Furthermore, as Tonegawa would remind the germ-line theorists some years later, how could the allotypic marker common to all gamma-globulin genes and segregating as a single Mendelian gene be maintained in the germ line while present in many thousands of gene copies?

As Edelman and Gally point out, there was also no direct evidence for a somatic recombination theory for antibody genes. Their conclusions allowed for the possibility of a single cell exhibiting pluripotency in respect of antibody production, recapitulating the uncertainty expressed by Talmage some eight years earlier. Molecular biology had not quite come of age in immunology.

But the genie was still in the bottle at the Rockefeller Institute and the lamp was being vigorously rubbed. The enormous efforts of Edelman and colleagues in protein sequencing led in 1969 to the complete amino acid sequencing of an entire human antibody. Employing the now internationally agreed nomenclature for antibodies,[27] Edelman

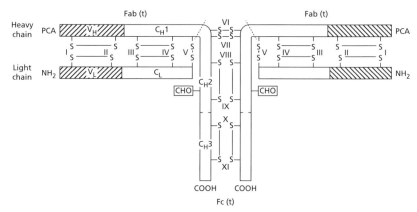

Fig. 6.7 Overall arrangement of chains in γG1 immunoglobulin Eu.

Reproduced from Edelman, G.M. et al., The covalent structure of an entire γG immunoglobulin molecule, *Proceedings of the National Academy of Science (PNAS)*, Volume 63, Number 1, pp. 78–85, Copyright © 1969, with permission from the author.

produced the first detailed 'plan' of an immunoglobulin (see Fig. 6.7) showing the locations of disulphide bonds, the chain structure of the variable sequences present in the V_H and V_L-regions, the location of carbohydrate and the sub-structural light chain and heavy chain 'homology regions' (C_L, C_H1, C_H2, and C_H3—now known as 'domains').[28]

The temptation was too great not to comment on the V- and C-region gene organization supporting the two-gene models already present in the literature. Edelman also speculated that the constancy of the C-region sequences even across species may be related to their effector functions such as complement activation. The momentum here however was building in other laboratories and soon the work of Milstein, Hood, Leder, Tonegawa, and others would release the genie, laying the foundation for a complete understanding of antibody genetics.

Acknowledgements

Text extracts reproduced from Edelman, G.M and Gally, J.A., A model for the 7S antibody molecule, *Proceedings of the National Academy of Sciences*, Volume 51, pp. 846–853, Copyright © 1964, by permission of the author.

Text extracts reproduced from Edelman, G.M. et al., The covalent strúcture of an entire gG immunoglobulin molecule, *Proceedings of the National Academy of Sciences*, Volume 69, pp. 878–85, Copyright © 1969, by permission of the author.

Text extracts reproduced from Edelman, G.M and Gally, J.A., Somatic recombination of duplicated genes: An hypothesis on the origin of antibody diversity, *Proceedings of the National Academy of Sciences*, Volume 57, pp. 353–358, Copyright © 1967, by permission of the author.

References

1. **Kunitz, M.** (1940). 'Crystalline ribonuclease.' *J. Gen.Physiol.*, **24**: 15–32.
2. **Kunitz, M.** (1950). 'Crystalline desoxyribonuclease.' *J. Gen. Physiol.*, **33**: 349–77.

3. **Porter, R. R., and Sanger, F.** (1948). 'The free amino groups of haemoglobins.' *Biochem. J.*, **42**: 287–94.

4. **Porter, R. R.** (1950). 'A Chemical Study of Rabbit Anti-ovalbumin.' *Biochem. J.*, **46**: 473–8.

5. **Porter, R. R.** (1950). 'The Formation of a Specific Inhibitor by Hydrolysis of Rabbit Anti-ovalbumin.' *Biochem. J.*, **46**: 479–84.

6. **Porter, R. R.** (1954). 'Chromatography of proteins.' *Brit. Med. Bull.*, **10**: 237–41.

7. **Sanger, F.** (1952). 'The arrangement of amino acids in proteins.' *Adv. Prot. Chem.*, **7**: 1–67.

8. **Porter, R. R.** (1955). 'The Fractionation of Rabbit γ-Globulin by Partition Chromatography.' *Biochem. J.*, **59**: 405–10.

9. **Humphrey, J. H, and Porter, R. R.** (1956). 'An investigation of rabbit antibodies by the use of partition chromatography.' *Biochem. J.*, **62**: 93–9.

10. **Porter, R. R.** (1957). 'The Isolation and Properties of a Fragment of Bovine-Serum Albumin which Retains the Ability to Combine with Rabbit Antiserum.' *Biochem. J.*, **66**: 677–85.

11. **Ouchterlony, Ö.** (1948). 'Antigen-antibody reactions in gels.' *Ark. Kemi. Min. Geol. B*, **26**: 14.

12. **Porter, R. R.** (1959). 'The Hydrolysis of Rabbit γ-Globulin and Antibodies with Crystalline Papain.' *Biochem. J.*, **73**: 119–26.

13. **Lederberg, L.** (1959). 'Genes and Antibodies.' *Science*, **129**: 1649–53.

14. **Edelman, G. M., and Poulik, M. D.** (1961). 'Studies on structural units of the γ-globulins.' *J. Exp. Med.*, **113**: 880.

15. **Porter, R. R.** (1962). 'The structure of gamma-globulin and antibodies', in A. Gellhorn and E. Hirschberg (eds), *Symposium on Basic Problems in Neoplastic Disease*. New York: Columbia University Press, p. 177.

16. **Fleischman, J. B., Porter, R. R., and Press, E. M.** (1963). 'The Arrangement of the Peptide Chains in γ-Globulin.' *Biochem. J.*, **88**: 220–28.

17. **Edelman, G. M., and Gally, J. A.** (1964). 'A model for the 7S antibody molecule.' *Proc. Natl. Acad. Sci.*, **51**: 846–53.

18. **Haber, E.** (1964). 'Recovery of antigenic specificity after denaturation and complete reduction of disulphides in a papain fragment of antibody.' *Proc. Natl. Acad. Sci.*, **52**: 1099–1106.

19. **Whitney, P. L., and Tanford, C.** (1965). 'Recovery of specific activity after complete unfolding and reduction of an antibody fragment.' *Proc. Natl. Acad. Sci.*, **63**: 524–32.

20. **White, F. H., and Anfinsen, C. B.** (1959). 'Some relationships of structure to function in ribonuclease.' *Ann. N.Y. Acad. Sci.*, **81**: 515–23.

21. **Noelken, M. E., Nelson, C. A., Buckley, III, C. E., and Tanford, C.** (1965). 'Gross conformation of rabbit 7S γ-immunoglobulin and its papain-cleaved fragments.' *J. Biol. Chem.*, **240**: 218–24.

22. **Edelman, G. M., and Benaceraff, B.** (1962). 'On structural and functional relations between antibodies and proteins of the gamma-system.' *Biochemistry*, **48**: 1035–42.

23. **Edelman, G. M., and Gally, J. A.** (1962). 'The nature of Bence-Jones proteins: Chemical similarities to polypeptide chains of myeloma globulins and normal g-globulins.' *J. Exp. Med.*, **116**: 207–27.

24. **Hilschman, N., and Craig, L. C.** (1965). 'Amino acid sequence studies with Bence-Jones proteins.' *Biochemistry*, **53**: 1403–9.

25. **Smithies, O.** (1963). 'Gamma-globulin variability: a genetic hypothesis.' *Nature*, **199**: 1231–6.

26. **Edelman, G. M., and Gally, J. A.** (1967). 'Somatic recombination of duplicated genes: An hypothesis on the origin of antibody diversity.' *Proc. Natl. Acad. Sci.*, **57**: 353–8.

27. **Agarwal, S. C.** (1964). 'Nomenclature for human immunoglobulins.' *Bull. World Health Organ.*, **30**: 447–50.

28. **Edelman, G. M., Cunningham, B. A., Gall, W. E., Gottlieb, P. D., Rutishauser, U., and Waxdal, M. J.** (1969). 'The covalent structure of an entire gG immunoglobulin molecule.' *Proc. Natl. Acad. Sci.*, **63**: 78–85.

Chapter 7

Uncovering the origins of antibody diversity

The gene as DNA

For much of the first half of the twentieth century, proteins dominated replication models while DNA and RNA were the poor cousins with little to offer genetics. Surprising as it may seem, the earliest concept of the gene did not require any understanding of its chemical composition at all. Genes were, as Mendel described them in 1866, 'elements' and their segregation and independent assortment could be described in the language of genetics without knowing what they consisted of. They were mere mathematical entities. Darwin's 'pangenes' were units of inheritance defining physiological macro-entities (e.g. organs), the required number of which would need, and from estimated molecular sizes were thought to be able to fit into, a germ cell (egg or sperm). In 1909 Johannsen (a professor of plant physiology at the University of Copenhagen) shortened Darwin's pangene to 'gene' and in doing so stated:

> Therefore, we will instead of the word 'Pangene' or 'Pangenes' simply say 'the Gene' or 'the Genes'. The word gene is fully void of any hypothesis; it merely expresses the confirmed fact that, at least many properties of an organism are determined by special and separable and therefore independent conditions, foundations or predispositions in the Gametes—in short, what we accordingly want to call Genes.[1]

The relationship of this classical, indivisible gene to a functional 'molecular' product was established through the work of Beadle and Tatum, and later that of Srb and Horowitz. Beadle and Tatum in their studies of Neurospora demonstrated that a single gene could account for a particular synthetic deficiency in this microorganism, stating:

> Inability to synthesize vitamin B6 is apparently differentiated by a single gene from the ability of the organism to elaborate this essential growth substance.[2]

Working with Neurospora in the same department at Stanford University, Srb and Horowitz showed some three years later that various enzyme deficiencies in specific steps of the ornithine cycle, required for the production of the essential amino acid arginine, could be linked to individual genes:

> Seven genetically and biochemically different arginineless strains in Neurospora crassa are described. In each, the arginineless character is inherited as a single gene... Different steps in the cycle are shown to be governed by the influence of particular single genes.[3]

The indivisibility of the gene as an inheritance unit was brought into question when Oliver, Lewis, and others showed that intragenic recombination could occur, but it was

Avery who first demonstrated in 1944 that the 'transforming principle' in the genetic material of pneumococcus was DNA rather than protein. At the time their claims were hotly debated due in no small part to the prevailing preoccupation of geneticists and immunologists with proteins. In fact Avery, MacLeod, and McCarty were not entirely convinced themselves or perhaps did not push their case strongly enough. In the event they mitigated their DNA claim somewhat by stating that their preparations may have contained small quantities of 'other substances' that were responsible for the transformation. Nevertheless, their work gave rise to a flurry of transformation activity. In 1947, at a Cold Spring Harbor conference, Boivin reported experimental support for Avery's claim by studies on human colon bacilli, going somewhat further than Avery in attributing the transformation activity to purified DNA:

> It resists the action of ribonuclease but disappears very rapidly under the effect of desoxy-ribonuclease (enzyme isolated from pancreas according to Fischer and collaborators and according to McCarty). Therefore it can be stated that the active principle in question is the desoxyribonucleic acid…[4]

Boivin continued with a rather more dogmatic statement:

> In bacteria—and, in all likelihood, in higher organisms as well—each gene has as its specific constituent not a protein but a particular desoxyribonucleic acid which, at least under certain conditions (directed mutations of bacteria), is capable of functioning alone as the carrier of hereditary character; therefore, in the last analysis, each gene can be traced back to a macromolecule of a special desoxyribonucleic acid.[4]

But Boivin's dogmatism did not convince all the opinion leaders. In a discussion of Boivin's paper and his assertions, Mirsky commented:

> In the present state of knowledge it would be going beyond the experimental facts to assert that the specific agent in transforming bacterial types is a desoxyribonucleic acid. It should also be stated that there is no need to believe that the specificity of the active principle must depend upon the presence in it of a specific protein. Discussions at these meetings have brought forward suggestions for experiments that may perhaps decide whether the transforming agent is a nucleic acid or a nucleoprotein.[5]

There has been a great deal of discussion about Mirsky's view of transformation and of the work of Avery in particular. It is clear that, as a chemist who grew up believing proteins to be the *primum mobile*, the acceptance by Mirsky of an entirely different code for dictating protein sequence would not be easy. He was not alone. In their 1952 publication on the T2 bacteriophage, Hershey and Chase surprisingly made no reference to the work of Avery, MacLeod, and McCarty, or of Boivin. While their now textbook discovery using radiolabelling (^{35}S for protein labelling and ^{32}P for DNA labelling) provided technically convincing evidence for the replicative role of DNA in the T2 bacteriophage, their respect for the lingering dogmatism that attributed the replicating role to proteins may have been the reason for their somewhat low-key conclusion:

> The sulfur-containing protein of resting phage particles… functions as an instrument for the injection of the phage DNA into the cell. This protein probably has no function in the growth of intracellular phage. The DNA has some function. Further chemical inferences should not be drawn from the experiments presented.[6]

In a 1968 retrospective entitled 'That was the molecular biology that was', Gunther Stent also omitted to mention the work of Avery and colleagues, and of Boivin. The influence of the newly formed bacteriophage 'group', founded by such great names as Max Delbrück, Salvador Luria, and Alfred Hershey, grew to dominate the molecular biology advances in the late 1950s and 1960s. Even allowing for the fact that bacterio-phages provided the ideal model for the study of replication, as Stent observed:

> The members of this group were united by a single common goal, the desire to understand how, during the brief half-hour latent period, the simple bacteriophage particle achieves its own hundredfold self-re-production within the bacterial host cell.[7]

Stent observed that the omission of the key pneumococcus discovery could be regarded as a symptom of the authoritarianism that often accompanies the formation of scientific 'clubs', particularly where leading opinion-makers are members. One is reminded of the scientific scepticism surrounding the *helicobacter pylori* discovery by Barry Warren in the late 1970s and 1980s as an etiological agent for gastritis and peptic ulcers. In this example the closed ranks of clinical prejudice observed, 'Just a secondary infection, due to the gastritis' and 'If it is true, why were they not recognized before?' This type of dogma-tism could have prevented the breakthrough were it not for the doggedness with which Warren and his clinical colleague Barry Marshall pursued their hypothesis to its dénoue-ment, resulting in their elevation to Nobel Laureate status almost two decades later.

Antibody diversity, protein sequences, and genetics

By the late 1950s the question of DNA as the genetic material directing antibody pro-duction was no longer in doubt among immunologists. What was uncertain was exactly how the observed variation in antibody chains could occur. Here were polypeptide chains with a significant amount of sequence variability in their N-terminal regions, with almost zero sequence variability (apart from allotypic changes) in the C-terminal regions, providing what Dreyer and Bennett[40] referred to as the 'genetic paradox'. The older hypermutation theories of Burnet, Lederberg, and others lacked credibility because no mutation mechanism was known that could alter one part of a gene while leaving the other unchanged. Fanciful epigenetic alternatives, reflecting the growing knowledge of bacterial genetics, were offered by Smithies and by Dreyer and Bennett. In Smithies'[41] model, rearranged antibodies formed in the primary response to antigen are packaged as viruses which exit the parent cells and introduce antibody-specific producing capability into other cells which are also 'transformed' by the viral DNA. Variable gene integration into the recipient genome would then require that the virally-carried antibody gene find and integrate with its cognate constant region gene. Subsequent exposure to antigen then engages these cells in the anamnestic response. In an attempt to resolve the genetic paradox, Dreyer and Bennett[40] describe a sort of mir-ror image of the Smithies' model in which episomal DNA carrying the constant region (what Dreyer and Bennett call the 'common gene') pairs with any one of a number of variable region genes carried in the chromosomal DNA. The analogy they draw on is the known fact that phage lambda can pair at various loci within the bacterial genome, leading to stable genomic incorporation of the lambda DNA. Of course, not to be outdone by the DNA-ists, the protein school made proposals that required enzymatic 'zipping' of the variable and constant sequences at the polypeptide stage.

While all these models were serious attempts to deal with the apparent gene mutation paradox, they lacked any experimental basis. By the mid 1960s the hypermutation theory dragged itself back into the current consciousness via a number of routes designed to resolve the problem. In 1966 Brenner and Milstein[8] invoked a DNA enzymatic process in which genes encoding the antibody light chain present in precursor cells are first cleaved at a recognition site positioned between the variable and invariant light chain sequences. During repair of this site after perhaps some nuclease trimming, a DNA repair enzyme closes the junction, introducing errors while doing so. After replication, in order to ensure that the error-strewn strand is present in the daughter cell, the process is repeated, leading to a number of stable antibody light chain variants present in different cells. There were a number of issues with the concept recognized by the authors, not least of which was that the same recognition sequence for cleavage would need to be present in the heavy chain gene. Furthermore, specific enzymes both for junctional cleavage and the mutagenic repair had not been demonstrated in antibody-producing cells, notwithstanding the fact that similar enzymatic activities were known in bacteria (e.g. exonuclease III) and bacteriophage (e.g. T4 encoded error-prone polymerase) replication.

Potter and colleagues proposed a mechanism in which variation would be introduced during translation of the RNA sequence.[9] This rather remote concept required that the genes for light and heavy chain genes contained certain sequences ('code words') in their variability regions (but not elsewhere) that would be recognized by enzymes that would translate the sequence differently depending on which of the small family of enzymes had been activated. Not only was this unlikely but, as with the chain paradox, it was also difficult to reconcile with any natural selection mechanism that would retain the code-word sequences in one part of the gene while other regions of the gene were undergoing mutation. This type of proposal was symptomatic of the race headlong toward resolution to the antibody gene paradox where limited, low-resolution data was all there was to fuel the sometimes exotic high resolution models.

In 1966, Lee Hood (see Fig. 7.1b) and colleagues at Caltech rejuvenated the germ line school by proposing a mechanism that could both resolve the genetic paradox and stand up in terms of genetic precedent. Hood's concept, supported by sequence results, was that multiple germ line genes code for the 'specificity' region and a single gene codes for the 'common' region and that the data:

> ... support the hypothesis that any one of **many** different genes may code for the first 105 amino acid residues ... Residues 106–212 are assumed to be encoded by a single 'common' gene, thus leading to the same sequence in each of the mouse light chains of the κ class.[10] (This author's bold emphasis.)

The genetic variation in the variable sequences would then be generated by a 'slow process of chemical evolution', a mechanism Hood surmised would be similar to that proposed for the cytochromes, where natural variation is seen in different species of this highly conserved protein but where only certain residue positions are able to accept change due to structural constraints. The joining of the variable and constant gene sequences would then be mediated either via a polypeptide chain 'zipping' mechanism post-translation or by fusion of the DNA (or RNA) during differentiation of the plasma cells. Whichever of these turned out to be correct, Hood and colleagues had taken a dramatic step forward towards a viable genetic explanation. The germ line model would now require experimental proof.

But the 'somaticists' were not yet finished. Edelman and Gally continued to plough the somatic furrow with a variation on the Smithies model. In 1967 they laid out the observed facts with which any hypothesis must be consistent. 1) There is high variability in the variable domain compared with the constant domain; 2) amino acid changes should typically be introduced parsimoniously via single base changes; 3) for light chains the variable and constant regions would be of similar length; 4) within the variable region there are stretches of polypeptide chain that are invariant and within the more variable segments certain positions and residues experience 'interchange' more frequently than others; 5) allotypes have a low recombination frequency; 6) individual plasma cells from tumours (myelomas) produce a single well-defined protein that has a constant sequence from one generation to the next. [11]

The model they proposed to explain facts 1–4 is purely somatic in concept. Antibody genes arose by tandem duplication of the constant region followed by somatic mutation. Recombination by somatic crossing over during maturation of the antibody-producing cell (the lymphocyte) then drives the variation. Edelman suggested that around 50 duplicated genes would be enough to drive the variation required for the observed antigen recognition. This model, while differing from Smithies in that it involves recombination of *duplicated* gene sets, failed to explain adequately how the constant region would be spared this variation, suggesting that:

> Mutations in cistrons corresponding to the constant regions of antibody polypeptide chains would be subject to stringent selection pressure. The selection would arise because of need to maintain structures capable of interchain bonding and physiologic functions such as complement fixation, opsonization, fixation to cells, etc. In contrast, individual mutations in variable regions are not necessarily selected for by interaction with any particular antigen in the environment. Instead, it is proposed that there is selective advantage for those mutations capable of generating the largest set of possible sequences by somatic crossing-over.[11]

In their *Science* paper of 1970, Hood and Talmage[12] essentially dismiss this and other somatic theories as requiring an 'ad hoc mutation mechanism' within what would probably need to be a much more complex hypermutation and recombination mechanism, or in other words 'unlikely'. Their germ line arguments, based on a relatively limited number of kappa light chain sequences, were perceptive and genetically convincing. The three kappa chain sequences discussed in detail are clearly not alleles and must therefore be encoded by three different germ line genes. In contrast the constant region sequences are so closely related as to be allelic. Thus, three germ line genes encode three variable region kappa sequences while one germ line gene encodes the constant region. A similar picture is proposed for lambda light chains, although two separate lambda constant region genes are proposed. The key now was to reconcile the multitude of specificities with a suitably large repertoire of variable region genes. Hood and Talmage made a simple calculation that went as follows:

- DNA content of human = $2.3 \times 10{-}11$ g (sperm cell (haploid))
- Molecular weight of one base pair = 6.2×10^2
- DNA content (per cell) = 3.7×10^9 base pairs
- One variable region = 107 amino acids
- One variable gene = 321 pairs
- 20 000 variable genes = 6.4×10^6 pairs
- 20 000 variable genes = 0.2% of genetic material of human haploid cells.

From this simplistic though logical calculation they concluded that each antibody chain 'subgroup' could have 1600 variable genes (distributed within ~12 kappa light chain subgroups). Their analysis was based on the sequences of 41 kappa chain and 223 lambda light chain sequences that could be separated by standard phylogenic 'tree' methods (e.g. Fitch and Margoliash[13]) into subgroups based on sequence similarity. So, assuming similar numbers and subgroups for the heavy chain variable genes, 3200 germ line genes would be required to service the full antibody response, representing only 0.2% of the genome. We now know the Hood and Talmage genome calculation to be a gross underestimate—using Hood's algorithm, the percentage of antibody gene DNA estimated from the human genome would be more like 13% of protein-encoding DNA, assuming a separate gene for every antibody. Had this been verifiable at the time, the 'one gene for every antibody variable region' version of the germ line theory would have already received its *coup de grâce*.

To verify their conclusions, Hood and Talmage proposed a number of experimental tests. First they suggested using a messenger RNA sequence (from a myeloma since that produces a single antibody) with germ line DNA to establish whether a large or small number of genes are present. RNA-DNA hybridization techniques were not yet developed, so this was a future hope rather than a test that could actually be carried out. The second test was more tractable. They suggested searching for kappa genes in a highly inbred mouse strain (e.g. Balb/c) and counting the frequency of identical kappa genes. On statistical grounds, they concluded that if, for example, only two identical kappa chains were found in the first 80 genes examined, this low frequency would eliminate or render highly unlikely a somatic theory with its requirement for a large number of different variable region sequences. Those tests would be done but by another great experimentalist in another place.

At about the same time the Hood and Talmage paper appeared, Elvin Kabat, now at Columbia University working together with a mathematician/engineering colleague at Cornell, Tai Te Wu, published a 40-page analysis of 77 different light chain sequences, derived from Bence-Jones proteins and various immunoglobulin kappa and lambda light chains. The results were exciting for the molecular immunologists but added genetic complexity to the antibody diversity models for both the germ line and somatic schools. What Kabat and Wu discovered was that sequence variability in the light chain variable regions was localized to three different segments (see Chapter 11).[14]

Two of these highly variable segments had been observed previously. In Milstein's analysis,[15] his proposed mechanism by which the variation was generated invoked the *in vogue* crossing-over mechanism. In contrast, Kabat postulated an episomal insertion mechanism but only for the first and third segment (designated as 'gaps' in Kabat and Wu's analysis) since these carried the largest number of substitutions observed. As he states:

> By hypothesis the complementarity-determining residues are considered to be the result of the insertion into the DNA of the two short linear sequences, 24–34 and 89–97, which specifically determine what kind of antibody site will be formed.[14]

Kabat continued:

> An insertion mechanism involving only short linear sequences provides a substantial simplification of the problem of providing a seemingly limitless number of complementary sites without the use of very large amounts of DNA.[14]

> Text extracts © 1970 Rockefeller University Press. Originally published in *The Journal of Experimental Medicine*, Volume 132: pp. 211–249

In a follow-on analysis published in 1971 in which data from a smaller number of heavy chain variable regions is also presented, with similar variability to that seen in the light chains, Kabat is more circumspect with respect to the exact genetic mechanism operating, concluding:

> The genetic mechanism of this variability and antibody complementarity is still not clear.[16]

In a 'numbers' discussion following presentation of this paper, Hood continues to argue the germ line cause while Kabat defended his somatic corner with some irascibility:

Dr. Hood: Right, but I think the point here is if one takes the kappa 1 sequences in human and mouse and says it's possible that there are a great many more genes here and starts correspondingly asking to compare the individual gene products in kappa 1 in mouse with the individual gene products in kappa 1 in human, then I think you are going to start expanding out the number of species specific residues. What I'm saying is, that there are in kappa 1 proteins, now there is good evidence that there are at least four sub-subgroups and I think most people would agree probably there are four additional germ line genes. And what one has to do is to compare these sequences at a much finer level and I think it's going to go from nine to 24 to I don't know what.

Dr. Kabat: It's never going to be 43.

Dr. Hood: Well no that's not true at all; I mean if we take the extreme and we say that each different sequence in fact represents a different gene, it could very easily be 43.

Dr. Kabat: No…[16]

Clearly, the germ-line–somatic debate was not finished. The respective protagonists were drawing clear lines in the sand. To resolve the debate a new direction and a new approach would be needed.

Gene-counting meets immunology

In the two years following the Hood and Talmage, and Kabat and Wu papers, Gelderman et al[17] and Bishop et al[18] demonstrated that if purified messenger RNA (mRNA) was used in a 'kinetic' DNA hybridization method, the amount of DNA—and if one knew the size of the gene, the number of genes—corresponding to the mRNA sequence could be estimated. The extensive study by Bishop established that where a specific mRNA is hybridized with a very large excess of DNA, the rate of hybridization will depend on the number of homologous DNA segments present. By plotting the amount of RNA-DNA hybrids as a function of DNA concentration and time for hybridization, so-called C_0T curves are obtained (C_0T is the product of total DNA concentration, C_0 and time T in seconds).

Further, if the hybridizing mRNA is radiolabelled and then challenged with increasing concentrations of mRNA from the same source, competition curves can be derived from which gene reiteration frequencies may be obtained.

At about the same time Bernard Mach described synthesis of a DNA copy of purified light chain mRNA, the first 'cloning' of an immunoglobulin gene cDNA.[19] Using an RNA-dependent DNA polymerase from avian myeloblastosis virus, Mach initiated the DNA synthesis with a dT-oligonucleotide which primed the synthesis via the poly-A tail of the mRNA. He presumed that any and all mRNAs could be copied to DNA in this way. Since the added nucleotides could be radiolabelled this would also be a powerful tool for gene dosage experiments since, as Mach points out, high specific activity cDNA could be generated resulting in high sensitivity in hybridization experiments.

In a small institute situated in the European city of Basel, application of these and other molecular biology methods to antibody genes was about to light the litmus paper of the antibody gene paradox and blow it apart. In 1970, Susumu Tonegawa, then at the Salk Institute, found himself en route to the Basel Institute of Immunology (BII) where Niels Jerne was Director. Tonegawa (see Fig. 7.1a) had worked on transcriptional control of SV40 viral genes under Dulbecco, continuation of which on his arrival in Basel did not trigger enormous excitement, populated as it was with hard core immunologists (see Tonegawa's own description of this[20]). In fact, his familiarity with techniques for the study of transcription—his 1968 paper on phage transcriptional control[21] employed DNA and RNA preparation, genomic DNA-RNA hybridization, and even in vitro transcription using DNA-dependent RNA polymerase—was the perfect experimental platform for the direction Tonegawa was to take when introduced by Askonas and Steinberg to the problem of antibody diversity.

Tonegawa's first attempts in 1973 and 1974 to isolate pure kappa light chain and gamma heavy chain messenger RNA from myeloma cells met with limited success.[22] Eukaryotic cells were not bacteria and the nucleic acid purification techniques were subject to a much more complex protein background. In the following study his conclusions still left open the question of the number of variable region genes:

At present our estimate must be between 1 and 200…[23]

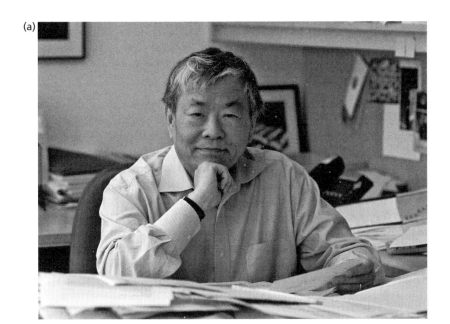

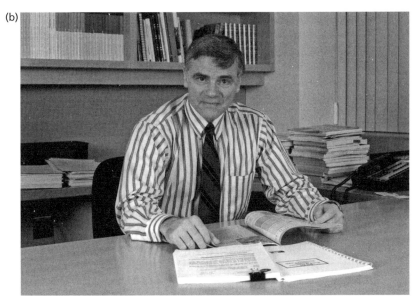

Fig. 7.1 (a) Susumu Tonegawa (b) Lee Hood.

(a) Reproduced with kind permission from tonegawalab.org and Susumu Tonegawa. (b) Reproduced with kind permission from Leroy Hood, MD, PhD.

However, they also raised the spectre of a much more interesting idea—a limited number of germ line genes plus a somatic diversification mechanism:

> … number of germ line genes seems to be too small to account for the observed variability of antibody V-regions.[23]

Around the same time, in what one might argue was a *volte face*, Hood and colleagues moved away from their previous estimates of the number of germ line genes in discussion of a study on the N-terminal sequences of gamma heavy chains.[24] While concluding that the sequence data supported the existence of multiple heavy chain branches (from phylogenetic analysis), the number of germ line genes required to explain the diversity observed in these sequences was either 16 or eight, depending on the extent of mutation activity allowable or possible during lymphocyte somatic development. This was far away from the earlier estimates of 1600 genes for each of the light and heavy chain groups. As a matter of interest, Tonegawa's (1974) *FEBS Letters* paper had been out for three months before the paper of Hood was submitted. Was the tide turning in favour of fewer germ line genes, requiring a more circumspect view of the antibody genome? The key open question, both for Hood and colleagues and for Tonegawa was: 'Exactly how many germ line genes were there, and if much lower than the germ line proponents were suggesting, what somatic mechanisms operated to generate the observed diversity in sub-sequences of variable region genes?' This was a time for fast experiments and rapid publishing, since there were significant prizes for first past the post!

Using improved methods, Tonegawa repeated his 1974 experiments using mRNA from myeloma tumours. He employed the competition hybridization method described in the 1974 paper and based on the previously described work of Bishop. Tonegawa's procedure was:

- Assume DNA-DNA binding has the same rate constants as RNA-DNA binding;

- Mix a large excess (50 000x) of DNA with a radiolabelled (^{125}I) RNA from the cells of interest (e.g. a light chain myeloma);

- Add increasing amounts of the unlabelled RNA;

- Plot the competition curves, estimate the half maximal hybridization ratio (where for each RNA molecule there would be exactly one homologous DNA copy), and calculate the gene reiteration frequency from:

$$N_k = R_{1/2}(M_m / M_k)$$

Where N_k is the nominal gene reiteration frequency, $R_{1/2}$ is the ratio of RNA to DNA at half maximal hybridization, and M_m and M_k are the molecular weights of the mouse haploid genome and the κ-chain mRNA molecule respectively.

The results were clear, controversial, and paradox shattering. In the concluding remarks to the 'Discussion', Tonegawa's message to the germ line and somatic theorists was:

> The germ line theory demands that for each chain there exists a germ line gene… we have previously concluded that the number of germ line Vκ genes is too small to account for the sequence diversity… The present results with λ and κ chains reinforce and extend this conclusion.[25]

In 1976, at what was becoming a mecca for molecular breakthroughs, a group of immunologists gathered at Cold Spring Harbor for a meeting on 'The origins of lymphocyte diversity'. In the session on 'Generation of diversity: 2. Structural aspects', a 'Who's Who' of immunology were gathered: Capra, Hood, Leder, Honjo, Weigert, Tonegawa, and others. While not diminishing the work of the others present, it was arguably the paper of Tonegawa that took the collective breath of the audience away. His contribution, 'Somatic changes in the content and context of immunoglobulin genes', would define the path forward. His experimental results allowed him to draw the following conclusions:[26]

1. Vκ and Cκ genes in mouse embryonic DNA are probably separated by some distance in the genome;

2. Hybridization of DNA from a homologous plasmacytoma suggests the Vκ and Cκ DNA sequences are brought together during differentiation;

3. Similar although not entirely unequivocal results are obtained using Vλ and Cλ probes;

4. The 'joining' mechanism is still compatible with the 'excision-insertion' model of Gally and Edelman, the 'deletion' model of Kabat, and the 'inversion' model of Steinberg, but incompatible with the 'copy-insertion' model of Dreyer et al;

5. Allelic exclusion operating to prevent multiple V genes being expressed by a single cell must involve some mechanism to avoid joining occurring on both chromosomes—why should the **same** V segment be joined on both homologs?

6. Examination of Vλ gene reiteration frequencies with Vλ-region specific probes confirms that only a few genes are present. From the nine Vλ sequences known and statistical arguments that the Vλ repertoire must be much larger, a somatic process must be operating on a small number of germ line genes in the differentiated cell;

7. Estimates of the total numbers of germ line genes remain uncertain but if the sub-group classifications based on available amino acid sequences holds true, 'the mouse genome contains from two to 100 Vκ genes.'

Despite the advances in hybridization methods, direct evidence for somatic rearrangement within the differentiated lymphocyte was still missing. During 1978 several groups made the breakthrough that established beyond doubt that somatic rearrangement of a limited number of germ line genes is the mechanism by which the observed antibody diversity can be generated. The first glimpse of the germ line was provided by Tonegawa, whose March report described the complete DNA sequence of a mouse lambda light chain germ line gene. Using the DNA sequencing method recently introduced by Maxam and Gilbert,[27] three clarifying observations were made. First, the DNA sequence contained both the variable region and the constant region sequence. Within the variable region the hypervariable sequences corresponded to the protein sequences previously observed. Second, the variable and constant region sequences were not contiguous but were separated by a long non-identifiable segment of DNA, a 'silent sequence' or 'intron' (for *intr*agenic regi*on*) as Tonegawa calls it. Third, an amino terminal 'leader' sequence is present, presumed to be important for transmembrane passage.

On the possibility that the hypervariable sequences are introduced by insertion of small DNA segments, as proposed by Kabat, Tonegawa is ambivalent though clearly uncomfortable with this notion:

> There are no features in these hypervariable regions that... define a mechanism by which these regions might be more labile than the rest of the DNA... it is not impossible that... an enzyme... would cleave or modify the DNA in order to make the sequence labile.[28]

The phrase 'it is not impossible' was perhaps a polite way of saying 'so unlikely as to be near impossible'. In May 1978 Tonegawa submitted what could be described as the *coup de siecle* in antibody genetics. Using a DNA transcript prepared from the mRNA of a lambda light chain myeloma as a probe to isolate homologous DNA sequences from mouse embryo DNA (the germ line), Tonegawa demonstrated exactly how a mature immunoglobulin gene is generated by somatic recombination in the differentiated antibody-producing cell.[29] He illustrated this in a cartoon (see Fig. 7.2) where the leader (L) and variable gene (V) sequences in the germ line DNA (upper line) recombine with

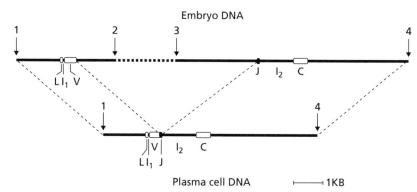

Fig. 7.2 Arrangement of mouse λ1 gene sequences in embryos and λ1 chain-producing plasma cells.

Reproduced with permission from *Cell*, Volume 15, Issue 1, Brack, C. et al., A Complete Immunoglobulin Gene Is Created by Somatic Recombination, pp. 1–14, Copyright © 1978, with permission from Elsevier, http://www.sciencedirect.com/science/journal/00928674.

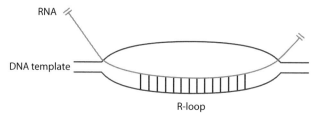

Fig. 7.3 R-loop formation. Complementary sequences in mRNA can displace one of the two DN strands in double-stranded DNA forming so-called 'R-loops' that are stable enough to be visualized by electron microscopy.

the right junction of the V translocating to the left junction of a small joining piece (or J region) located close to the constant region gene, generating the somatically recombined structure in the lower line.

A similar recombination would be required to translocate the V-J sequence to the constant region DNA with excision of the intervening intron or introns since the exact number of intervening sequences in the C region sequences was not yet known. How then could Tonegawa be certain of the non-contiguity of the V and C sequences in the germ line DNA? By using R-loop mapping (see the cartoon in Fig. 7.3), in which mRNA from either the V or C region sequence is used to hybridize to embryonic DNA which can then be visualized by electron microscopy.

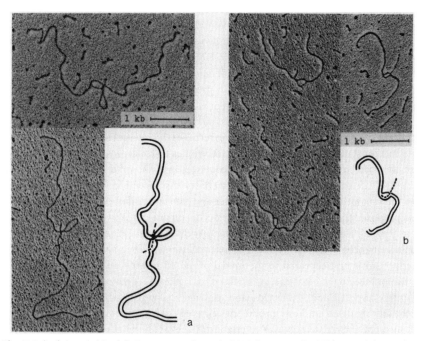

Fig. 7.4 (Left hand side, (a)) A mouse embryonic DNA fragment (Ig 25λ) containing only the constant region sequence (Cλ₁) is hybridized to mRNA from a λ₁ producing mouse myeloma (HOPC 202) containing both constant and variable region sequences. The mRNA displaces one of the DNA strands where it finds its complementary sequence of Cλ₁ DNA forming an R-loop structure as shown in Fig. 7.4. On the right hand side a different DNA fragment (Ig99λ) is shown hybridized with the same mRNA but this time the DNA only contains the λ variable sequences so that the R-loop formed contains only the Vλ-complementary sequences and a long tail containing the constant region and untranslated (polyA) tail.

The locations of complementary sequences in the cloned DNA fragments from embryonic antibody gene DNA are clearly visible in the electron micrographs in Fig. 7.4.

In commenting in the 'Discussion' on the evidence presented in this study, Tonegawa made his position on germ line versus somatic theories clear and without equivocation:

> The heteroduplex analysis of the three λ1 DNA clones combined with the gel blotting analysis of the total cellular DNAs demonstrated beyond a doubt the occurrence of somatic rearrangements of immunoglobulin gene sequences.[29]

In a follow-on study published in the same month,[30] Tonegawa confirmed that the order of recombination is V (variable)-J (joining)-C (constant) and further that mutations observed in the hypervariable regions of the V-gene DNA sequences, when compared with the germ line sequence, must have been somatically introduced and may occur via an enzymatic mechanism that targets mutations to these hypervariable sequences, as Brenner and Milstein had suggested in 1966.[8]

In September and December of the same year, Phil Leder's group at the NIH published similar results on kappa light chain DNA sequences, while Leroy Hood's group at Caltech reported results from 22 different kappa chain protein sequences. Both Leder and Hood had already seen an 'in press' version of the Tonegawa *Cell* paper (they referred to it) and would have been anxious to get their own data into the public domain.

Leder's study[31] was even more explicit in terms of the intergenic relationship of variable and constant regions. Using similar techniques to Tonegawa, Leder demonstrated that the variable and constant region sequences in embryonic DNA present on the same DNA fragment are as much as 3700 bases apart (see Fig. 7.5) and also showed that the J segments lie between the variable and constant region genes (not shown). He also proposed that this arrangement only occurs on one of the two light chain alleles.

In parallel, Hood and colleagues, using protein sequence data from murine kappa chain sequences, arrived at a similar set of conclusions.[32] Their somatic rearrangement mechanism is best captured in the model proposed in their 1978 *Nature* paper and shown in Fig. 7.6.

In this respect Hood was as close to the actual mechanism of light chain formation in the differentiated antibody-producing cell as any of his contemporaries. All that was left for light chain assembly was to establish the exact number of germ line encoded variable region genes, the number of J region segments, and to establish the exact mechanism by which combinatorial joining takes place. This would not be trivial and it would require hard work with little opportunity for grand mechanistic breakthroughs. That would not be the case for heavy chain genes however.

Two years after the light chain rearrangements were verified, the larger more complex heavy chain recombination mechanism was revealed. When sequences at the junction of the V and J regions were examined it was found that somewhere between one and 12 codons were present that were neither part of the V gene nor the J segment. In his *Nature* paper of February 1980 (submitted October 1979), Hood described the recombination of a V region, J segment and an alpha chain constant region, a constant region gene related to but not identical to the gamma heavy chain. In doing so, Hood revealed

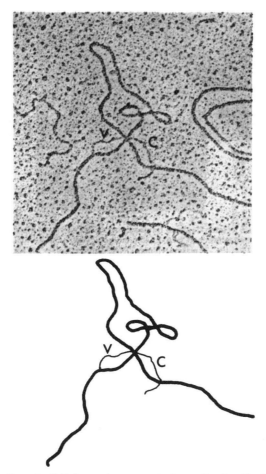

Fig. 7.5 Hybridization of mRNA from a kappa-producing antibody cell with a large embry-onic DNA fragment showing the R-loops indicating the relative disposition of variable and constant region genes in a single DNA fragment.

Reprinted by permission from Macmillan Publishers Ltd: *Nature,* Seidman, J.G. and Leder, P., The arrangement and rearrangement of antibody genes, Volume 276, pp. 790–795, Copyright © 1978.

one aspect of the additional internal complexity in heavy chain constant regions. While for IgG molecules a single gamma constant region was known, other immunoglobulin classes (see Chapter 8) must also be present, characterized by their particular constant region genes. What Hood proposed was that DNA rearrangement and constant region selection, followed by deletion of unwanted constant region class sequences, were the most likely somatic 'switching events' enabling the correct constant region pairing with the VJ region to make the relevant antibody.[33] Such switching events had been hypoth-esized previously by Hood[34] and Smithies,[35] but here was the first direct evidence.

Two months later, Hood followed up this study by a comprehensive attack on the heavy chain rearrangement problem, in some respects 'trumping' the field. In this

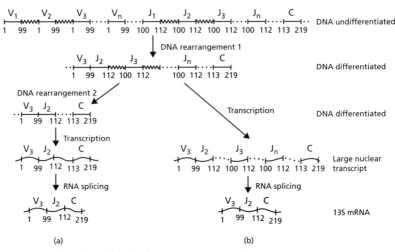

Fig. 7.6 Hypothetical models for the DNA segments of mouse κ-genes.

Reprinted by permission from Macmillan Publishers Ltd: *Nature*, M.Weigert et al., Rearrangement of genetic information may produce immunoglobulin diversity, Volume 276, pp.785–790, Copyright © 1978.

later paper,[36] the presence of an additional gene, the D segment, was discovered that explained the additional sequences observed in antibody protein sequences between the V and J regions, but that were encoded by neither V genes nor J segments. Here then was a fourth genetic element in the heavy chain construction, summarized from Hood's paper in Fig. 7.7.

Two months after Hood's paper, Tonegawa elaborated on the class-switching event with a comprehensive study in which he proposed that a VH and JH region would first recombine, followed by recombination of the VJ fusion with a mu heavy chain constant region 'exon' giving an IgM antibody, expressed on the surface of the B lymphocyte.[37] After antigen binding, the differentiating B cell would be triggered to undergo a class-switching cycle. In Tonegawa's system the switch was to a γ_{2b} heavy chain constant region. This rearrangement, referred to by Tonegawa as the 'Cμ–Xγ_{2b} switch recombination', occurred by an, as yet, unknown mechanism.

While Hood had discovered the D segment in antibody sequences from differentiated cells, its exact location, presence, and if there, copy number in the immunoglobulin germ line and mechanism of insertion was still unexplained. Exactly one year later, Tonegawa would put the mystery to rest. Not only were germ line D segments identified but they were flanked by conserved sequences in inverted orientations that suggested a recombinase enzyme recognition site, as had been seen for V and J joining sequences. In his 1983 review article for *Nature*, Tonegawa cemented his position as the cornerstone of the new immunogenetic edifice, the person most likely to wear the laurel.[38] In Fig. 7.8 his model for organization of the antibody genes is reproduced.

While he was not responsible for discovery of all the elements of the kappa and lambda light chain and heavy chain genetic arrangements, he arguably made the breakthroughs that opened up the critical path to the true structure while constantly

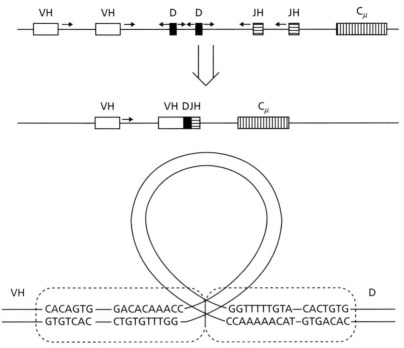

Fig. 7.7 Hood's model for rearrangement of heavy chain genes. In the upper part of the diagram possible germ line D segments with arbitrary distances from other segments of the gene are shown (the starting position). In the next stage V, D and J joining takes place with deletion or rearrangement of intervening DNA pieces, by as yet an unknown mechanism. In the lower part of the figure a possible mechanism is shown for bringing VJ and D segments together. The dotted areas might entertain DNA-joining proteins.

Reproduced with permission from *Cell*, Volume 19, Early, P. et al., An Immunoglobulin Heavy Chain Variable Region Gene Is Generated from Three Segments of DNA: VH, D and JH, pp. 981–992, Copyright © 1980, with permission from Elsevier, http://www.sciencedirect.com/science/journal/00928674

correcting other wayward models along the way. Were the contributions of Leder and in particular Hood major enough to warrant equal recognition? Together with Tonegawa, Hood and Leder shared the 1987 Albert Lasker Prize in Basic Medical Research, an award that counts 50% of its recipients as Nobel Prize winners. Whatever the relative contributions of his contemporaries, Tonegawa made the critical breakthroughs that laid the foundations for the general principle of somatic rearrangement of a limited number of germ line genes in differentiated antibody-producing cells. It is notable that on receipt of his Nobel Prize in 1987 another great immunologist, Hans Wigzell, said of Tonegawa in his opening address:

> When Tonegawa did his experiments at the Basel Institute of Immunology in Switzerland other scientists had already generated a considerable amount of knowledge regarding the features and functions of antibodies. But this knowledge had also led to uncertainty and even confusion.[39]

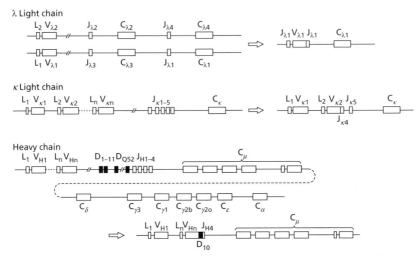

Fig. 7.8 Organization of various mouse immunoglobulin gene segments, before (left of arrows) and after (right of arrows) somatic rearrangement.

Reprinted by permission from Macmillan Publishers Ltd: *Nature,* Tonegawa, S., Somatic generation of antibody diversity, Volume 302, pp.575–581, Copyright © 1983

Here then was scientific greatness at work: creating a path of scientific fact with clear, clever, and beautifully executed experiments, leaving in its wake the uncertainties and the confused models they had spawned.

Acknowledgements

Text extracts from Boivin, A., Directed mutation in colon bacilli, by an inducing principle of desoxyribonucleic nature: its meaning for the general biochemistry of heredity, *Cold Spring Harbor Symposia On Quantitative Biology*, Volume 11, pp. 7–17 © 1947, reproduced with permission from Cold Spring Harbor Laboratory Press.

Text extracts from Kabat, E. A. and Wu, T. T., Attempts to locate complementarity-determining residues in the variable positions of light and heavy chains, *Annals of the New York Academy of Sciences*, Volume 190, pp. 382–393, Copyright © 1971 John Wiley and Sons.

Text extracts reproduced from Edelman, G.M and Gally, J.A., Somatic recombination of duplicated genes: An hypothesis on the origin of antibody diversity, *Proceedings of the National Academy of Sciences*, Volume 57, pp. 353–358, Copyright © 1967, by permission of the author.

References

1. **Johannsen, W.** (1909). *Elemente der exakten erblichkeitslehre.* Jena: Gustav Fischer, p. 124. (Translated by E.Yilmaz, 2012).

2. **Beadle, G. W., and Tatum, E. L.** (1941). 'Genetic control of biochemical reactions in *Neurospora*.' *Proc. Natl. Acad. Sci.*, **27**: 499–506.

3. **Srb, A. M., and Horowitz, N. H.** (1944). 'The ornithine cycle in *Neurospora* and its genetic control.' *J. Biol. Chem.*, **154**: 129–39.

4. **Boivin, A.** (1947). 'Directed mutation in colon bacilli, by an inducing principle of desoxyribonucleic nature: its meaning for the general biochemistry of heredity.' *Cold Spring Harbor Symp.*, **11**, 7–17.

5. **Boivin, A.** (1947). 'Directed mutation in colon bacilli, by an inducing principle of desoxyribonucleic nature: its meaning for the general biochemistry of heredity.' *Cold Spring Harbor Symp.*, **11**: 16.

6. **Hershey, A. D., and Chase, M. J.** (1952). 'Independent functions of viral protein and nucleic acid in growth of bacteriophage.' *Gen. Physiol.*, **36**: 39–56.

7. **Stent, G. S.** (1968). 'That Was the Molecular Biology That Was.' *Science*, **160**: 390–5.

8. **Brenner, S., and Milstein, C.** (1966). 'Origin of antibody variation.' *Nature*, **211**: 242–3.

9. **Potter, M. E., Apella, E., and Geisser, S.** (1965). 'Variations in the heavy polypeptide chain structure of gamma myeloma immunoglobulins from an inbred strain of mice and a hypothesis as to their origin.' *J. Mol. Biol.*, **14**: 361–72.

10. **Hood, L. E., Gray, W. R., and Dreyer, W. J.** (1966). 'On the Mechanism of Antibody Synthesis: A Species Comparison of L-Chains.' *Proc. Natl. Acad. Sci.*, **55**: 826–32.

11. **Edelman, G. M., and Gally, J. A.** (1967). 'Somatic recombination of duplicated genes: an hypothesis on the origin of antibody diversity.' *Proc. Natl. Acad. Sci.*, **57**: 353–8.

12. **Hood, L., and Talmage, D. W.** (1970). 'Mechanism of Antibody Diversity: Germ Line Basis for Variability.' *Science*, **168**: 325–34.

13. **Fitch, W. M., and Margoliash, E.** (1967). 'Construction of phylogenetic trees.' *Science*, **155**: 279–84.

14. **Wu, T. T., and Kabat, E. A.** (1970). 'Analysis of the sequences of variable regions of Bence Jones proteins and myeloma light chains and their implications for antibody complementarity.' *J. Exp. Med.*, **132**: 211–49.

15. **Milstein, C.** (1967). 'Linked groups of residues in immunoglobulin κ chains.' *Nature*, **216**: 330.

16. **Kabat, E. A., and Wu, T. T.** (1971). 'Attemps to locate complementarity-determining residues in the variable positions of light and heavy chains.' *Ann. N.Y. Acad. Sci.*, **190**: 382–93.

17. **Gelderman, A. H., Rake, A. V., and Britten, R. J.** (1971). 'Transcription of nonrepeated DNA in neonatal and fetal mice.' *Proc. Natl. Acad. Sci.*, **68**: 172–6.

18. **Bishop, J. O., Pemberton, R., and Baglioni, C.** (1972). 'Reiteration frequency of haemoglobin genes in the duck.' *Nature New Biol.*, **235**: 231–4.

19. **Diggelmann, H., Faust, C. H., and Mach, B.** (1973). 'Enzymatic Synthesis of DNA Complementary to Purified 14S Messenger RNA of Immunoglobulin Light Chain.' *Proc. Natl. Acad. Sci.*, **70**: 693–6.

20. **Tonegawa, S.** (1987). *Somatic generation of immune diversity*. Nobel Lecture. Stockholm: The Nobel Foundation, pp. 381–2.

21. **Tonegawa, S.** (1968). 'Genetic transcription directed by the b2 region of λ bacteriophage.' *Proc. Natl. Acad. Sci.*, **61**: 1320–7.

22. **Tonegawa, S., Bernadini, A., Weimann, B. J., and Steinberg, C.** (1974). 'Reiteration frequency of antibody genes. Studies with k-chain mRNA.' *FEBS Lett.*, **40**(1): 92–6.

23. **Tonegawa, S.** (1974). 'Evidence for somatic generation of antibody diversity.' *Proc. Natl. Acad. Sci.*, **71**: 4027–31.

24. **Barstad, P., Farnsworth, V., Weigert, M., Cohn, M., and Hood, L.** (1974). 'Mouse Immunoglobulin Heavy Chains Are Coded by Multiple Germ Line Variable Region Genes.' *Proc. Natl. Acad. Sci.*, **71**: 4096–4100.

25. **Tonegawa, S.** (1976). 'Reiteration frequency of immunoglobulin light chain genes: Further evidence for somatic generation of antibody diversity.' *Proc. Natl. Acad. Sci.*, **73**: 203–7.

26. **Tonegawa, S., Hozumi, N., Matthyssens, G., and Schuller, R.** (1977). 'Somatic Changes in the Content and Context of Immunoglobulin Genes.' *Cold Spring Harbor Symp. Quant. Biol.*, **41**: 877–89.

27. **Maxam, A., and Gilbert, W.** (1977). 'A new method for sequencing DNA.' *Proc. Natl. Acad. Sci.*, **74**: 560–4.

28. **Tonegawa, S., Maxam, A. M., Tizard, R., Bernard, O., and Gilbert, W.** (1978). 'Sequence of a mouse germ-line gene for a variable region of an immunoglobulin light chain.' *Proc. Natl. Acad. Sci.*, **75**: 1485–9.

29. **Brack, C., Hirama, M., Lenhard-Schuller, R., and Tonegawa, S. A.** (1978). 'Complete Immunoglobulin Gene Is Created by Somatic Recombination.' *Cell*, **15**: 1–14.

30. **Bernard, O., Hozumi, N., and Tonegawa, S.** (1978). 'Sequences of Mouse lmmunoglobulin Light Chain Genes before and after Somatic Changes.' *Cell*, **15**: 1133–44.

31. **Seidman, J. G., and Leder, P.** (1978). 'The arrangement and rearrangement of antibody genes.' *Nature*, **276**: 790–5.

32. **Loh, E., Schilling, J., and Hood, L.** (1978). 'Rearrangement of genetic information may produce immunoglobulin diversity.' *Nature*, **276**: 785–90.

33. **Davis, M. M., Calame, K., Eraly, P. W., Livant, D. L., Joho, R., Weissman, I. L., and Hood, L.** (1980). 'An immunoglobulin heavy chain gene is formed by at least two recombinational events.' *Nature*, **283**: 733–9.

34. **Sledge, C., Fain, D. S., Black, B., Krieger, R. G., and Hood, L.** (1976). 'Antibody differentiation: apparent sequence identity between variable regions shared by IgA and IgG immunoglobulins.' *Proc. Natl. Acad. Sci.*, **73**: 923–7.

35. **Smithies, O.** (1970). 'Pathways through networks of branched DNA.' *Science*, **169**: 882–3.

36. **Early, P.,** Huang, H., Davis, M., Calame, K., and Hood, L. (1980). 'An lmmunoglobulin Heavy Chain Variable Region Gene Is Generated from Three Segments of DNA: VH, D and JH.' *Cell*, **19**: 981–92.

37. **Maki, R., Traunecker, A., Sakanao, H., Roeder, W., and Tonegawa, S.** (1980). 'Exon shuffling generates an immunoglobulin heavy chain gene.' *Proc. Natl. Acad. Sci.*, **77**: 2138–42.

38. **Tonegawa, S.** (1983). 'Somatic generation of antibody diversity.' *Nature*, **302**: 575–81.

39. **Wigzell, H.** (1987). Award ceremony speech by Hans Wigzell at The Nobel Prize in Physiology or Medicine, awarded to Susumu Tonegawa. Stockholm: The Nobel Foundation.

40. **Dreyer, W. J., and Bennett, J. C.** (1965). 'The Molecular Basis of Antibody Formation: A Paradox.' *Proc. Natl. Acad. Sci. USA*, **54**: 864–9.

41. **Smithies, O.** (1963). 'Gamma-globulin variability: A genetic hypothesis.' *Nature*, **199**: 1231–5.

Chapter 8

Immunoglobulin constant regions

A classification of immunoglobulins arrives

The early years of immunoglobulin discovery attempted to delineate different 'globulin' types according to their separation behaviour during electrophoresis. Protein 'bands' seen by staining or other visualization methods and containing multiple protein species of varying molecular weights that happened to have the same mobilities after electrophoretic separation were designated with a mixture of Greek letters, Arabic numbers, and Latin letters leading eventually to a complex codified system that even today's immunologists would find baffling. When Svedberg enabled the multiglobulin bands to be separated by ultracentrifugation on the basis of molecular weight, new descriptions became necessary. In 1964, WHO convened a meeting on nomenclature of human immunoglobulins in Prague[1] at which some semblance of order was introduced into the naming system with the following results (see Table 8.1):

Further, a convention for the naming of individual chains was also agreed for the different immunoglobulin classes (see Table 8.2):

At this time the remaining D and E classes of immunoglobulin had not yet been discovered although the WHO allowed for such, indicating that new classes may be required when:

> ... molecules containing a novel heavy chain are discovered.[1]

Table 8.1 Naming based on heavy chain differences

Existing names	New names proposed by WHO
γ, 7Sγ, 6.6Sγ, γ2, $γ_{ss}$	γG or IgG
β2A, γ1A	γA or IgA
$γ_1$M, $β_2$M, 19Sγ, γ-macroglobulin	γM or IgM
Naming based on light chain differences	
Type I, 1, B	Type K
Type II, 2, A	Type L

Table 8.2 Immunoglobulin classes

Immunoglobulin	Heavy chain	Light chain
γG or IgG	γ (gamma)	
γA or IgA	α (alpha)	
γM or IgM	μ (mu)	
Type I	Type K	κ (kappa)
Type II	Type L	λ (lambda)

Adapted with permission from World Health Organization, Memorandum from WHO Meeting on Nomenclature of Human Immunoglobulins, *Bulletin of the World Health Organization*, Volume 30, Number 3, pp. 447–450, Copyright © 1964 World Health Organization.

Furthermore, the possibility that new 'immunoglobulins' may be discovered led to the suggestion of *subclasses*, a designation retained today.

> … which can be recognized as members of presently known classes… even though they may differ in some significant detail…[1]

Immunoglobulin classes: light chains

The earliest description of proteins now classified as light chains goes back to Henry Bence Jones who in 1848 described 'A new substance in the urine of a patient with *Mollities Ossium*'.[2] The Latin name *Mollities Ossium*, now known as osteomalacia or bone softening, is associated with myeloma cell activation of osteoclasts which increases bone resorption and 'softening'. As a chemical pathologist Bence Jones attempted to identify the 'substance', carrying out an extraordinarily comprehensive chemical analysis, finally concluding that the urine contained:

> … the hydrated deutoxide of albumen.[2]

Bence Jones' chemical analysis gave albumen as $C_{48}H_{37}N_6O_{15}$ and the 'substance' as $C_{48}H_{38}N_6O_{18}$. This led to the conclusion that there was an excess of three oxygen atoms and one hydrogen atom for every 48 carbon atoms, hence the 'hydrated deutoxide' or hydrated dioxide of albumen. In fact many proteins would have been present in late-stage myeloma due to their passage from blood through damaged kidneys. He further calculated that the 'albumen', a recently described protein substance, represented 67 parts per 1000 of the patient's urine and that:

> … therefore there was as much of this peculiar albuminous substance in the urine as there is ordinary albumen in healthy blood.[2]

In 1982, on the occasion of the Eastman Kodak lectureship award, Frank Putnam commented[3] that Bence Jones must have been intimately involved in the diagnosis of the first recorded death from *Mollities Ossium* in 1846. The patient died on 2 January, 1846 in St Georges Hospital, London where Bence Jones was a physician. The death certificate records 'Atrophy from Albumenuria, certified' (see Fig. 8.1). Bence Jones records:

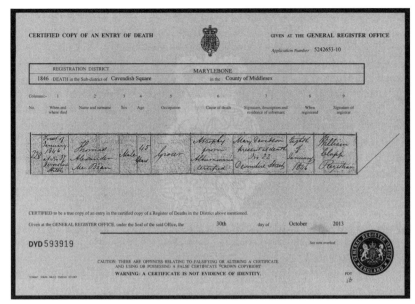

Fig. 8.1 Death certificate of the first recorded case of Bence-Jones proteinuria.
Death Certificate © Crown Copyright, reproduced under Open Government Licence v.2.0.

The following day I saw that the bony structure of the ribs was cut with the greatest ease, and that the bodies of the vertebrae were capable of being sliced off with a knife.[2]

A more complete history of this patient and of Bence Jones' involvement in the diagnosis can be found in Robert Kyle's short historical review of Henry Bence Jones[4] (see Fig. 8.2). Here then was the first example associating what Rustizky would later describe as 'multiple myeloma'[5] (this form of cancer results in 'multiple' punched-out areas of bone destruction) with a protein substance. Surprisingly, further elaboration of this relationship had to wait until the late 1940s, with only seven new cases of Bence

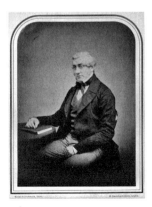

Fig. 8.2 Portrait of Henry Bence Jones.
Reproduced with permission from the Wellcome Library, London.

Jones proteinuria being recorded in the 50 intervening years after the initial description. A possible catalyst for further intensive investigation of myeloma proteins was the discovery of the syndrome 'macroglobulinemia' by Waldenström[6] in 1944, characterized by a large serum excess of a 19S immunoglobulin now known to be IgM (M for macroglobulinemia).

The realization that Bence Jones proteins were actually over-produced normal light chains (and not albumen as Bence Jones had incorrectly thought) would dawn as a result of the biophysical and amino acid compositional studies of Edelman and Gally and the pugnacious attacks on myeloma chemistry by Frank Putnam, who in 1962 demonstrated that myeloma proteins and normal immunoglobulins were similar if not identical. In concluding his study using proteolytic enzymatic methods Putnam observed:

> ... when disease processes elicit changes in the production of γ-globulin, the new proteins produced must reflect the genetic makeup of the clone of cells in which they are synthesized... normal γ-globulin and myeloma γ–globulins... will be found to possess the same underlying structure...[7]

Edelman and Gally's conclusions were similar:

> ... the amino acid analyses of chromatographically isolated L chains and Bence-Jones proteins were similar or identical. Until exhaustive studies are done... their complete identity cannot be considered proven. Consideration of the physicochemical similarities of these proteins, however, would favor the notion that they are identical. [8]

They had also suggested that the Bence Jones light chains existed as non-covalent dimers that could be dissociated by exposure to high concentrations of urea. Putnam confirmed Edelman's suggestion one year later but took the concept one step further by demonstrating via peptide mapping that the dimers were of *identical* light chains. In a discussion of sequence data for kappa light chains in 1966, Putnam may also have pre-empted Kabat and Wu on the significance of variability in different regions of the amino-terminal half of the chain, commenting:

> The clustering of interchanges [sequence substitutions] in three localized areas of sequence is immediately evident... It is tempting, therefore, to think that all the major areas subject to variation in sequence are part of a single topographical region, which... may define a portion of the antigen-combining site.[9]

At the time of Putnam and Edelman's studies there was still limited amino acid sequence data on either normal or Bence-Jones light chains so that their equivalence, although likely, was not proven. In 1967 Putnam produced the first complete sequence of a Bence-Jones lambda light chain and by comparison with known kappa chain sequences suggested a high degree of structural identity—40% identity at the amino acid sequence level with conserved disulphide bridge positions and identical sequences immediately adjacent to the cysteine residues. In a second paper in the same year two further lambda light chain sequences were published, allowing some comparisons and observations on conservation in certain regions of the light chain. In this second paper Putnam commented:

Like κ-chains, human λ-chains differ in many positions in the NH2-terminal portion of the molecule… The positions of variation are distributed in a seemingly random fashion through the first half of the λ-chains; yet there are two short peptide stretches where the amino acids differ in all three λ-chains (residues 48–51 and 91–95). [10]

Putnam also commented on the mutation frequencies in different λ-chains and in addition the evolutionary significance of the large regions of sequence homology:

These structural relations which are evidence for a common evolutionary origin of the light and heavy chains of immunoglobulins are in accord with our suggestions that κ- and λ-chain specialization preceded interspecies differentiation and that the sequence variation in light chains results from an accumulation of mutations through many separate genes for κ- and λ-chains rather than through some novel method of somatic hypermutation.[10]

In a series of later papers the complete amino acid sequences and disulphide bridge locations of both kappa[11] and lambda[12] Bence-Jones proteins were published by Putnam in 1969 and 1970. His conclusions drawn from the studies of the kappa chain confirmed what many in the field had speculated on with regard to the dualistic nature of light chain structure:

… these proteins differ in many positions in the amino-terminal or variable half of the molecule but appear to have an identical sequence in the carboxy-terminal or constant half except for a substitution at position 191 that is correlated with the Inv genetic factor.[11]

For the lambda chain similar conclusions were drawn and additionally, Putnam speculated that since human lambda chains were homologous to both human and mouse kappa chains that there must have been a common ancestral gene. While getting it right on the question of Bence-Jones light chain equivalence to normal light chains, Putnam clearly nailed his colours to the germ line mast on the genetics of immunoglobulin diversity. In just three short years he and others would experience the beginning of the demolition of the germ line model by Tonegawa.

Here then was a convergence of data that clarified the antibody light chain story: Bence-Jones proteins were normal light chains that were secreted by aberrant (myeloma) plasma cells and could be either kappa or lambda chains (but not both from the same cell). In normal plasma cells two identical copies of single kappa or lambda light chains would be paired with the cognate heavy chain pair to form a complete antibody, as finally established in 1969 by Edelman whose sequencing of the IgG four-chain molecule (see Chapter 6) put an end to any doubts about the light chain-heavy chains relationship in the antibody molecule.

Immunoglobulin isotypes and sub-types

Immunoglobulin G (IgG)

From the earliest studies of Tiselius and later Svedberg the predominance of γ-globulins in the gamma migrating region during electrophoresis and their 7S size in ultracentrifugation firmly established this antibody class, or *isotype* as IgG. Porter's sequencing of this fraction from rabbit sera provided the molecular details while both Porter and Edelman established the exact relationship of gamma chains and light chains in the complete antibody molecule. The current view of the IgG molecule in terms of its chain organization has not changed since those early studies. As we shall see in a later chapter the arrival of three-dimensional structural information for this immunoglobulin isotype catapulted forwards our understanding of the mechanisms of antibody-mediated biological effects.

While the presence of two linked heavy chains and two heavy chain-light chain pairings was an established organizational structure for IgG, the behaviour of γ-globulin in serological experiments indicated that a single isotype was an over-simplification. While Porter and Edelman were communicating the results of their chain-sequencing work, others were investigating the heterogeneity of the γ–globulin fraction, both in mice and humans. During 1964 several groups arrived at similar conclusions on IgG isotype diversity. In January of 1964 Lichter and Dray used primate antisera to delineate serologically distinct patterns in various serum proteins. In Fig. 8.3 the results of their analysis of γ-globulin from normal human serum using the Ouchterlony method are shown. Inspection of the bottom three wells clearly indicates distinct immunoprecipitation 'arcs' which Dray labels as γA, γB, and γC.[13] Dray also observed multiple arcs with the IgA (β_2A) and IgM (β_2M) fractions and suggested that these isotypes might also exist in 'at least two antigenically different forms in human serum'.[13] Here then was a first indication that multiple forms of IgG may exist in normal human serum.

Parallel studies by Putnam's team made use of antisera raised against pathological heavy-chain species from two different patients (Cr and Zu) with a lymphoma-like disorder. The anti-Cr and anti-Zu rabbit antisera cross-reacted with normal 7S γ-globulin allowing the following conclusion to be drawn:

> These findings are consistent with the assumption that in normal human serums at least two populations of 7S γ-globulins are present which differ in part of the antigenic structure of their H chains.[14]

Later that same year Henry Kunkel added to the body of knowledge with a study of 13 myeloma proteins and was able to identify three separate heavy chain antigenic responses also suggesting the existence of three separable sub-groups of the γ-globulin isotype which he named Vi, We, and Ge.[15] Two months after Kunkel's study appeared, Terry and Fahey reported a similar set of serological studies but this time using monkey antisera raised against normal human sera. Using Ouchterlony techniques and fragmentation of the γ-globulin fraction they described three different sub-classes associated with the heavy chain constant regions which they named $\gamma^{2\alpha-}$, $\gamma^{2\beta-}$, and γ^{2c-} globulins. Were these related to the sub-groups reported by Terry and Fahey? Exchange of proteins between the two groups clearly showed that the Vi and We sub-groups of Kunkel corresponded to the γ^{2c} and γ^{2b} sub-groups respectively of Terry and Fahey while the third sub-group reactivity from each laboratory appeared to be different. Here then was at least a partial agreement suggesting that IgG was not a single species but existed as a family of probably three sub-isotypes, the antigenic differences of each being located within the constant regions of the heavy chain. Confirmation that this was not a special feature of human γ-globulins was provided by Fahey with the identification of similar sub-classes in mouse determined by the same serological procedures.[16]

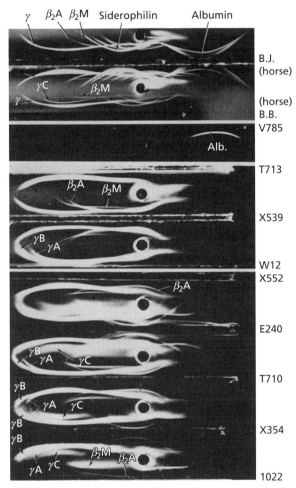

Fig. 8.3 The image shows a number of immunoelectrophoresis experiments in which protein constituents of normal human sera are visualized by the presence of precipitin arcs when challenged with different primate antisera.

Reproduced with permission from Lichter, E. A. and Dray, S., Immunoelectrophoretic characterization of human serum proteins with primate antisera, *The Journal of Immunology*, Volume 92, Number 1, pp. 91–99, Copyright © 1964, The American Association of Immunologists, Inc.

To provide a clear, universal nomenclature Kunkel, Fahey, Terry, and others evaluated the existing results and proposed a system of identification that was approved in 1966 and published via the WHO Bulletin 'Notation for immunoglobulin subclasses'.[17] Their proposal was as follows (Table 8.3).

In their 1973 review[18] Natvig and Kunkel provided a more comprehensive measure of the percentage subclass distribution in both normal human serum and the known myeloma proteins, confirming that data generated via myeloma patients reflected the inter-subclass distribution in normal human sera (Table 8.4).

Table 8.3 WHO notation for IgG subclasses

Current	Occurrence as myeloma proteins (%)	Proposed	Polypeptide heavy chain (γ-chain)
We or γ2b or C	70–80	IgG1 or γG1	γ1
Ne or γ2a	13–18	IgG2 or γG2	γ2
Vi or γ2c or Z	6–8	IgG3 or γG3	γ3
Ge or γ2d	3	IgG4 or γG4	γ4

Reproduced with permission from Kunkel, H.G. et al., Notation for human immunogobulin subclasses, *Bulletin of the World Health Organization*, Volume 35, Number 6, p. 953, Copyright © 1966 World Health Organization.

Table 8.4 Percentage values of IgG subclasses*

IgG1	IgG2	IgG3	IgG4	
66[a] ± 8	23 ± 8	7.3 ± 3.8	4.2 ± 2.6	Normal values, 145 Caucasian sera
64[b]	28	5	3	Mean values for 10 adults
69[c]	18	8	5	Myeloma incidence; 144 cases
72[d]	17	7	4	Myeloma incidence; 368 cases

*See original article for complete reference list

Reproduced from *Advances in Immunology*, Volume 16, J.B. Natvig and H.G. Kunkel, Human Immunoglobulins: Classes, Subclasses, Genetic Variants, and Idiotypes, pp. 1–59, Copyright © 1973, with permission from Elsevier, http://www.sciencedirect.com/science/bookseries/00652776

A decade after Kunkel's review, the genetic origins and structural differences of IgG subclasses would begin to be understood. In the first of many studies that would employ DNA cloning techniques, Terry Rabbitts and colleagues drew attention to the significant difference in length of the hinge region of the γ3 constant region compared with the other subclasses.[19] Four copies of the classical 'core hinge' sequence (CPPC in IgG1 and IgG4—two disulphide bonds separated by a short proline segment; CCVECPPC in IgG2 giving additional disulphide bonds) are present in IgG3 (CPRCP(EPKSCDTPPPCPRCP)$_3$) giving this IgG a much longer separation between the antigen recognition Fab regions and the functional constant domains, at the same time conferring flexibility and *parri passu*, proteolytic susceptibility. As we shall see in later chapters, these differences between hinge regions play a key role in determining the observed functional behaviour of the different IgG subclasses.

Immunoglobulin A (IgA) and 'Secretory IgA'

In 1953 Grabar and Williams at the *Institut Pasteur* described a combined serum electrophoresis with the Ouchterlony method using horse anti-human serum and identified a number of discrete globulin fractions in the γ-, β-. and α-regions.[20] They named the new fraction β2A-globulin. Some six years later the first detailed analysis of this material was made by Heremans and colleagues in a joint study between the St Pierre University Clinic in Louvain and the pharmaceutical company Behringwerke in Marburg (the first company in Europe to begin fractionating human plasma proteins on an industrial scale). In a carefully executed purification of *normal* human serum Heremans demonstrated a clear difference between the gamma globulins and β2-macroglobulin, later to be called IgM. He suggested that the β2A fraction had significantly more carbohydrate than γ-globulin and the observation of some cross-reactivity between γ-, β2-M, and the β2A precipitin curves using anti-human sera allowed him to conclude:

> It is tempting to interpret the above findings as indicative of partial correspondence.[21]

Of particular importance in proving the identity of the β2A fractionated protein was the fact that when the anti-human serum was pre-adsorbed with a known β2A secreting myeloma protein, precipitin lines with the normal β2A were reduced or abolished. Heremans reported a size of 7S in the ultracentrifuge for his purified material but dismissed a second fraction of size ~11S as:

> much less important... artifact... such as a polymerized form....[21]

Some years after Heremans' studies Thomas Tomasi took the IgA story one step further, firstly by demonstrating that γA was predominantly of the 7S form (the size of IgG) in both normal serum and in serum from patients with Laennec's cirrhosis and secondly by discovering a secretory form of γA present in 'certain external secretions' such as saliva, colostrum, lacrimal secretions, and nasal and bronchial fluids. This secretory γA existed as a dimer, similar but not identical to the ~11S form seen by Heremans in serum since it was unaffected in its ultracentrifuge behaviour when subjected to disulphide bond reducing agents. In addition, it appeared to contain an additional 'piece' since it exhibited an immunological specificity not present in the serum γA material. Tomasi speculated on the origin of this addition to γA:

> Whether that portion of the γ1A which is immunologically specific is a piece incorporated during the local synthesis of γ1A in the gland or is added by the epithelial cell in the process of transport remains to be determined.[22]

> Text extract ©1965 Rockefeller University Press. Originally published in *The Journal of Experimental Medicine*, Volume 121: pp. 101–124.

In concluding his paper he further commented on the possible role of this secretory antibody system:

> There appears to be an immunological system which is characteristic of certain external secretions. Its properties including the local production of a distinctive type of antibody separate it from the 'systemic' system responsible for the production of circulating antibody. This system may play a significant role in the body's defense mechanisms against allergens and microorganisms.[22]

> Text extract ©1965 Rockefeller University Press. Originally published in *The Journal of Experimental Medicine*, Volume 121: pp. 101–124.

In 1966 three almost simultaneous studies published by Vaerman and Heremans,[23] Feinstein and Franklin,[24] and Prendergast and Kunkel[25] described serological studies of myelomas in which anti-IgA antisera were used to characterize IgA myelomas and normal human sera. All three studies separated the myelomas into two antigenic types, experimentally established by pre-absorption of the antisera with the two distinct myeloma specificities to produce derivative antisera that were now specific for either one or other myeloma type. Testing of pooled normal human sera suggested that the normal IgA population exhibits two subclasses but with significantly different normal serum concentrations. Two years later Henry Kunkel and colleagues produced an even more bizarre picture of the IgA family, whose subclasses were now designated γA1 and γA2. When monomeric human IgA prepared from colostrum (polymeric IgA was separated from the monomeric material) was subjected to electrophoresis under denaturing conditions but without disulphide reducing agents, the γA2 subclass appeared to show disulphide bonds between the light chains but not the heavy chains.[26] This non-classical immunoglobulin structural arrangement would later be shown to be typical only for a particular IgA human *allotype* (allotypy will be discussed later in this chapter). Importantly, what Kunkel's study also showed was that while IgA2 was much lower in concentration than IgA1 in serum it was much higher in colostrum samples (by three to ten times), confirming other proposals of a protective role for IgA2 in external secretions. Later studies by Putnam[27,28] on the differences in the hinge regions of IgA1 and IgA2 would provide a rationale for the subclass differences. IgA1 has a hinge sequence 13 amino acids longer than in IgA2, is glycosylated, and protease sensitive. The IgA2 hinge in contrast is short and shows greater stability to microbial proteases, a property essential for survival in the hostile external secretory compartments.

The exact manner in which IgA was assembled in its secreted form was examined by several parallel studies. In a study on rabbit immunoglobulins published in 1967, Cebra and Small described a γA immunoglobulin from rabbit colostrum having a size of 370 000 Daltons, a heavy chain easily distinguishable from either γ– or μ-chains and containing a third chain which they named T for transport.[29] This third 'piece' had a molecular weight of 50 000 Daltons but could be halved by chemical reduction. They postulated that the T piece was required to hold together the γA dimers and was either non-covalently associated with the α-chain (since most could be removed by denaturing agents) or partially disulphide bonded. Tomasi and Bienenstock had a slightly different picture of this transport protein. In their studies on human IgA, they concluded that the majority of the secretory piece was covalently bound via disulphide bonds and that further this could not be reduced in size by chemical reduction.[30] Was this an example of species differentiation or doubtful experimentation?

Three years later, Halpern and Koshland clarified the rabbit versus human discrepancy but also added yet a further component, the 'J'- (for joining) chain, to what was now called 'secretory IgA'. In a series of smart experiments they confirmed that the secretory, or 'S' component is a single chain that cannot be chemical reduced, as erroneously suggested by Tomasi. Furthermore, the J-chain was not a renegade light chain—this was demonstrated by studies of three different myeloma IgAs in which the J component was present but was shown by comparative amino acid composition to be clearly different from either the expressed κ or λ light chains. Here then was a set of defining conclusions but not quite the *denouement*. As Halpern and Koshland observed:

> The role of J in the final assembly of the dimer and the S component is intriguing. J may provide the binding site for S, either directly through the contribution of groups to the site, or indirectly through an induced conformation change in the α chains. J may further provide the recognition for interaction between the plasma cell synthesizing the J-dimer complex and the epithelial cell synthesizing the S component.[31]

> Text extract reprinted by permission from Macmillan Publishers Ltd: *Nature*, Halpern, M.S. and Koshland, M.E., Novel subunit in secretory IgA, Volume 228, pp.1276–1278, Copyright © 1970.

Further explanation was to arrive via a series of protein chemistry experiments by Chapuis and Koshland in 1975.[32] The J-chain, known to be rich in cysteine, was shown to be disulphide-bonded between the C-terminal extensions (an 18 amino-acid extension present in α-chains, often referred to as the 'tailpiece') of two α-chains, its assembly occurring in the IgA-producing plasma cell. This gave a picture which Koshland referred to as the 'dimer clasp' (see Fig. 8.4).

While Koshland's model gave an explanation of how two IgA monomers became linked together, it did not provide (or even attempt) an explanation of how this dimer is transported from its site of synthesis in plasma cells to the multiple secretory sites in the body (colostrum, tears, saliva, and the major mucosal surfaces) via the mucosal epithelium and furthermore, how its stability is controlled at those sites, exhibiting as they do uncharitable chemical environments (e.g. the GI tract) for proteins. This would turn out to be somewhat more complicated than the simple identification of a transport (T)-piece that Cebra and Small had suggested. In fact, the secretory component would be shown to be part of a much more complex receptor located in the basolateral membrane of mucosal epithelial cells. IgA would first bind to this receptor (now known as the polyIg receptor, or pIgR) and would be transported into the epithelial cell where the receptor would be proteolytically processed, allowing release of the IgA molecule bound to a part of the pIgR receptor at the apical membrane and from there into the mucous milieu.[33] The role of this secretory component (SC) derived from the pIgR has been shown to mediate the transcytosis of IgA through the epithelial cell and to have a protective effect on the immunoglobulin dimer in the hostile

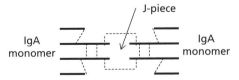

Fig. 8.4 The dimer clasp model of IgA.

protease environments it operates in. It now seems likely that using its five-domain structure it forms a protective association with the constant regions of the IgA dimer.[34] There are in fact two forms of IgA dimer, only one of which (IgA1) has a covalent link between the SC and the CH_2 domain of one IgA monomer, the other (IgA2) forming a non-covalent and hence proteolytically more sensitive association. A simple picture of the epithelial path to generate the SIgA complex (as understood in 1990) and the structural relationship of the IgA, J, and S components (as proposed in 2009) is shown in Fig. 8.5a and b respectively.

With a total surface area of ~400m², human mucosal surfaces present the most important interfacial barrier against potentially harmful organismal invasion (skin surface area is ~1.8m²). The evolution of a specific secretory antibody family to trap and remove viruses, bacteria, and other invasive pathogens 'at the doorstep' has been of great importance for human survival, particularly at the stage of neonatal development. Despite this, IgA, which is produced at levels greater than all the other immunoglobulins together, has been the 'poor relation' when it comes to detailed structural studies, and even at the time of writing, high resolution x-ray structural information for the SIgA complex remains elusive.

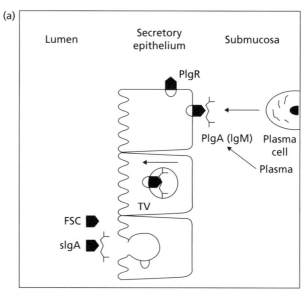

Fig. 8.5 (a) A model of the translocation of IgA from the plasma cell to the lumen of mucosal epithelial membrane barriers; [PIgR, polymeric immunoglobulin receptor; SIgA, secretory IgA; FSC, free secretory component; TV, transport vesicle; PIgA, polymeric IgA]. (b) A structural plan for the manner in which dimeric IgA, J-piece, and secretory component derived from the polyIg receptor may be associated.

(a) Reproduced with permission from Goldblum, R.M., The role of IgA in local immune protection, *Journal of Clinical Immunology*, Volume 10, Issue 6 Supplement, pp. 64S–71S, Copyright © 1990, Plenum Publishing Corporation; (b) Reproduced with permission from Bonner, A., et al., The Nonplanar Secretory IgA2 and Near Planar Secretory IgA1 Solution Structures Rationalize Their Different Mucosal Immune Responses, *The Journal of Biological Chemistry*, Volume 284, pp. 5077–5087, Copyright © 2009 by the American Society for Biochemistry and Molecular Biology.

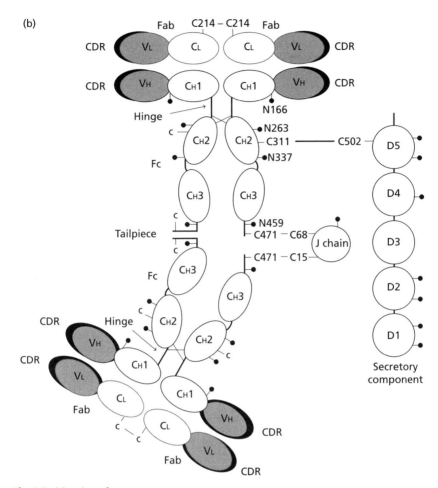

Fig. 8.5 (*Continued*)

Immunoglobulin M (IgM) or 'macroglobulin'

The predominant species in serum was long known to be the 'γ-globulin' fraction in electrophoresis with a size of 7S in the ultracentrifuge, but it was not alone. It had also been observed by Kabat in 1938 that a heavier fraction was present between the gamma and beta regions, particularly evident in horse serum (see Chapter 4). This fraction had an estimated size of 900 000 Daltons and was termed the 'heavy band'. At this time its relationship to gamma globulin was unclear.

In 1944, Jan Waldenström described the clinical profile of two male patients who showed fatigue, bleeding from the gums and nasal mucosa, lymphadenopathy, normochromic anaemia, low serum fibrinogen and a high serum viscosity evidently due to a high concentration of a macroglobulin, characterized by electrophoresis and having a mass by ultracentrifugation of about 1M Daltons. The patients showed no typical signs of myeloma, even on post-mortem examination. The name Waldenström gave to this euglobulin (Greek *eu*, normal; euglobulins were insoluble in water but soluble in dilute salt solution) was 'macroglobulin', and the condition was designated macroglobulinaemia. A decade later Henry Kunkel carried out more extensive ultracentrifugation studies of normal human serum, producing a beautiful three-dimensional representation of the serum proteins (see Fig. 8.6) allowing deconvolution of the components of the gamma, beta, and alpha electrophoretic regions.[35] The dominance of albumin (Alb) in serum is also evident. From this analysis and other studies published around the same time Kunkel drew attention to the fact that the 19Sγ material was different from γ-globulin, in size, in immunological reactivity, and in having considerably more carbohydrate.

It is ironic that, as with the light chains, detailed molecular descriptions of antibody chains relied on pathological disease states providing the over-production of immunoglobulin to facilitate their characterization. This was to some extent a reflection of the limited scope of the physical methods of purification. With the further development of chromatographic purification methods this changed rapidly, as Chaplin, Cohen, and 'Betty' Press observed in the introduction to their analysis of normal 19S γ-globulin (IgM) in 1965, drawing attention to the fact that because of:

> ... the difficulty of isolating this fraction from normal serum, chemical studies of IgM have been carried out mainly on the γ-macroglobulins that occur in high concentration in pathological sera. The isolation of normal IgM has, however, been greatly simplified by the recent introduction of gel filtration methods...[36]

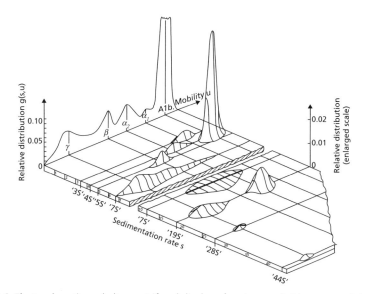

Fig. 8.6 Electrophoretic and ultracentrifugal display of major non-lipid serum proteins.

Reproduced with permission from Wallenius, G., et al., Ultracentrifugal studies of major non-lipide electrophoretic components of normal human serum, *The Journal of Biological Chemistry*, Volume 225, pp. 253–257, Copyright © 1957 by the American Society for Biochemistry and Molecular Biology.

During this analysis the chromatographic properties of the B (light) 19S chains were shown to be closely similar if not identical to those of IgG light chains, confirming the view that light chains from individual antibodies of different 'classes' are identical in type, that is they are either kappa or lambda chains. In contrast, the A- (heavy) chains of the 19S material showed differences to the 7S IgG heavy chains in electrophoresis. At the level of amino acid and carbohydrate composition this difference was more marked. When subjected to reduction of disulphide bonds and stabilization by alkylation, the 19S IgM dissociated into 7S units, suggesting prior to this chemical modification it existed in a polymeric form. Press speculated that in IgM the heavy A-chains must be disulphide-bonded together to generate the high molecular weight observed in the ultracentrifuge (19S ≈ 900 000 Daltons). This was wholly prophetic if lacking a detailed description of exactly how the interconnectivity might occur, the variation in published molecular weights size allowing for tetrameric and hexameric IgM molecules.

The precision of many of these earlier molecular weight determinations for IgM was questionable, as Metzger points out in his defining 1965 study. Using a highly purified preparation of Waldenström's IgM, Metzger established a benchmark size for the IgM monomer of 185 000 Daltons and a size for the natural polymeric macroglobulin of 890 000 Daltons, using carefully controlled ultracentrifugation measurements. The structure of the polymeric IgM was then obvious to Metzger as he points out:

> It has been widely assumed that the similar sedimentation constant of γM, and γG… reflected an identity of molecular size and… that γM contained six subunits. The present data indicate that there are only five subunits, with each γM, having a molecular weight significantly higher than that of γG.[37]

In 1971 Mestecky, Zikan, and Butler began to fill in more of the gaps and in so doing raised the possibility of a unified structural basis for polymeric immunoglobulins. Their study on IgM, also from patients with Waldenström's macroglobulinaemia, established that IgA and IgM share a common polypeptide chain, the J-chain, unrelated to normal light chains and involved in holding the polymeric structures together. As they concluded:

> The apparent identity of J chains from S-IgA and IgM is interesting in view of their presence in two classes of immunoglobulins… permissible to speculate that the J chain with its unusually high cysteine content may aid in maintaining the tertiary structure of the polymeric immunoglobulin molecule.[38]

Text extract reproduced from Mestecky, J. et al., Immunoglobulin M and secretory immunoglobulin A: presence of a common polypeptide chain different from light chains, Science, Volume 171, Issue 3976, pp. 1163–1165, Copyirght © 1971. Reprinted with permission from AAAS.

In 1973, Putnam and colleagues published the complete amino-acid sequence of the human IgM μ-chain (see Fig. 8.7).[39] This threw up some confirmations of previous observations but also some puzzles. The μ-chain was different to the γ-chain in several respects. Firstly, it showed evidence of having five structurally homologous

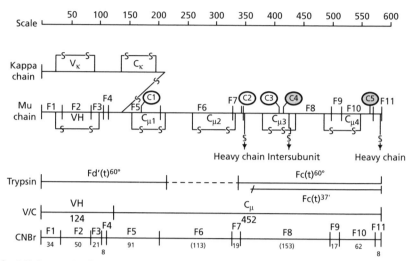

Fig. 8.7 Putnam's schematic structure of the IgM heavy chain (μ) organization. The F1–11 labels refer to fragments obtained by chemical cleavage of the chain which helped assemble the sequence in the correct order. The various domains are shown as VH, Cμ, etc. and the positions of carbohydrate as C1, C2 etc. while inter- and intrachain disulphide bonds are also marked.

Reproduced with permission from Putnam, F.M., et al., Complete Amino Acid Sequence of the Mu Heavy Chain of a Human IgM Immunoglobulin, *Science*, Volume 182, Issue 4109, pp. 287–291, Copyright © 1973.

'domains'—V_H and constant region domains Cμ1 to Cμ4—rather than the four of IgG molecules (V_H and Cγ1, Cγ2, and Cγ3), as well as having a 19 residue peptide 'tail'. This explained the higher molecular weight shown earlier by Metzger. Secondly, Putnam showed that the region between the first and second constant domains (the hinge region) was quite different to that in IgG and IgA in lacking multiple proline residues and extensive disulphide bonding, both thought to impart flexibility between the antigen-binding and Fc regions of IgG and IgA. Thirdly, IgM was extensively glycosylated, particularly in its Cμ3 domain.

It was later shown that IgM is able to form both hexameric and pentameric structures in the absence of the J-chain, both of which are able to activate complement more effectively than the normal J-chain containing IgM pentamer (J[-minus] hexamer >100x more effective than J[plus]pentamer).[40] In the most abundant species, pentameric IgM, the role of the J-chain is now thought to be to link two monomer μ-chains together during polyIgM formation such that a sixth chain is barred from entry.[41] The role of non-J-chain IgM molecules has seen much debate but clearly the low level of non-J polymers in normal serum suggests it is 'not a good thing' to have highly active complement-activating immunoglobulins circulating freely. In addition, it has been shown that without the J-chain present, polymeric IgM cannot interact with the pIg receptor and that these non-J pentamers and hexamers cannot therefore be transported across epithelia to antigen-rich mucosal secretions. Lacking the elevated complement-activating capacity, such effective antigen-trapping polymeric immunoglobulins are then able to engage in passive antigen exclusion without activation of those inflammatory responses accompanying complement activation.[42] Today we still await a definitive x-ray structure for IgM, although many medium-resolution structures based on x-ray and/or neutron scattering have been published.

Immunoglobulin D (IgD)

During 1964, David Rowe and John Fahey, working at the NIH (US) described a protein from a patient with multiple myeloma showing the usual high concentration typical of multiple myelomas (3.9g/100mL) but with unusual electrophoretic, ultracentrifuge, and immunological patterns.[43] It was unusual in that its heavy chain was slightly smaller than IgG or IgA, and furthermore it failed to react with anti-IgG, anti-IgM, or anti-IgA heavy chain antisera in Ouchterlony analyses (see Fig. 8.8a and b). In contrast, reaction with anti-λ light chain antisera was evident and furthermore, pre-absorption with the anti-λ chain antiserum obliterated the precipitin line, confirming that the protein was an immunoglobulin carrying a normal light chain (see Fig. 8.8b).

Was this an aberrant IgG or a new immunoglobulin? After papain digestion and electrophoresis Rowe and Fahey declared:

> Three features of the S. J. myeloma protein helped to distinguish it from G myeloma proteins, A myeloma proteins, or M macroglobulins of Waldenström. The first of these was immunochemical; i.e., the absence of specific IgG, IgA, or IgM determinants. The second feature was the unusually rapid electrophoretic mobility of the Fc fragment obtained by papain digestion. Most, but not all, G myeloma proteins yield Fc fragments of slower mobility... The third was the lack of effect of this myeloma protein on the rate of catabolism of normal IgG... All three of the atypical features of the S.J. myeloma protein [S.J. was the patient] reflect specific properties of the heavy polypeptide chains.... might represent the quantitative increase of a previously unrecognized normal class of immunoglobulins.[43]

In a parallel study, published back-to-back with the myeloma story, these authors demonstrated the presence of the new molecule in normal human sera and named it IgD (allegedly D for 'distinctive' when compared with the other known G, A, and M heavy chains).[44] Both λ-light and κ-light chains were found to be present in the normal IgD. In an analysis of 72 normal adult males and 28 normal adult females, Rowe and Fahey measured IgD levels using specific anti-IgD sera and found a large range (>100 fold) of concentrations, from <0.3mg/100 mL to 40mg/100mL, representing less than 1% of total serum immunoglobulin. Furthermore, the new IgD was present at the same levels in children between the ages of two years to 11 years, but was undetectable in two healthy infants of four months.

But why did the immune system require a separate circulating antibody isotype that appears to mimic IgG in many respects but fails to activate complement and was unreactive with skin, mast cells, or neutrophils. As Rowe commented eight years later in 1973:

> The function of immunoglobulin D (IgD) in the immune response is not yet clear...[45]

We shall return later to the functional significance of IgD as a lymphocyte receptor, a property it shares with IgM.

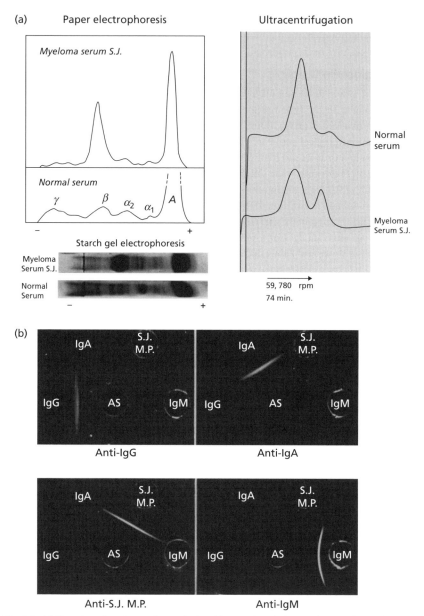

Fig. 8.8 (a) Showing the elevated protein level in starch gel electrophoresis from the multiple myeloma patient plus the abnormal Schlieren pattern in the ultracentrifuge; (b) Showing the Ouchterlony analysis and the unreactivity of the new Ig protein with any of the conventional antisera.

Figure reproduced with permission © 1965 Rockefeller University Press. Originally published in Rowe, D.S. and Fahey, J.L, A new class of human immunoglobulins. I. A unique myeloma protein, The *Journal of Experimental Medicine*, Volume 121, Number 1, pp. 171–184.

The last of the isotypes: immunoglobulin E (IgE)

The rich immunological discovery landscape of the 1960s and 1970s was an exciting place to walk. It was also highly competitive. The search for new antibody types or sub-types was relentless, but sometimes studies from earlier generations were either lost or ignored. The role of IgE in allergy was no exception.

The earliest observation of a hypersensitivity reaction was documented by Prausnitz in 1921 in which serum from one of his patients (Küstner) who was allergic to fish, when injected intradermally into Prausnitz' own forearms followed by injection 24 hours later by fish extract, produced an immediate weal and erythema.[46] The skin reaction was exactly as seen by Küstner and other fish-sensitive patients. However, it was not that simple. Prausnitz was sensitive to pollen hay fever, but the reverse proce-dure on Küstner using Prausnitz' serum followed by pollen challenge did not transfer sensitivity. In commenting on this and other observations on hypersensitivity transfer, Coca and Grove made a number of prognostic observations following their 1925 study (reproduced in part below):

1. The atopic reagins, discovered by Prausnitz and Küstner, have been found to be demon-strable in the blood of all subjects of hay fever and asthma in whom the cutaneous reac-tion to the injection of the atopen is positive.
2. Not all normal skins are susceptible to local passive sensitization. About 84% of normal skins are receptive; about 11% are non-receptive; and about 5% are slightly receptive.
3. The duration of the local passive sensitiveness is at least four weeks.
4. Heating for one-half hour at 56°C injures the atopic reagins.
5. The normal human skin could not be passively sensitized with an anti-egg precipi-tating serum or an anti-ragweed pollen precipitating serum, both from an injected rabbit.
6. The atopic reagin is neutralizable in the test tube or in the tissues. It does not produce a visible precipitate nor complement fixation, when mixed with the related atopen…
7. The atopic reagin is unable to sensitize the guinea-pig, confirming Prausnitz and Küster, or the guinea-pig uterus.
8. Atopic reagins could not be demonstrated in 5 cases of drug idiosyncrasy, nor in a case of hypersensitiveness to green pea, without asthmatic symptoms.
9. The atopic reagin is specific. In the blood of individuals sensitive to more than one sub-stance, more than one reagin can be demonstrated.
10. With the method of desensitization of the passively sensitized skin site, the identity or non-identity of atopens of different origin can be determined…[47]

Text extract reproduced with permission from Coca, A.F. and Grove, E.F., Studies in hypersentitiveness XIII. A study of the atopic reagins, *The Journal of Immunology*, Volume 10, Number 2, pp. 455–464, Copyright © 1925, The American Association of Immunologists, Inc.

In short, Coca and Grove were reluctant to ascribe the observed hypersensitivities to an 'immune globulin' since the 'atopic reagin' as they preferred to call it lacked the ability to form precipitates with antigen, a characteristic of known serum globulins. Again, while it could be neutralized by the atopen (from the Greek word *atopia* mean-ing 'unusualness') the reagin was unable to activate complement and it was sensitive to heat. They speculated that a number of reagins with different specificities would exist and cross-species sensitization was not always observed, a further characteristic that diverged from the known immune gamma globulins where cross-reactivity was common if not always complete. Of particular interest was the suggestion that the method of Prausnitz and Küstner (the PK test) could be used in a diagnostic context using skin sensitization to identify different atopens.

Without dismissing as unimportant the enormous body of work on allergy in the intervening years, it must be said it was not until the early 1960s that the nature of the 'atopic reagin' began to be understood. As late as 1963, Stanworth, while reviewing the field in the *British Medical Bulletin*, drew attention to the lacunae in structurally convincing data on the nature of the reagin material. Reagin-like material was associated with the 'fast' gamma region in electrophoresis but its exact size in ultracentrifugation was unclear, largely due to its extremely low concentrations in normal serum. Unlike 7S γ-globulins it was unable to cross the placenta, a property which was initially thought to be a function of size. Others had associated the sensitization property with IgA while some studies suggested that 'configurational changes' in γ-globulin might mediate such responses. In commenting on one of such studies, Stanworth observed:

> This implies that PK reactions can be stimulated directly as a response to configurational changes in the human γ-globulin molecule...[48]

Stanworth further observed the following in his conclusions, illustrating the embryonic understanding at this time of allergic responses:

> In explaining the mechanism of the PK reaction, however, account must be taken of the part played by the allergen in the elicitation of a wheal and erythema response at passively sensitized sites. Could it be that, in this case, an interaction between allergen and adjacent cell-bound reagin molecules results in configurational changes in the antibody molecules that are responsible for the ensuing tissue damage? This question cannot be answered yet, nor is it possible to say definitely whether complement plays any part in the PK reaction.[48]

Similar uncertainties were present in the mind of Bridget Ogilvie, working at the NIMR in London, as she attempted to explain the observed reagin response to helminths in rats, observing that '... it may well be that reagin-like antibodies are responsible for immunity to helminths in many species of animal.'[49]

While the allergy world was speculating, the group of Ishizaka in Colorado was at work attempting to identify the nature of reagin molecules. They had already shown that reaginic activity in serum was not diminished after γG, γA, and γD globulins were removed by adsorption and precipitation. Others had shown that the size of the reagin molecule was about 8S in the ultracentrifuge and coupled with the fact that its activity did not co-precipitate with the γM fraction, the association with γM globulins was unlikely. In their 1966 paper, Ishizaka and colleagues proposed that reaginic reactions must be mediated by a 'unique immunoglobulin'.[50] In summarizing their findings in studies with the ragweed allergen and dismissing the reaginic activity association with IgA they concluded:

> Precipitation of γE-globulin anti-ragweed antibody in the reagin containing fraction was accompanied by the loss of reaginic activity, whereas the precipitation of the γA-globulin antibody in the fraction did not result in any decrease of reaginic activity. The results highly suggest that the reaginic activity is associated with γE-globulin.[50]

Ishizaka's antigen from ragweed pollen was 'antigen E', hence his tentative designation γE for the new antibody class. In a detailed follow-up study he confirmed that the γE globulin contained light chains and would thus fit into the general requirements for an immunoglobulin. Despite confidence in their own results, doubts raised by the potential heterogeneity within reaginic responses (differential anaphylactic responses observed by others suggested multiple antibody types) led Ishizaka and his group, in a follow-up study, to allow for the possibility that:

> … human reaginic antibody may well be composed of multiple classes of immuno globulins.[51]

About a year later, on the other side of the Atlantic, Johansson and Bennich, working in Uppsala, described the immunological characterization of an 8S myeloma protein from a patient (ND) with myelomatosis that had no antigenic determinants in common with human α-, δ-, γ-, or μ-polypeptide chains.[52]

This new protein was immunologically distinct from all other known heavy-chain classes and was shown to contain lambda light chains. It was therefore a myeloma protein of the 'complete immunoglobulin class'. In concluding their study the authors proclaimed that:

> … the myeloma protein ND described in the present report is structurally related to normal immunoglobulins and carries unique antigenic determinants on its heavy polypeptide chains.[52]

However, since they observed a lack of reactivity of antisera raised against the myeloma protein with the sera of normal healthy individuals, they were also forced to conclude:

> … that if a normal counterpart to protein ND exists, it must be present in a concentration lower than 1–10 µg/ml serum.[52]

Surprisingly, Johansson and Bennich made no mention of the work of Ishizaka. There may have been a good reason for that omission. Although they concluded protein ND was a new immunoglobulin and was present at very low concentrations in serum, they did not appear to make the association at that time with the reagin immunoglobulin of Ishizaka. In what is a remarkable story of serendipity and collaborative inventiveness (beautifully reminisced by Stanworth[53]), it was suggested by a visiting scientist in Bennich and Johansson's laboratory that they provide protein samples to Stanworth in Birmingham UK who would test the ability of protein ND to block basophil sensitization *in vitro*. The results, though not entirely convincing, were presented by Stanworth at the British Society of Immunology in early 1967. John Humphrey, chairing the symposium, asked whether the ND protein had been tested for its ability to block sensitization in a standard PK test. It had not. The experiment was rapidly carried out (using Humphrey's skin as the guinea pig!) and reported in *The Lancet* in the same year. Here was the *coup de maître*, the defining moment for the allergy field. Total inhibition to a horse dander allergen response was seen after pre-injection of ND protein and subsequent sensitization of the same site with serum from an allergen-sensitive patient followed by challenge with the allergen.[54] The mechanism of this inhibition was later elegantly teased out by the same two groups when they demonstrated that the Fc region of protein ND was alone able to block the response, by competing with the Fc receptors on skin mast cells, thereby preventing access of the 'reagin' antibody.[55] In February of 1968, the three pioneering groups of Ishizaka, Johansson, and Stanworth gathered in Lausanne at a WHO immunoglobulin-reference-laboratory-sponsored meeting where IgE was formally declared as 'a new class of immunoglobulin'.[56]

Immunoglobulin allotypes

The observation that immunoglobulins from one animal may exhibit antigenicity in another animal *of the same species* was first proposed by Oudin in 1956. In his presentation to the French Academy of Sciences on 14 May 1956, Jacques Oudin reported the following observation: antiserum and antigen precipitates from rabbits immunized with various antigens were injected into non-immune rabbits in the presence of Freund's adjuvant. The non-immune rabbit sera then showed precipitation behaviour with the donor sera and displayed particular recognition patterns. To Oudin this was extraordinary since as he stated in the first sentence of his paper:

> Il est généralement admis que l'on ne peut pas immuniser un animal contre une protéine du sérum d'un animal de la même espèce.[57]

> [It is generally accepted that one cannot immunize one animal with a protein from the serum of an animal of the same species.]

Of 57 rabbits injected with the priming rabbit serum, 50 showed a positive response. Further, Oudin showed that the recipient's serum proteins precipitated by the donor sera were 'sometimes an antibody'. Oudin named these reactive serum components *allotypes* and further concluded that it is reasonable to suppose that allotypy is not an unusual phenomenon, particularly with regard to certain rabbit serum proteins, that it might also be expected to occur in other species, and that the phenomenon may have a genetic basis, a proposition arising from the individual rabbit diversity of allotypic reactivity (see Table 8.5).

On the basis of these and later more extensive data[58,59] Oudin proposed seven different allotypes (a–g) where no serum protein appeared to contain more than one allotypic pattern. Further he proposed that allelic relationships exist between the genes that control the allotypes, evidenced by:

> ... (1) the absence of certain kinds of groupings of the allotypes, ... (2) dosage effects ... The concentration of certain allotypes ... being smaller in supposed heterozygotes than in supposed homozygotes ... (3) the results of the analysis of the sera of a number of rabbits and their parents.[59]

The situation in humans was different. In the same year of Oudin's first publication (1956), Rune Grubb, working in Lund, Sweden examined the ability of sera of various

Table 8.5 Responses of 45 non-immune rabbits to immunization with sera from immune rabbits

Immune rabbit donor number	Pattern of reactivity observed in 45 non-immune rabbits								
	2	**18**	**8**	**3**	**5**	**5**	**1**	**2**	**1**
295	++	0	++	++	0	0	+	0	++
497	++	0	++	++	0	0	+	0	++
194	0	0	0	+++	+++	+++	+++	0	+++
411	0	0	0	++	+++	++	+++	0	+++
195	0	++	++	+++	++	+++	++	0	++
196	0	++	++	+++	+++	+++	+++	0	+++

patients to agglutinate red blood cells that had been coated with 'incomplete' anti-Rh antibodies (antibodies that bind to the Rh antigen but do not agglutinate the rbc's) and found that certain sera were able to induce agglutination while others were not. Further, the positive sera were of more than one type and a particularly high percentage of such sera were found in patients with rheumatoid arthritis (RA). Using the positive RA sera Grubb found it was possible to group the human sera. He also found that the serum groups were transmitted as dominant autosomal Mendelian traits.[60,61] During a collaborative study published in 1964, the groups of Kunkel and Grubb established a clear relationship between the primitive IgG subclasses already described (three of the four only since none were found for what is now IgG4) and the Gm (for **G**amma chain **m**arker) haplotypes.[15] Their data were clear-cut and delineated three different Gm phenotypes (Grubb nomenclature): a⁻ b⁺ f⁻; a⁺/a⁻b⁻ f⁻/f⁺; a⁻ b⁻ f⁻. In 1965 the WHO established a new naming procedure whereby numbers were allocated rather than letters. At that time 14 Gm factors and three Km factors had been described.

A substantial body of work over the following 20 years firmly established that allotypes are unique antigenic determinants recognized by specific antibodies and correspond to serologically determined amino acid changes that characterize the polymorphism of a chain within a given isotype. In his excellent monograph in 1970 Grubb analyses the three most studied allotypic markers, the Gm family, the Am family (for alpha chain marker but with limited data available in 1970) and the Inv family (for kappa chain marker, later renamed Km).[62] Since all humans have the immunoglobulin subclasses (e.g. IgG1–4) they cannot be used as haplotype sets, but it turned out that allotypic differences could however. Grubb summarized the correlation between IgG subclasses and the Gm markers known at the time of his monograph, using the WHO notation method (see Table 8.6).

Extensive studies during the 1980s established that certain Gm haplotypes were differently represented in the Negroid, Caucasoid, and Mongoloid populations. Summarizing the extensive data accumulated, Marie-Paule and Gérard Lefranc

Table 8.6 Correlation between IgG subclass and Gm factors in myeloma proteins

Subclass	Gm factors
γG1	1, 2, 3, 4, 17
γG2	23
γG3	5, 6, 10, 11, 13, 14, 21
γG4	None of the known

Reproduced from *Molecular Biology, Biochemistry and Biophysics series, No.9.*, Genetic Markers of Human Immunoglobulins, Grubb, R., Table III-2, Springer-Verlag, New York, USA, Copyright © 1970, with kind permission from Springer Science and Business Media.

point out in their recent comprehensive and excellent review of allotypes that certain Gm haplotype combinations are shared between populations while other combinations are unique.[63] For example, Gm 5, 10, 11, 13, 14, 26, and 27 on IgG3 is a specific Caucasoid haplotype while Gm 5, 10, 11, 13, 14, 26, and 27 on IgG1 is a haplotype only found in the Negroid population. Further illustrating the power of allotypic markers, these same authors remind us that prior to DNA fingerprinting techniques, Gm haplotypes were used in bone marrow transplantation, forensic medicine, and even paternity testing.

At the time of writing, 26 human allotypes are known: 20 Gm, three A2m (IgA1 has no allotypes) and three Km. No formal allotypes are known for IgG4. Gm and Am haplotypes are inherited in fixed combinations (Gm-Am haplotypes), now explained by the linkage of the constant region genes on chromosome 14. We shall return to the importance of allotypic responses later, in the context of antibody-mediated immune therapy. However, as early as 1963 some warning signals had already been suggested by Allen and Kunkel in a short communication to *Science* in which they reported the presence of anti-Gm agglutinating antibodies in 71% of the sera from a group of 24 children who had received multiple blood transfusions.[64]

Epilogue: antibodies as membrane-bound receptors

The discovery of IgD by Rowe and colleagues at the University of Lausanne was exciting and at the same time perplexing. Not only was this isotype unable to activate complement, react with skin cells, mast cells or neutrophils, it was at a very low concentration in normal serum (~0.2% of total antibody). Some years after its discovery by Rowe, Ira Green, William Paul, and colleagues at the NIH made the key observation in 1972 that IgD was actually membrane associated:

> The finding that IgD-bearing cells account for approximately 1/5 of all circulating lymphocytes with demonstrable surface immunoglobulin was very surprising in view of the fact that serum IgD comprises only about 1/500 of all serum immunoglobulin.[65]

In speculating on the origin of its membrane location, Green concluded:

> In view of the low serum concentration of IgD and the relatively large number of cells bearing surface IgD, it is possible that IgD or its Fc fragment is highly cytophilic for a subset of lymphocytes.[65]

One year later, Rowe reported an enhanced level of IgD on lymphocytes in the umbilical cord blood of newborns and in the same year provided evidence that discounted the 'cytophilic IgD' idea which would have required passive acquisition of IgD from serum and further, demonstrated that it is normally associated with membrane-associated IgM on the lymphocyte surface. An important result was that IgD and IgM are not only both present on the same cell but also present a single light chain type. In drawing conclusions from these findings Rowe and colleagues made the following interpretive leap, full of immunological insight:

> The finding that both IgD and IgM are simultaneously present in a high proportion of lymphocytes is remarkable and does not follow the pattern of previous reports concerning other immunoglobulins where restriction to one class is the general rule... It seems more probable that both receptors have the same combining site, consistent with the presence of light chains of one type only... The class of the receptor determines the signal to the cell. For example, tolerance and induction may be dependent on the heavy chain class of the receptor... IgD constitutes the first antigen receptor. The appearance of IgM (potentially a secreted immunoglobulin) as a receptor indicates a step in differentiation towards a plasma cell... In any event, we consider that the simultaneous presence of two receptors on the same cell indicates a remarkable genetic event of fundamental significance for immune responsiveness.[66]

Reprinted with permission from Macmillan Publishers Ltd: *Nature New Biology,* Rowe, D.S., et al. IgD on the surface of peripheral blood lymphocytes of the human newborn, *Nature New Biology,* Volume 242, pp.155–156,Copyright © 1973.

Further evidence that IgD and IgM were on the same cells was produced by Uhr in 1976 by showing that if IgM-bearing cells were ablated by anti-IgM plus complement and the dead cells removed, IgD-bearing cells were lost also.[67] Since both IgM and IgD are also found in the serum as soluble antibodies, the question of their role when membrane bound (since apparently not related to any cytotoxic action) and furthermore, how the membrane form differs from the soluble form was a puzzle that would only slowly be pieced together. The ontogeny of the two membrane forms provided a rich forum for debate during the 1970s. Primitive (pre-B cell) lymphocytes from bone marrow appeared to express mainly membrane-bound IgM while the arrival of IgD expression accompanied lymphocyte maturation. Furthermore, cross-linking of surface IgM on neonatal cells resulted in growth inhibition that was absent when maturation and appearance of IgD occurred. Uhr and colleagues showed that when IgM$^+$/IgD$^+$ B-cells were treated with papain to specifically degrade the IgD molecule, the cells became susceptible to tolerance induction.[68] This led to the suggestion that IgM played a role in tolerance induction in thymus-derived lymphocytes. In the same year as the studies of Uhr were reported, Nossal and colleagues at the Walter and Eliza Hall Institute described a more physiological approach:

> A more direct way of determining the role of IgD is by attempting to induce tolerance in vitro by pretreatment of adult B cells with an anti-d serum before culture with tolerogen... Our results suggest that d$^+$ m$^-$ cells do become susceptible to tolerance induction if the d-receptor is blocked or modulated, and that mice suppressed for the d-allotype remained susceptible to tolerance in vitro into adult life.[69]

Text extract © 1977 Rockefeller University Press. Originally published in *The Journal of Experimental Medicine,* Volume 146. pp.1473–1483.

Similar results were obtained by Vitetta, Uhr, and colleagues using a slightly different protocol but arriving at the same conclusions: δ^+/μ^+ adult B cells are resistant to thymus-dependent tolerance while cells with ablated IgD or immature B cells not yet expressing IgD were easily tolerized.[70] Subsequent to these studies many groups sought to explain this differential influence of IgD and IgM on the lymphocyte membrane. How could two antibodies with the same apparent antigenic specificity give such different cellular responses? The answer would come in two parts. David Scott's group showed that the internal signaling from these two isotypes was different. They further suggested that the immature B-cell phenotype, known to be susceptible to tolerization, could not be changed by simply putting IgD into the cells and that *ipso facto* the immature B cell was phenotypically 'different' to the adult B cell in some functional manner.[71] The second part of the answer came some years later when, in 1990 Michael Reth and his group at the Max-Planck Institut für Immunbiologie in Freiburg carried out some clever molecular biology and protein chemistry in myeloma cells.[72] First they expressed the membrane-bound form of IgM in the cells but it failed to appear at the membrane surface even though it was present within the cells. Then they isolated cell variants that carried two new proteins which when introduced into the myeloma along with the IgM placed the IgM on the cell surface. Here was a eureka moment for the field. IgM could only be expressed on the cell surface if it was associated with these two proteins (as an IgMα–Iγβ heterodimer). Similar results were obtained for IgD although in this case a different alpha protein was seen (IgDα). At last a possible explanation of the differential signaling by IgM and IgD was possible. The fact that the alpha proteins were different and each had a long polypeptide tail in the cytoplasm was a veritable feast for the mechanistic cell biologists over the following decade.

In 2006 Geisberger, Lamers, and Achatz published a review on the IgM/IgD story with the title 'The riddle of the dual expression of IgM and IgD'.[73] In 2011, Chen and Cerutti reviewed the same area stating in their introduction:

> While the function of IgM, IgG, IgA and IgE is relatively well known, the function of IgD has remained obscure since... 1965... IgD is co-expressed with IgM on the surface of the majority of mature B cells prior to antigenic stimulation and functions as a transmembrane antigen receptor.[74]

Since this is a history of antibodies no attempt will be made to say when an understanding of the duality of membrane-bound IgM and IgD will be resolved. To misquote Neils Bohr, 'Prediction is very difficult, especially if it is about immunology'.

Acknowledgements

Text extract reproduced with permission from Van Boxel, J.A. et al., I. IgD-bearing human lymphocytes, *Journal of Immunology*, Volume 109, pp. 648–651, Copyright © 1972 The American Association of Immunologists, Inc.

Text extract reproduced with permission from Rowe, D.S., et al., IgD on the surface of peripheral blood lymphocytes of the human newborn, *Nature New Biology*, Volume 242, pp.155–156, Copyright © 1973 Macmillan Publishers Ltd.

References

1. **WHO** (1964). Memorandum from WHO Meeting on Nomenclature of Human Immunoglobulins, 29/30 May, 1964, Prague. *Bull. Wld Hlth Org.*, **30**: 447–50.

2. **Bence Jones, H.** (1848). 'On a New Substance Occurring in the Urine of a Patient with Mollities Ossium.' *Phil. Transac. Roy. Soc.*, **138**: 55–62.

3. **Putnam, F. W.** (1983). 'From the first to the last of the immunoglobulins: perspectives and prospects.' *Clin. Physiol. Biochem.*, **1**: 63–91.

4. **Kyle, R. A.** (2001). 'Henry Bence Jones—physician, chemist, scientist and biographer: A man for all seasons.' *Brit. J. Haematology*, **115**: 13–18.

5. **Rustizky, J.** (1873). 'Multiple Myeloma.' *Ztschr. Chir.*, **1**: 161.

6. **Waldenström, J.** (1944). 'Incipient myelomatosis or "essential" hyperglobulinemia with fibrinogenopenia — a new syndrome?' *Acta. Med. Scand.*, **117**: 216–47.

7. **Fried, M., and Putnam, F. W.** (1962). 'Peptide Chromatograms of Normal Human and Myeloma γ-Globulins.' *Biochemistry*, **1**: 983–7.

8. **Edelman, G. M., and Gally, J. A.** (1962). 'The nature of Bence Jones proteins: Chemical similarities to polypeptide chains of myeloma globulins and normal γ-globulins.' *J. Exp. Med.*, **116**: 207–27.

9. **Putnam, F. W., Titani, K., and Whitley, E.** (1966). 'Chemical Structure of Light Chains: Amino Acid Sequence of Type K Bence-Jones Proteins.' *Proc. Roy. Soc. Lond. B.*, **166**: 124–37.

10. **Putnam, F. W., Shinoda, T., Titani, K., and Wikler, M.** (1967). 'Immunoglobulin Structure: Variation in Amino Acid Sequence and Length of Human Lambda Light Chains.' *Science*, **157**: 1050–3.

11. **Titani, K., Shinoda, T., and Putnam, F. W.** (1969). 'The amino acid sequence of a kappa type Bence-Jones protein. 3. The complete sequence and the location of the disulfide bridges.' *J. Biol. Chem.*, **244**: 3550–60.

12. **Titani, K., Wikler, M., Shinoda, T., and Putnam, F. W.** (1970). 'The amino acid sequence of a lambda type Bence-Jones protein. 3. The complete amino acid sequence and the location of the disulfide bridges.' *J. Biol. Chem.*, **245**: 2171–6.

13. **Lichter, E. A., and Dray, S.** (1964). 'Immunoelectrophoretic characterization of human serum proteins with primate antisera.' *J. Immunol.*, **92**: 91–9.

14. **Ballieux, R. E., Bernier, G. M., Tominaga, K., and Putnam, F. W.** (1964). 'Gamma globulin antigenic types defined by heavy chain determinants.' *Science*, **145**: 168–70.

15. **Kunkel, H. G., Allen, J. C., Grey, H. M., Mårtensson, L., and Grubb, R.** (1964). 'A relationship between the H chain groups of 7S gamma globulin and the Gm system.' *Nature*, **203**: 413–14.

16. **Fahey, J. L., Wunderlich, J., and Mishell, R.** (1964). 'The immunoglobulins of mice. I. Four major classes of immunoglobulins: 7S gamma-2, 7S gamma-1, gamma-1A (beta-2A) and 18S gamma-1M-globulins.' *J. Exp. Med.*, **120**: 223–42.

17. **Kunkel, H. G., Fahey, J. L., Franklin, E. C., Osserman, E. F., and Terry, W. D.** (1966). 'Notation for human immunogobulin subclasses.' *Bull.Wld. Hth. Org.*, **35**: 953.

18. **Natvig, J. B., and Kunkel, H. G.** (1973). 'Human Immunoglobulins: Classes, Subclasses, Genetic Variants and Idiotypes.' *Adv. Immunol.*, **16**: 1–59.

19. **Krawinkel, U., and Rabbits, T. H.** (1982). 'Comparison of the hinge-coding segments in human immunoglobulin gamma heavy chain genes and the linkage of the gamma 2 and gamma 4 subclass genes.' *EMBO J.*, **1**: 403–7.

20. **Grabar, P., and Williams, C. A.** (1953). 'Method permitting the combined study of the electrophoretic and the immunochemical properties of protein mixtures: application to blood serum.' *Biochim. Biophys. Acta*, **10**: 193–4.

21. **Heremans, J. F., Heremans, M. T., and Schultze, H. E.** (1959). 'Isolation and description of a few properties of the beta 2A-globulin of human serum.' *Clinica Chimica Acta*, **4**: 96–102.

22. **Tomasi, T. B., Jr., Tan, E. M., Soloman, A., and Prendergast, R. A.** (1965). 'Isolation and description of a few properties of the beta 2A-globulin of human serum.' *J. Exp. Med.*, **121**: 101–24.

23. **Vaerman, J-P., and Heremans, J. F.** (1966). 'Subclasses of Human Immunoglobulin A Based on Differences in the Alpha Polypeptide Chains.' *Science*, **153**: 647–9.

24. **Feinstein, D., and Franklin, E. C.** (1966). 'Two antigenically distinguishable subclasses of human A myeloma proteins differing in their heavy chains.' *Nature*, **212**: 1496–8.

25. **Kunkel, H. G., and Prendergast, R. A.** (1966). Subgroups of gamma-A immune globulins.' *Proc. Soc. Exptl. Biol. Med.*, **122**: 910.

26. **Grey, H. M., Abel, C. A., Yount, W. J., and Kunkel, H. G.** (1968). 'A subclass of human gA-globulins (gA2) which lacks the disulphide bonds lining heavy and light chains.' *J. Exp. Med.*, **128**: 1223–6.

27. **Torano, A., and Putnam, F. W.** (1978). 'Complete amino acid sequence of the alpha 2 heavy chain of a human IgA2 immunoglobulin of the A2m (2) allotype.' *Proc. Natl. Acad. Sci.*, **75**: 966–9.

28. **Putnam, F. W., Liu, Y-S., and Low, T. L. K.** (1979). 'Primary structure of a human IgA1 immunoglobulin. IV. Streptococcal IgA1 protease, digestion, Fab and Fc fragments, and the complete amino acid sequence of the alpha 1 heavy chain.' *J. Biol. Chem.*, **254**: 2865–74.

29. **Cebra, J. J., and Small, P. A.** (1967). 'Polypeptide Chain Structure of Rabbit Immunoglobulins. III. Secretory γA-Immunoglobulin from Colostrum.' *Biochemistry*, **6**: 503–12.

30. **Tomasi, T. B., and Bienenstock, J.** (1968). 'Secretory immunoglobulins.' *Adv. Immunol.*, **9**: 1–96.

31. **Halpern, M. S., and Koshland, M. E.** (1970). 'Novel subunit in secretory IgA.' *Nature*, **228**: 1276–8.

32. **Chapuis, R. M., and Koshland, M. E.** (1975). 'Linkage and assembly of polymeric IgA immunoglobulins.' *Biochemistry*, **14**: 1320–6.

33. **Goldblum, R. M.** (1990). 'The role of IgA in local immune protection.' *J. Clin. Immunol.*, **10**: 64S–71S.

34. **Bonner, A., Almogren, A., Furtado, P. B., Kerr, M. A., and Perkins, S. J.** (2009). 'The Nonplanar Secretory IgA2 and Near Planar Secretory IgA1 Solution Structures Rationalize Their Different Mucosal Immune Responses.' *J. Biol. Chem.*, **284**: 5077–87.

35. **Wallenius, G., Trautman, R., Kunkel, H. G., and Franklin, E. C.** (1957). 'Ultracentrifugal studies of major non-lipide electrophoretic components of normal human serum.' *J. Biol. Chem.*, **225**: 253–7.

36. **Chaplin, H., Cohen, S., and Press, E. M.** (1965). 'Preparation and Properties of the Peptide Chains of Normal Human 19s γ-Globulin (IgM).' *Biochem. J.*, **95**: 256–61.

37. **Miller, F., and Metzger, H.** (1965). 'Characterization of a Human Macroglobulin. I. The molecular weight of its subunit.' *J. Biol. Chem.*, **240**: 3325–33.

38. **Mestecky, J., Zikan, J., and Butler, W. M.** (1971). 'Immunoglobulin M and secretory immunoglobulin A: presence of a common polypeptide chain different from light chains.' *Science*, **171**: 1163–5.

39. **Putnam, F. M., Florent, G., Paul, C., Shinoda, T., and Shimizu, A.** (1973). 'Complete Amino Acid Sequence of the Mu Heavy Chain of a Human IgM Immunoglobulin.' *Science*, **182**: 287–91.

40. **Wiersma, E. J., Collins, C., Fazel, S., and Shulman, M. J.** (1998). 'Structural and Functional Analysis of J Chain-Deficient IgM.' *J. Immunol.*, **160**: 5979–89.

41. **Brewer, J. W., and Corley, R. B.** (1997). 'Late events in assembly determine the polymeric structure and biological activity of secretory IgM.' *Mol. Immunol.*, **34**: 323–31.

42. **Johansen, F.-E., Braathen, R., and Brandtzaeg, P.** (2000). 'Role of J chain in secretory immunoglobulin formation.' *Scand. J.Immunol.*, **52**: 240–8.

43. **Rowe, D. S., and Fahey, J. L.** (1965). 'A new class of human immunoglobulins. I. A unique myeloma protein.' *J. Exp. Med.*, **121**: 171–84.

44. **Rowe, D. S., and Fahey, J. L.** (1965). 'A new class of human immunoglobulins. II. Normal serum IgD.' *J. Exp. Med.*, **121**: 185–99.

45. **Rowe, D. S., Hug, K., Forni, L., and Pernis, B.** (1973). 'IgD as a lymphocyte receptor.' *J. Exp. Med.*, **138**: 965–72.

46. **Prausnitz, C., and Küster, H.** (1921). 'Studien über die überempfindlichkeit.' *Zentr. Bakteriol. Paraiteuk.*, Abt. I, **86**: 160–9.

47. **Coca, A. F., and Grove, E. F.** (1925). 'Studies in hypersentitiveness XIII. A study of the atopic reagins.' *J. Immunol.*, **10**: 445–64.

48. **Stanworth, D. R.** (1963). 'Reagins.' *Brit. Med. Bull.*, **19**: 235–40.

49. **Ogilvie, B. M.** (1964). 'Reagin-like antibodies in animals immune to helminth parasites.' *Nature*, **204**: 91–2.

50. **Ishizaka, K., Ishizaka, T., and Hornbrook, M. M.** (1966). 'Human reaginic antibody IV. Presence of a unique immunoglobulin as a carrier of reaginic activity.' *J. Immunol.*, **97**: 75–85.

51. **Ishizaka, K., Ishizaka, T., and Hornbrook, M. M.** (1966). 'Physicochemical properties of reaginic antibody V. Correlation of Reaginic Activity with γE-Globulin Antibody.' *J. Immunol.*, **97**: 840–53.

52. **Johansson, S. G. O., and Bennich, H.** (1993). 'Immunological Studies of an Atypical (Myeloma) Immunoglobulin.' *Immunology*, **13**: 381–94.

53. **Stanworth, D. R.** (1993). 'The discovery of IgE.' *Allergy*, **48**: 67–71.

54. **Stanworth, D. R., Humphrey, J., Bennich, H., and Johansson, S. G. O.** (1967). 'Specific inhibition of the Prausnitz-Küstner reaction by an atypical human myeloma protein.' *The Lancet*, **2**: 330–2.

55. **Stanworth, D. R., Humphrey, J. H., Bennich, H., and Johansson, S. G. O.** (1968). 'Inhibition of Prausnitz-Küstner reaction by proteolytic-cleavage fragments of a human myeloma protein of immunoglobulin class E.' *The Lancet*, **2**: 17–18.

56. **Bennich, H., Ishizaka, K., Johansson, S. G. O., Rowe, D. S., Stanworth, D. R., and Terry, W. D.** (1968). 'Immunoglobulin E: A new class of human immunoglobulin.' *Bull. WHO*, **38**: 151–2.

57. **Oudin, J.** (1956). 'L'allotypie de certains antigènes protéidiques du sérum.' *Compt. Rend. Acad. Sci. France.*, **242**: 2606–8.

58. **Oudin, J.** (1960). 'Allotypy of rabbit serum proteins I. Immunochemical analysis leading to individualization of seven main allotypes.' *J. Exp. Med.*, **112**: 107–24.

59. **Oudin, J.** (1960). 'Allotypy of rabbit serum proteins. II Relationships between various allotypes: their common antigenic specificity, their distribution in a sample population, genetic implications.' *J. Exp. Med.*, **112**: 125–42.

60. **Grubb, R.** (1956). 'Agglutination of erythrocytes coated with "incomplete" anti-RH by certain rheumatoid arthritic sera and some other sera.' *Acta Pathol. Microbiol. Scand.*, **39**: 195–7.

61. **Grubb, R., and Laurell, A. B.** (1956). 'Hereditary serological human serum groups.' *Acta Pathol. Microbiol. Scand.*, **39**: 390–8.

62. **Grubb, R.** (1970). 'The Genetic Markers of Human Immunoglobulins.' In A. Kleinzeller, G. F. Springer, and H. G. Whitman (eds.), *Molecular Biology, Biochemistry and Biophysics*, No. 9, pp. 1–152. New York: Springer-Verlag.

63. **Lefranc, M-P., and Lefranc, G.** (2012). 'Human Gm, Km, and Am Allotypes and their Molecular Characterization: A Remarkable Demonstration of Polymorphism.' In Frank T. Christiansen and Brian D. Tait (eds.), *Immunogenetics: Methods and Applications in Clinical Practice*, pp. 635–80. New York: Springer Science and Business Media.

64. **Allen, J. C., and Kunkel, H. G.** (1963). 'Antibodies to Genetic Types of Gamma Globulin after Multiple Transfusions.' *Science*, **139**: 418–19.

65. **van Boxel, J. A., Paul, W. E., Terry, W. D., and Green, I.** (1972). 'IgD-bearing human lymphocytes.' *J. Immunol.*, **109**: 648–51.

66. **Rowe, D. S., Hug, K., Page Faulk, W., McCormick, J. N., and Gerber, H.** (1973). 'IgD on the surface of peripheral blood lymphocytes of the human newborn.' *Nature New Biol.*, **242**: 155–6.

67. **Vitella, E. S., and Uhr, J. E.** (1976). 'Cell surface immunoglobulin. XV. The presence of IgM and an IgD-like molecule on the same cell in murine lymphoid tissue.' *Eur. J. Immunol.*, **6**: 140–3.

68. **Cambier, J. C., Vitetta, E. S., Kettman, J. R., Wetzel, G., and Uhr, J. W.** (1977). 'B-cell tolerance. III. Effect of papain-mediated cleavage of cell surface IgD on tolerance susceptibility of murine B cells.' *J. Exp. Med.*, **146**: 107–17.

69. **Scott, D. W., Layton, J. E., and Nossal, G. J. V.** (1977). 'Role of IgD in the immune response and tolerance.' *J. Exp. Med.*, **146**: 1473–83.

70. **Vitetta, E. S., Cambier, J. C., Ligler, F. S., Kettman, J. R., Wetzel, G., and Uhr, J. W.** (1977). 'B-cell tolerance: IV. Differential Role of Surface IgM and IgD in Determining Tolerance Susceptibility of Murine B Cells.' *J. Exp. Med.*, **146**: 1804–8.

71. **Alez-Martinez, J. E., Warner, G. L., and Scott, D. W.** (1988). 'Immunoglobulins D and M mediate signals that are qualitatively different in B cells with an immature phenotype.' *Proc. Natl. Acad. Sci.*, **85**: 6019–923.

72. **Hombach, J., Tsubata, T., Leclercq, L., Stappert, H., and Reth, M.** (1990). 'Molecular components of the B-cell antigen receptor complex of the IgM class.' *Nature*, **343**: 760–2.

73. **Geisberger, R., Lamers, M., and Achatz, G.** (2006). 'The riddle of the dual expression of IgM and IgD.' *Immunology*, **118**: 429–37.

74. **Chen, K., and Cerutti, A.** (2011). 'The Function and Regulation of Immunoglobulin.' *D. Curr. Opin. Immunol.*, **23**: 345–52.

Chapter 9

Effector functions of constant regions

Cellular and molecular interactions of the antibody constant region

In Chapter 8 we have explored a little of the structural complexity and organizational variation in the different immunoglobulin isotypes and how these properties were unravelled by careful application of serology, protein chemistry, and later molecular biology. Discovering and understanding the *functional* consequences of antigen binding, revealed eventually through isotype constant region structural variations that allow engagement to a variety of molecular or cellular partners, were no less daunting. The discovery of the key roles to be played by the antibody Fc region opened a 'Pandora's box' of effector biology that required careful study and today even greater diligence in exploiting such biology for therapeutic good.

Antibody constant regions and the complement system

The first indication that whole blood possessed the ability to kill bacteria came from the work of George Henry Falkiner Nuttall, an anglo-american by birth but working in Carl Flügge's laboratory in Göttingen in the late 1880s. Nuttall already knew from the work of Fodor and Wyssokowitsch that bacteria injected into an animal disappeared from the animal, but by an unknown mechanism. At the same time he was fascinated by the developing European debate between the humoral and cellular immunologists—Metchnikoff had recently published his provocative paper on the apparent protective role of blood corpuscles when challenged with fungi (see Chapter 2). Using defibrinated rabbit blood, Nuttall showed that exposure of the anthrax bacilli to the treated blood resulted in a bactericidal response.[1] The effectiveness of the response was lost by heating the blood to 55°C, or over time in stored blood samples. Nuttall's observations of 1888 were confirmed by others, who further showed that the strength of the bactericidal effect varied with the bacteria employed. The following year, von Buchner, working in Munich, questioned Nuttall's experimental procedure in which cells were not removed from the plasma, thereby in his opinion rendering the experiments indecisive. Using primitive centrifugation Buchner removed the cells and demonstrated that the effect could be obtained with cell-free serum, raising doubts about a cellular mechanism.[2] Furthermore, as Nuttal had described, the serum effect was abolished by heat treatment (55°C for one hour).

Buchner named the substance 'alexine' (from the Greek 'to ward off' or 'protect'). As Metchnikoff himself observed:

> Buchner determined the conditions under which alexine acts best as a bacterial poison and developed the humoral theory of natural immunity according to which the latter is reduced to the bactericidal property of the body fluids.[3]

Between 1894 and 1901 Jules Bordet was at work in Metchnikoff's laboratory in Paris. He was aware of the work of Nuttall and Buchner, but another set of rather unexplained results appeared in 1894 from the work of Richard Pfeiffer, working at Koch's Institute for Infectious Diseases in Berlin. Pfeiffer had immunized guinea pigs against cholera vibrios (bacteria) and then challenged the guinea pig by injection of live vibrios into the peritoneal cavity. The vibrios lost their normal motility, assuming a spherical granular form and soon died, but only in the immunized guinea pigs *unless* the non-immunized animals simultaneously received anti-cholera antiserum along with the live vibrios. Pfeiffer presumed that the source of the bactericidal effect was the peritoneal endothelium.[4] This observation, known as the 'Pfeiffer phenomenon' was followed up by Metchnikoff, who demonstrated that the same effect could be seen *in vitro* if live vibrios were exposed to serum from an immunized guinea pig mixed with a leucocyte-containing peritoneal exudate from a non-immunized animal. Metchnikoff, quite reasonably continuing to plough the phagocytosis furrow he had so elegantly started, attributed the bacterial changes to:

> ... *une substance bactéricide, échappée des leucocytes morts ou avariés.*[5]
>
> [... a bactericidal substance, released either from dead or damaged leucocytes.]

Metchnikoff did express doubt that the Pfeiffer phenomenon fell into his phagocytosis theory, although he was convinced that the bactericide substance originated from cells. In a piece of scientific arm-wrestling he asked his associate Gengou to compare the bactericidal effectiveness of exudations rich in either macrophages or microphages (polymorphonuclear leucocytes (PMNs)) with that of serum. The PMNs, perhaps not surprisingly, won the day:

> The result of these experiments leaves no room for doubt. The microphages, collected in the aseptic exudations of the dog and rabbit, contain more bactericidal substance than does the blood serum of these animals. Nor can there be a doubt that this bactericidal substance is the same whether it appears in the microphages or in the blood serum: in both cases it is destroyed by heating to 55°C...[6]

As a result of this suggestion he kept open the possibility that the vibrio-killing substance was cellular in origin, although later admitted that the secretion was only likely to originate from damaged cells.

From the same laboratory, in the same year, in a paper following immediately that of Metchnikoff in the Annals of the Pasteur Institute, Jules Bordet published a large series of experiments that suggested a radically different explanation of the Pfeiffer phenomenon. Bordet described experiments in which he was able to transform the virulent cholera vibrions to their 'killed' (spherical granule) form with guinea pig antiserum plus the defibrinated serum from non-immune guinea pigs, provided the non-immune serum was freshly prepared. So, whatever factor was in the peritoneum was also in the serum. Furthermore, sera from multiple species were able to exert the same effect, with guinea pig and human sera the most effective. Of greater importance was Bordet's logical conclusion of the experimental results from heat treatment. While temperatures of 55°C or higher inactivated the cholera killing effect, it did not affect the agglutinating effect of the immune sera. In concluding his report Bordet declared:

> Le choléra-sérum, on le sait, n'est pas antitoxique; les animaux vaccinés n'ont eux-mêmes, d'ailleurs, aucune immunité réelle contre la toxine que fabrique le vibrion. Le sérum ne produit donc que l'immunité vis-à-vis du microbe lui-même. Il contient, lorsqu'il est frais, deux substances, une substance bactéricide, une substance préventive... on doit admettre qu'à côté de la stimulation cellulaire, un **phénomène purement chimique**, que l'on peut reproduire in vitro, joue un grand rôle dans la production de l'immunité passive.[7]

> [It is a known fact that immune sera raised against the cholera vibrio are not antitoxic. Moreover, animals vaccinated with *Vibrio cholerae* do not develop antitoxin immunity either. Thus the serum induces immunity only against the microbe itself. When fresh, such sera contain two substances: a bactericidal substance, and a preventive substance... one should therefore admit that besides the cellular stimulation, a purely chemical phenomenon that can be reproduced *in vitro*, plays a critical role in the production of passive immunity.]

What then was the connection between antibodies and the agglutinating or hemolysing 'alexine'? With the hemolysis effect, studied in one key experiment by immunizing guinea pigs with rabbit red cells and then challenging the rabbit red cells with the guinea pig antiserum, Bordet observed that the rabbit cells were both agglutinated and then lysed within a few minutes of exposure to the serum. The alexine effect was abolished by heating at 55°C but restored by addition of a fresh source of alexine. His conclusion was that the heat resistant antibody sensitized the red cells in such a way that the heat-sensitive alexine could then exert its effect directly on the cells.[8] As we have seen in Chapter 2, Bordet was convinced that direct interaction of antibody and alexine was not required to give rise to the bactericidal or hemolysis effects. This was in stark contrast to Ehrlich and his colleague Morgenroth who firmly believed that the amboreceptor (immune body plus complement receptor) and complement must interact directly to produce hemolysis and that there were a number of different alexines, or 'complements' as they renamed them. Metchnikoff attempted to reconcile the different views of Bordet and Ehrlich by supposing that there may be a single alexine but that different hemolyzing factors which he named cytases (he supposed they were enzymatic by analogy with the enzymatic 'ferments from the digestive system') might have different specificities for animal cells (macrocytase) and bacteria (microcytase).[9]

While Bordet and Ehrlich may have differed in interpretation of their respective extensive experimental data, with Metchnikoff taking a more expansive view of immune mechanisms, here were the fragments of an early model for antibody-mediated complement fixation: antibodies, complement (now the adopted term rather than alexine) receptors either on the antibody or the cell and the possibility of enzymatic activity. But it was not that straightforward and no real understanding would emerge until the different elements of the complement system had been uncovered. It would be further complicated by the discovery of a complement-like substance that was heat stable!

The first clue that complement contained multiple fractions came from the work of Ferrata[88] in 1907, followed by that of Sachs and Altmann[89] (1909), and Liefmann[90] (1909). Ferrata showed that if fresh guinea-pig serum was dialysed against running water two complement fractions were identifiable, one associated with the precipitated globulin (antibody) fraction and a second in the soluble fraction. Neither was active alone but when recombined complement-lysing activity was restored. Sachs generated similar results using gentle acid precipitation while Liefmann obtained the same fractionation by saturating the serum solution with carbon dioxide (this would have generated the weak acid, carbonic acid). The early nomenclature of complement fractions was a little clumsy, the globulin associated and precipitated fraction being called 'middle piece' and the soluble or albumin fraction 'end piece'. The chemical identity of neither fraction was understood. Even as late as 1920 it was proposed by Brooks that complement was lecithin-derived[10] and that serum proteins may only play an indirect role, despite results from various laboratories that complement activity could be destroyed by exposure to proteolytic enzymes.[11] By the mid-1920s it became clear that not all complement components were heat sensitive. Wormall and colleagues at the universities of Leeds and Newcastle (UK) described a new, 'third component' that was heat stable but inactivated by exposure to yeast or zymin (dehydrated yeast). As Wormall states:

> No definite chemical or physical relationship appears to exist between this third component and the mid-piece and end-piece.[12]

To add to the complexity, Wormall added yet another piece to the puzzle, with a description of a fourth component.[13] The new factor was identified by its sensitivity to treatment of serum by ammonia. It was however heat stable and seemed to fractionate along with the soluble ('end piece' or albumin) serum fraction. It was different to the third component since it was not sensitive to exposure to yeast or zymin.

Here then was a complement substance having four identifiable components with different heat stabilities and some evidence for enzymatic activity at least with some of the components. Given the combinatorial complexity that would arise, the Ehrlich and Morgenroth view of the hemolysis world where a different complement would exist for every antigen was fast becoming unsustainable. The more likely explanation was that a single set of 'substances' worked together to provide a common hemolysis package in an antibody-mediated process. However, it should not be taken to mean that in 1926 the compositional chemistry of complement was understood. There were still segments of the scientific community who believed in a non-protein model, exemplified by the work of Liebermann[14] who postulated a lipidic mechanism operating via calcium oleic acid salts (in fact, soaps). Even as late as 1929 Eagle and Brewer, working at the Johns Hopkins Medical School, declared in their introduction:

> Despite an enormous literature which has accumulated since the discovery of the bactericidal, bacteriolytic and hemolytic properties of fresh serum, the terms alexin and complement still denote unexplained properties of serum rather than a chemical entity.[15]

Text extract ©1929 Rockefeller University Press. Originally published in *The Journal of General Physiology*, Volume 12, pp. 845–862.

Following on from this introductory pessimism, Eagle and Brewer described a series of elegant and quantitative experiments that established a direct relationship between the level of hemolysis induced by complement and the amount of antibody bound to the cells. With regard to the functional role of antibodies vis-à-vis complement they concluded:

> If this mobilization of complement is the sole function of immune serum (and there is as yet no reason to assume any other), then the accepted terminology, in which amboceptor, immune body, and hemolysin are used synonymously, is erroneous. The immune body would function only as an 'amboceptor', mobilizing the effective hemolysin, complement, upon the surface of the cell.[15]

> Text extract ©1929 Rockefeller University Press. Originally published in *The Journal of General Physiology*, Volume 12, pp. 845–862.

This was a pro-Ehrlich statement in part since the antibody (amboceptor) was asserted as the anchoring component for the complement 'mid-piece' on the cell surface. However, there was still as yet no progress on the interrelationship between the different complement components and which of them interacted directly with antibody-antigen complex on the cell surface to initiate the hemolysis process. As with many subjects but particularly immunology, nomenclature tended to escalate into an unnecessary complexity that either obscured the reality or suggested erroneous conclusions. In 1941, Pillemer and Ecker, working at the Western Reserve University and University Hospitals in Cleveland, proposed the following simplification of the complement nomenclature[16] after discussion and agreement with Michael Heidelberger:

$C'1$ = mid-piece
$C'2$ = end-piece
$C'3$ = third component
$C'4$ = fourth component

This naming system has survived until today although the numbering bears no direct relationship to the actual order of activation in the classical complement pathway.

In making his proposal Pillemer showed electrophoretic analyses of whole serum, mid- and end-piece preparations and complement deprived of either its third or its fourth component, arising from a more extensive investigation of complement protein fractionation using ammonium sulphate precipitation.[17] This drew attention to the fact that each of the named components may not be a single species—the end- and middle-piece components, for example, appeared to have at least four distinct proteins each.

A year later Pillemer published a comprehensive study of complement and its components in two related papers.[18,19] Some rather important conclusions were made that reinforced the Ehrlich view of mechanism but somewhat radicalized Bordet's contention that complement did not interact directly with antibody. Pillemer's conclusions in his second paper were:

> Anti-sheep cell rabbit serum by itself does not combine with complement or any of its components, or at least does not inactivate them. Nevertheless, when the specific antibody enters into the primary combination with the red cell, the surface pattern of the antiserum molecule or the antiserum-cell aggregate changes and in turn different groups are in contact with the complement complex. This alteration in the surface pattern increases the affinity for $C'4$, $C'2$, and $C'1$. The adsorption of these complement components on the red

cell-antibody complex then renders the red cell amenable to the action of the unadsorbed C'3 and hemolysis results. Since C'3 is not fixed by the sensitized cell and is apparently not used up in the process of hemolysis, it appears to have certain enzymic qualities.[19]

Text extract © 1942 Rockefeller University Press. Originally published in *The Journal of Experimental Medicine*, Volume 74, pp. 421–435.

Pillemer further concluded that C'4 was unable to bind in the absence of C'1 and that:

the data … warrant classification of C'3 as a catalyst … [19]

As we shall see later, some of Pillemer's conclusions for the few complement species known were more or less correct and given the primitive purification methods available in 1942, rather clever. However, insight is not always enough and progress sometimes requires hard, sometimes repetitive research using less eye-catching methods. For example, measuring the weight of antibody-antigen immune complex precipitates after fixation of complement (measured by nitrogen content) was routinely used by those groups attempting to establish which C' components were directly associated with the immune complex and which were not. Progress was slow, so much so that in 1950, Michael Heidelberger attempted to bring all the complement groups together in a National Academy of Sciences sponsored conference at the Ram's Head Inn, Shelter Island, New York to discuss how to take the field forward. In a summary of the conference published the following year and emphasizing the importance of the subject, Heidelberger drew attention to the fact that clinical diagnostic tests, such as the Bordet-Wassermann test for syphilis which relied on determination of complement activity, were in 'enormous use'. The Bordet-Wassermann test relied on depletion of rabbit complement when added to patient serum that had been pre-treated at 55°C. If syphilis was present the patient's serum would contain circulating cardiolipids and anti-cardiolipin antibodies that would 'fix' the rabbit complement. Subsequent addition of anti-red cell antibodies and red cells would then measure any remaining complement activity, the diagnostic indicators being: no observed hemolysis = +ve for syphilis; observed hemolysis = -ve for syphilis. This test unfortunately gave many false positives (of concern among pre-marital couples in the United States where a medical certificate was required prior to marriage, a practice still maintained by a small number of states although now using a more reliable method) and results varied from laboratory to laboratory, probably because of release of cardiolipids into the circulation from infections other than *Treponema pallidum*.

A measure of the still fledgling state of the field can be seen in Heidelberger's own conference summary on the 'Definition of complement':

Particularly for the benefit of those present who had not actually worked with C' an attempt was made to define C' but agreement could not be reached. This was mainly because independent, functionally different methods of measurement lead to conflicting results.[20]

The situation had not improved markedly eight years after Heidelberger's conference with its 'Who's Who' of complement science. As Rowley and Wardlaw conclude from their laboratory in St. Mary's Hospital Medical School in London:

If, in conclusion, one compares the present state of knowledge of serum bactericidal action with that existing around 1900, it is apparent that we yet know little more about the actual mechanism of the reaction.[21]

As with antibodies, the complement proteins were in a complex matrix (serum) and unless the individual components were isolated and characterized, rather than hitherto where complement was studied by investigating whole serum from which various complement factors had been depleted, mechanism would still evade definition.

By 1961, a new name had appeared in the field. Hans Joachim Müller-Eberhard was clinically trained in Göttingen, spent two post-doctoral years at the Rockefeller Institute in New York working with Henry Kunkel, moved to Uppsala for two years finally settling back at the Rockefeller for the remainder of his career. Müller-Eberhard published a series of breakthrough studies in 1960 and 1961 describing work carried out partly in Uppsala and completed at the Rockefeller. He was the first to break the existing complement sequence rule by suggesting that a newly identified component with a size of γ-globulin (11S by ultracentrifugation) formed direct interactions with antibody.[22] At the time it was known that C'1 required divalent ions (e.g. Ca^{2+} or Mg^{2+}) to express its activity but the 11S protein did not. His conclusion was that this protein, which was heat labile, was distinct from any of the known classical components of complement and 'is involved in the initial stage of complement action'.[23]

Two years later Irwin Lepow at Western Reserve University Medical School in Cleveland, carrying forward the pioneering complement work of Louis Pillemer (whose untimely death, aged 49 years, was a considerable blow to the field; although his work was initially challenged it was subsequently proved correct), showed that C'1 was actually three proteins, the first of which was analogous to the 11S protein of Müller-Eberhard (see Fig. 9.1). He named the three components C1q, C1r, and C1s.[24]

This was a significant breakthrough. It suggested that before any hemolytic activity could be initiated, a membrane complex mediated by antibody should be formed. This initial event would involve a sub-component of C'1 (C1q) binding to antibody followed by activation of certain enzymes. Müller-Eberhard (see Fig. 9.2) and Kunkel had already suggested that the 11S protein binding to antibody may be the first event to occur in complement activation.[22] Whether C1q was able to bind free antibody or only after it had formed a membrane-bound antigen complex was not yet addressed. This was an important question if complement activation leading to cell lysis was not to be a profligate biological weapons system.

By 1971–2 an understanding of C1q and its associated activities began to emerge. Müller-Eberhard showed that C1q bound most strongly to aggregated antibody[25] and in a more comprehensive analysis of C1q by protein chemistry proposed that it bore some resemblance in part to collagen since it contained unusually high levels of glycine, hydroxylysine, and hydroxyproline, certain signals of fibrous protein character. It also contained a significant amount of carbohydrate and appeared to have a structure in which six non-covalently linked subunits assembled to form the native molecule.[26] Svehag and colleagues, encouraged by Müller-Eberhard, subjected the preparation to electron microscopy (EM) and deduced that C1q had either a disc or a rod form.[27] In parallel the group of Robert Stroud at the University of Alabama, using similar

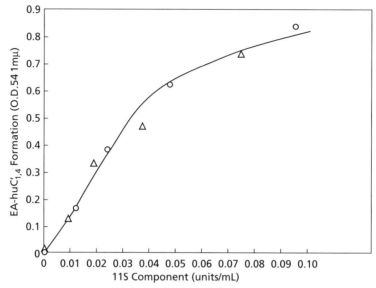

Fig. 9.1 Lepow shows here the titration of a purified 11S protein preparation, after Müller-Eberhard's procedure, against a preparation of sheep red blood cells sensitized with antibody and containing complement lacking the C'1 component. When C1q was present (circles) the binding complex (EAhuC'$_{1,4}$) was formed from the non-binding complex EAhuC'$_4$. The same result was obtained when EAhuC'4 was supplemented by C1r, C1s, and the 11S protein in place of C1q (triangles).

Figure reproduced with permission © 1963 Rockefeller University Press. Originally published in Lepow, I.H. et al., Chromatographic resolution of the first component of human complement into three activities, *The Journal of Experimental Medicine*, Volume 117, pp. 983–1008.

techniques, extracted a slightly different set of ultrastructural features of C1q that have better stood the test of time.[28] Stroud's analysis differed from that of Svehag in two respects. Firstly, he proposed a quaternary structure in which C1q can be separated into three distinct covalently-bonded subunits or into two non-covalent subunits of unequal molecular weight that are in the ratio of 3:1 (60kDa:42kDa). This was consistent with the second proposal on the structure of the molecule, proposed as a set of globular 'heads' linked by fine strands to a central rod-like core, rather like a 'bunch of tulips' (see Fig. 9.3).

At about the same time Ken Reid and Rodney Porter, in a comparison of rabbit and human complement and differing from Stroud on the detailed chain and subunit composition, proposed a chain structure of C1q consisting of six copies each of three different types of chain (A, B, and C), the N-terminal region of each chain containing a significant collagen-like composition. Digestion of the C1q molecule with collagenase caused a rapid loss of hemolytic activity while the undigested 'heads' were still able to bind to antibody.[29] It was later shown by Reid and Porter that the antibody-binding activity of C1q is lost when C1q is exposed to pepsin, suggesting a more conventional globular protein structure for the heads.[30] The structural features proposed by Stroud

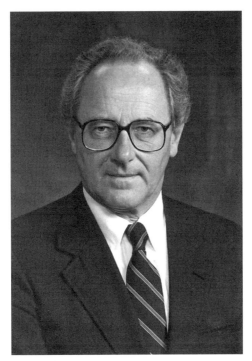

Fig. 9.2 Hans Müller-Eberhard.

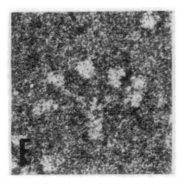

Fig. 9.3 The structural features of the C1q molecule, showing a 'bunch of tulips'-like morphology, as revealed by electron microscopy.

were later confirmed and extended by Knobel who, using a mixture of protein chemistry and electron microscopy, established that:

> … all C1q preparations had six peripheral subunits connected by fibrillar strands to a central subunit.[31]

By 1980, Porter had gathered together the extensive studies from a number of groups into a model explaining the assembly and activation of complement. He delivered his analysis in the Royal Society Croonian Lecture, May 1980.[32] After several decades of intensive investigation the role of the antibody in the activation of the classical complement pathway was now becoming clear. Porter's illustration of the antibody C1q interaction as the first step in complement activation (see Fig. 9.4) provided the molecular answer to Bordet and Ehrlich's early observation that formation of a cell surface immune complex was a necessary step for subsequent lytic activity.

Porter's model was much more than a pictorial condensation of already-published observations, many by his own research group. It was a predictive model that explained the required presence of multiple Fc regions of bound antibodies in order to elicit C1q-mediated activation of C1s and C1r, which in the absence of antibody possessed only a weak association affinity for C1q. This suggested the exposure of the tetrameric $C1s_2$-Ca-$C1r_2$ binding sites on C1q that were only revealed after multiple interactions of the C1q heads with antigen-bound antibody. However, while it was attractive by virtue of its simplicity, it was not the whole story. Müller-Eberhard had shown that a small molecule hapten (dinitrophenyl-) linked to either end of an oligo-lysine chain

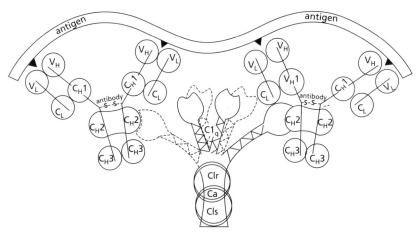

Fig. 9.4 Suggested assembly of early component of complement onto antibody molecules bound to cell surface antigens. The heads of the C1q molecules bind to the CH_2 domain of several antibody molecules and a tetramer of $C1r_2$-Ca-$C1s_2$ binds to the collagen stems of C1q (Ca = calcium).

(10-mer) was able to fix complement when an antibody bound monovalently to each of the haptens, probably initiated by binding of C1q to either the Fc region, the polylysine chain, or both.[33] This was clearly not an aggregation of antibodies on a cell surface but would have been a soluble circulating di-antibody complex. Of more concern was his observation that a single hapten on the oligo-lysine triggered a similar activation, although others had shown that single hapten-antibody complexes were unable to fix complement. The question of how activation of the downstream enzymatic components of complement by C1q binding is controlled to mitigate collateral damage to normal tissues was also still an open question.

While allosteric theories were popular for a time, requiring IgG to change conformation in its Fc region after binding antigen thus exposing a C1q binding site, they were unproven and eventually fell out of favour. The answer appeared to be in the relative affinity of the $C1s_2$-Ca-$C1r_2$ complex for C1q in the immune complex state versus the non-aggregated IgG state with or without antigen bound. Hughes-Jones and colleagues showed that the association constant of $C1s_2$-Ca-$C1r_2$ for C1q increases tenfold when C1q is part of an immune complex.[34] This was consistent with the results of Ziccardi, working at the Scripps Research Institute, who in the closing paragraph of his paper stated:

> In conclusion, under physiologic conditions, C1q and C1r2s2 are two weakly interacting proteins. Immune complexes provide a site for the assembly of a stable C1 complex, in which C1q and C1r2s2 remain associated long enough for C1q to activate C1r2s2.[35]

Here then was a model for biological control. C1q could bind to a single IgG, but only when multi-IgG complexes or IgM complexes (exploiting the intrinsic pentavalency of IgM) were formed at the cell surface would a biologically effective level of complement activation occur. But was it safe enough to prevent even low-level activation of a massively dangerous 'membrane attack complex', as the late stage cell-punishing enzyme systems would become known. The considerable research activity on complement control mechanisms during the 1980s and 1990s led to the discovery of specific fluid-phase and membrane-associated inhibitors that could intervene at various stages of the classical complement cascade (for example the C1 inhibitor, C1-INH, that causes inactivation of the C1s and C1r components at the level of the antibody immune complex). A detailed explanation of the development of this work, as well as the non-antibody mediated, or 'alternative complement' pathways and the clinical relevance of pathologically important complement abnormalities, is beyond the scope of this book and the reader is directed to excellent reviews and references[36,37] or standard textbooks.[38]

Antibody isotypes and complement

While γ-globulin was known to be distinguishable on size, sequence of the constant region, serum concentration, and diversity of antigen specificity, it was also known to be a multi-isotype class and as we have seen earlier, diversified even further via allotypic differences. In humans four isotypes were known, IgG1, 2, 3, and 4. The first attempt to measure the binding strength of these four different IgG isotypes for C1q was carried out by Müller-Eberhard in 1976, working with human myeloma proteins and using the analytical ultracentrifuge to quantitate complex formation with C1q. This study established C1q binding affinity differences in the order IgG3>IgG1>IgG2>IgG4 with no binding seen for IgA due, it was presumed, to its reduced 'segmental flexibility'. While interesting as a stand-alone study, Müller-Eberhard's study addressed only the question of the possible stoichiometry of C1q-IgGx interactions derived from the ultracentrifuge analysis, leading him to suggest that as many as 18 IgG1 molecules might be bound by a single C1q molecule. This seemed excessive and in any case what was lacking was the correlation of isotypic variation in C1q binding with cell lysis. This was not fully explored until the elegant work of Michael Neuberger, Hermann Waldmann, and colleagues in Cambridge (UK). In their 1987 paper they describe the construction of a series of chimeric antibodies in which the variable region of a mouse anti-hapten (4-hydroxy-3-nitro-phenacetyl or NP or its iodinated version, NIP) antibody was joined to each of the human IgG isotypes, IgM, IgE, and IgA2 constant regions and then expressed in a lambda chain-secreting plasmacytoma cell line. The resulting full-length antibodies were shown to display quite marked differences in their C1q binding and complement-mediated cell lysis behaviour.[39] The binding efficacy appeared to confirm in part Müller-Eberhard's observations some nine years earlier: IgG3 (two different allotypes)>IgG1>IgM with no observed binding for IgE, IgG2, or IgG4. When the lytic efficiency however was measured on NIP-coated red blood cells, the results reversed the order of C1q binding with IgG1≥IgM >IgG3 (with rather different behaviour of the two allotypes) and no or almost no lysis by IgG2, IgG4, or IgE. The prediction of these authors, that IgG1 may be the most interesting isotype to consider for therapeutic intervention, was yet to be put to the test!

One year later Hermann Waldmann and his group pushed this study one step further by providing an explanation for the 'C1q binding-cell lysis' reversal paradox.[40] By measuring the next step in the complement cascade, the activation of C4 by C1s after C1q binding to the cell surface immune complex, Waldmann was able to resolve the paradox. The IgG1-C1q complex appeared to be much more efficient than the IgG3-C1q complex at activation of the $C1r_2$-$C1s_2$ protease tetramer, binding of C4 (ten times greater with IgG1), and attachment of one of the C4 cleavage product (C4b) to the cell surface as a receptor for the next protein in the complement cascade. The explanation for the greater IgG3 binding to C1q is still not fully understood but is possibly due to the much longer hinge region of IgG3 allowing perhaps better accessibility of C1q binding sites. Whatever the structural basis for this difference, the usefulness of the IgG1 isotype in later clinical applications of antibody technology would become quite important.

The wider functions of antibody constant regions

We have explored a little in earlier chapters how differentiation of the antibody regions into distinct functional domains was revealed through protein chemistry and later molecular biology. The Fab region contained the elements for antigen recognition and some ideas on the mechanisms used by the immune system to build a vast specificity repertoire were revealed through the cloning of antibody variable region genes. Not all aspects of 'real-time' variability generation were known when Tonegawa and his contemporaries unveiled the structure and organization of immunoglobulin genes but we shall explore this later. The constant regions were known to do 'something else'. Some of those something else functions were worked out in some detail for the IgG-complement defense system, as we have seen. The special functions of IgM and IgD would also need explanations, in particular their membrane association and how this was coupled to their immunological functions. The allergic responses of IgE, while well known for most of the last century, begged a detailed description of how an antigen binding to IgE could trigger a cascade of inflammatory reactions.

For the complement system, the prevailing view before 1960 was that somehow IgG and various components of the complement family assembled on the target cell. The question of how the initial binding of the antibody-antigen triggering complex to the cell surface occurred was unknown. It would be the cellular immunologists who would start to unveil the molecular origins of the cell-antibody interactions, returning full circle to the concepts of Metchnikoff but providing answers that would turn his microscopic observations into detailed molecular mechanisms.

Specificity in antibody-cell interactions

It was well known that cells of various types were able to adsorb antigens, including whole bacteria. For immunological responses this was considered to be the *sine qua non* for antigen-mediated antibody production and the presence of antigens on spleen cells after immunization was believed to be one means of identifying antibody-producing cells. While not entirely incorrect, these observations lacked the molecular detail that would be necessary to explain the many other antibody-mediated cellular responses.

In 1942, Coons established a fluorescent antibody-staining method that allowed visualization of antibody, antigen, and cell ensembles. In describing this technique he observed:

> It is obvious that a technic for the demonstration of antigens in situ in the animal body is highly desirable for the investigation of many conditions which have been attributed to tissue-damage resulting from the localized union of antigen and antibody.[41]

Coons' subsequent studies, interrupted by the war, were extensive but somewhat monothematic in that they focused on establishing the association of many different sorts of antigens with cells. The preoccupation with how antibodies were produced by antigen-cell interactions was the obvious driver. This was still the period in which antigen drove antibody production by either templating or the more favoured new instructional theory of Pauling (see Chapter 4). By the 1950s, Coons and others were still concerned with cellular association of antigens. Of course, antigen interaction with tissues was understood to be part of the underlying cause of the observed pathology and associated tissue damage. Direct antigen interaction with cells in antibody-producing tissues was demonstrated in rabbits by Coons in 1955 using a 'sandwich' method in which dilute antigen would be added to cells (frozen tissue sections), allowing interaction with any antibody in the tissue and formation of insoluble immune complexes, followed by development with a fluorescent antibody that would detect the immobilized antigen. In describing this phenomenon after introduction of antigen *in vivo* followed by various tissue examinations, Coons' interpretation was as follows:

> A study of the hyperimmune rabbit on the first few days after the last of a series of intravenous antigen injections reveals that antibody against human γ-globulin or ovalbumin is present in groups of plasma cells in the red pulp of the spleen...[42]

So, Coons observed that a spleen-cell extract containing putative antibody-producing (plasma) cells, when exposed to antigen and then followed up with a second antibody, a 'precipitation' on the cell surface occurred giving rise to the punctate fluorescence. This was an important first step and the fluorescence-marker technique a significant addition to the armamentarium of the cell biologist. Visualization with an antibody conjugate could now move away from the visible dye chemistry used for more than 50 years which suffered from the difficulty of distinguishing experimental from background signal.

But the second step would take another half decade, with the observations of Boyden and Sorkin in 1960 who were working at the Statens Seruminstitut, Copenhagen.[43] First they exposed rabbit spleen cells (and other cells; see Table 9.1) to rabbit anti-human serum albumin (HSA) or normal rabbit serum, washed and added HSA that had been radio-iodinated. To their surprise they observed a behaviour that required explanation since it flew in the face of the current dogma—antigen was more effectively bound to cells that had previously been exposed to an antibody that bound that antigen.

Boyden and Sorkin's observations led to the following suggestion:

> The factor in the antiserum responsible for the adsorption of antigen appears to be firmly bound to the cells. For convenience, this substance will be referred to hereafter as 'cytophilic antibody'.[43]

This phenomenon was not peculiar to soluble antigens. Boyden, now back in Australia, repeated his earlier work using sheep red blood cells as antigens in the guinea pig and showed a similar 'cytophilic antibody' effect but this time clarified his earlier confusion about the cell type involved, confirming that it was indeed the macrophage that

Table 9.1 Exposure of rabbit spleen cells to antibody followed by antigen showing greater adsorption of antigen to cells if the cells had previously been exposed to the cognate antibody.

Type of cell	Treated with normal serum and washed four times	Treated with anti-serum and washed four times
Rabbit spleen cells	2	556
Methanol-treated RSC	5	267
Guinea-pig spleen cells	3	648
Rabbit red cells	17	18

Source: data from Boyden, S.V. and Sorkin, E., The Adsorption of Antigen by Spleen Cells previously treated with Antiserum in vitro, *Immunology*, Volume 3, Issue 3, pp. 272–283, Copyright © 1960.

displayed the antibody-antigen mediated opsonization.[44] Further work by Uhr in 1965 took the story one step further.[45] Uhr repeated Boyden's work with macrophages. Using bacterial antigens he demonstrated that after sensitization the macrophages were triggered to phagocytose the bacteria. However, in order to achieve passive sensitization of lymphocytes derived from lymph nodes by antigen-antibody complexes it appeared to require the presence of one or more components of complement. Where heat treatment of the guinea-pig serum before sensitization was performed or ions known to be critical for complement activity (Ca^{2+} and Mg^{2+}) were sequestered with EDTA, the sensitization of lymphocytes was abolished but with no effect on macrophage behaviour. As Uhr speculated, somehow the complement protein(s) were involved in stabilization of the antigen-antibody complex on the lymphocyte surface perhaps involving direct interaction of antibody and complement proteins (treatment of the IgG with either pepsin or a disulphide bond-reducing agent abolished the effect). The following year in a presentation to the NY Academy of Sciences on transplantation biology, Uhr proposed two hypotheses, the first of which he clearly preferred:

> After interaction with antigen, the change in the configuration of the antibody molecule results in exposure of a binding site for phagocytes on the Fc fragment of antibody. The binding site interacts with a complementary receptor on the surface of the phagocyte as a preliminary step for phagocytosis.[46]

In the same year Berken and Benacerraf recapitulated and extended Boyden's observation using the guinea-pig model in the first real breakthrough study that brought together cell biology and protein chemistry in some rigorous and wide-ranging experimentation. They were not in total agreement with Uhr's conclusions. Cytophilic antibodies were simply antibodies in the IgG population that had encountered antigen and then been bound by macrophages after which phagocytosis occurred. Free antibodies had a much lower affinity for the macrophage receptor as shown by the high concentrations required to displace antigen-antibody complexes from macrophage surfaces at temperatures low enough to inhibit phagocytosis. Critically, Berken and Benacerraf showed that in this model complement was not required for the binding and phagocytosis functions although they were polite enough to suggest that there may be instances where complement is required. Here then were preliminary indications that IgG had a cognate partner on the surfaces of cells of the immune system but that interaction with that 'receptor' gave rise to different biological responses in different cells. In summarizing, Benacerraf proposed a molecular explanation for the earlier observations of Boyden, adducing the first real evidence for the role of the Fc region in binding reversibly to macrophage cell surface membranes:

> γ_2-Globulins bind to macrophages because of the presence of a receptor for the macrophage cell membrane on their Fc fragment... The binding reaction is reversible with a high rate of dissociation at 37°C.[47]

While the macrophage interaction he had observed was also shown by Uhr to be present in polymorphonuclear leucocytes, lymphocytes from the blood, and plasma cells from lymph nodes, he cautioned drawing the conclusion that antigen-driven association of antibodies with target cells did not mean the cells themselves produced the antibody. In tying down more clearly the exact cells in lymph-node tissues that were responsible for this passive sensitization effect, Nussenzweig took the cell biology further. In the 1970 study, he and his colleagues mapped the cell types involved in sensitized red cell adherence. Some of his conclusions were:

> … follicular localization of sensitized sheep erythrocytes on tissue sections is mediated by complement … tissue adherence of EAC is restricted to the 'thymus-independent' regions … predominant cells in the areas that bind EAC are lymphocytes … antibody-mediated follicular localization of antigen in vivo … attributed to trapping by dendritic reticular cells …[48] (EAC = sensitized erythrocytes)

So, Nussenzweig observed that the guinea-pig thymocytes were unable to engage in the complement-associated immune complex binding but that both lymphocytes and dendritic cells were. In commenting on the follicular association he suggested this may be a mechanism for antigen localization by specialized lymphocytes. In the same year, Brown et al demonstrated that soluble aggregates of IgG (normal IgG treated at 63°C for 15 minutes and centrifuged) also distributed to the germinal centres and remained associated with dendritic and other cell types for many days. This behaviour was identical to that shown by injection of immune complexes. Brown speculated that a role for the germinal centres might be to remove altered antibody from the circulation. Seven months later the same group showed that lymphocytes are able to take up this aggregated IgG without the intervention of any complement component, acknowledging that the mouse system may behave differently to guinea pigs in which Uhr had established the complement requirement, and further that the role of the IgG-receptor-bearing lymphocytes may be to concentrate antigen in the germinal centres where it would impact regulation of an immune response, a possible function of the process that had also been suggested by Nussenzweig. The origin of the lymphocytes involved was inferred from blockade of the germinal transfer by anti-lymphocytic serum suggesting to Brown that they are part of the circulating pool of lymphocytes requiring an 'intact thymus'.[49]

The phenomena observed by Boyden, Uhr, Benaceraff, Brown, Nussenzweig, and others were exciting for cellular immunologists but at the same time frustratingly short of mechanistic insight and in some areas, contradictory. It would require someone to design the right experiments and at the same time suspend the belief that the observed interactions were solely to do with regulation of antibody responses to antigen. In 1972 Paraskevas and colleagues did just that, using a clever technique that enabled them to measure the presence of IgG on the surfaces of mouse and human lymphocytes while eliminating direct Fc interactions with the cell. Two different antibodies were generated in rabbits with specificity for either mouse IgG or ferritin. They were treated with pepsin to produce $F(ab')_2$ fragments, mixed in the presence of reducing agents to produce free Fab' fragments and then reoxidized to generate hybrid $F(ab')_2$ reagents containing both anti-IgG and anti-ferritin binding activities. Using this reagent Paraskevas screened cells from lymph nodes, spleen, bone marrow, peripheral blood, thymus, and lymphomas. First, the cells were exposed to the hybrid anti-$F(ab')_2$, washed and then challenged with ferritin-coated red cells. Any rosettes formed should then be due to pre-existing antibody on the cell surface. Paraskevas found all tissues examined *except* thymus and lymphoma cells carried IgG on the cell surfaces and suggested that 'this technique detects a γ-globulin which forms an integral part of the cell surface and may represent the antigen receptor γ-globulin'.[50] The following year Paraskevas extended his work using the hybrid antibody approach, demonstrating that mouse-spleen lymphocytes have IgG on their surface, that both mouse and rabbit antibody-antigen complexes are able to bind, that purified rabbit Fc fragments are able to interfere with the hybrid F(ab')$_2$ binding in a dose-dependent manner while Fab fragments have no effect, and that Fc from immune rabbit antibodies was more potent than Fc from normal rabbit IgG. This last observation was a rather odd result and perhaps reflected the prevailing 'allosteric Fc' activation model bias, although as Paraskevas notes 'More work is needed to substantiate further this result'. What was also observed was that a fraction of spleen cells bearing no antibody on their surface were able to bind antigen-antibody complexes giving a positive result in the hybrid test. This suggested that some spleen cells do not carry pre-existing antibody and that the cells must *ipso facto* bear a receptor that recognizes the Fc region. This conclusion was complicated a little by the results of Alan Williams in Oxford who, working with a rat system, showed that non-thymus derived lymphocytes had expressed antibody (IgG) on their surface from internal synthesis while thymus-derived cells only adsorbed immunoglobulin from the serum and further that this immunoglobulin was IgM.[51] Williams equated these two cell types as B cells and T cells respectively. The results Paraskevas obtained led him to propose that spleen lymphocytes and the other positive cells observed must carry a receptor specific for the Fc region. He provisionally called this the 'Fc receptor' (FcR).[52] Thereafter the name would remain although the Fc receptor would turn out to be much more complicated than these early experiments suggested. Of particular note in Paraskevas' work was the smart assembly method for generating hybrid antibodies carrying two different specificities, a theme that would return in later decades as an important therapeutic tool for the clinical immunologist.

In his review in 1981 Jay Unkeless, working at the Rockefeller, described some aspects of the Fc receptor 'complication'.[53] The difficulty in defining the Fc receptor landscape was for two reasons. Firstly, the molecular analysis tools available to the immunologists in the 1960s and early 1970s were not discriminating enough to allow absolute differentiation between different types of receptor should they exist on different cell types or more importantly, coexist on the same cell type. For example, the possibility of two different Fc receptors residing on macrophages relied on their relative proteolytic sensitivity after treatment of cells with trypsin, an approach fraught with interpretive difficulties given the fact that the membrane surface was replete with many different kinds of protein, some of which might have been essential protein partners for Fc receptor function. Other methods used the quantitative difference in Fc receptor binding shown by different IgG subclasses although this was complicated to explain without any knowledge of the FcR binding sites on the different IgG isotypes. By 1981 Unkeless had exploited the new technique of monoclonal antibodies (see Chapter 12) and obtained an antibody specific for the trypsin-resistant receptor in mouse macrophages. Armed with this high resolution analytical tool he mapped the receptor distribution in a large number of cell types, analysed its subclass preferences, and used it to affinity purify an Fc receptor candidate from a murine macrophage cell line. Unkeless's receptor had multiple polypeptides, was glycosylated, and because it required detergents for solubilization was considered to be an integral (trans-) membrane protein. In his review Unkeless places the challenge of identifying *bona fide* Fc receptors firmly in the court of the immunologists who to date had perhaps jumped to quick and often erroneous conclusions.

In contrast to murine and guinea-pig studies, human studies were less advanced. Huber and Fudenberg[54] had shown binding of IgG to blood monocytes while binding to neutrophils was shown by Messner and Jelinek.[55] In both these studies different binding behaviour was seen with different isotypes, IgG1 and IgG3 being the most strongly bound, matching the equivalent subclass behaviour seen in mice (IgG1 and IgG2a). However, immune complexes formed with bacterial antigens allowed differentiation of binding sites on monocytes and neutrophils, again suggesting multiple receptor types. In studies of a human lymphoma cell line with monocyte and macrophage properties, Anderson and Abraham quantified the subclass binding question using reciprocal inhibition methods and showed that the Fc receptor on this cell line was trypsin resistant and appeared to represent the only receptor present, with IgG1 and IgG3 having similar affinities while IgG4 and particularly IgG2 had lower affinities.[56] This was consistent with the results of McNabb who observed the same subclass behaviour on cells from the human placenta.[57] Having seen the work of Crabtree[58] on a human promyelocytic cell line just before the 1980 publication went to press, Anderson and Abraham repeated some of his experiments and confirmed that on their human macrophage cell line there were in fact two types of receptor, one having high affinity for monomeric IgG (IgG1, IgG3> IgG4 >> IgG2) and low avidity for complexes or aggregated IgG and a second receptor with the reverse selectivity.

The research on Fc receptors up to the early 1980s was hampered by the fact that they were widely distributed on many cell types, were clearly functionally and probably structurally heterogeneous, and their detailed characterization would have benefited from tools that were not yet available to the immunologist. Where sometimes conflictual, sometimes overlapping results poured into the world's scientific journals, simplistic models were proposed that contained kernels of truth but would require continuous modification because of the vast amount of data being generated. Resolution of the complexity, at least in structural terms, arrived with the application of DNA cloning techniques that would allow analysis of the Fc receptor phenotype of the many cell lineages implicated in Fc-mediated functions.

The molecular biologists entered the fray in the mid-1980s. The first cloning results were published in 1986 by the joint groups of Jeffrey Ravetch (see Fig. 9.5) at the Sloan Kettering Cancer Centre, New York and Jay Unkeless at Rockefeller University, New York.

Using the monoclonal antibody Unkeless had developed to purify Fc receptor protein from a mouse macrophage cell line, Ravetch applied the following cloning protocols:

- Obtain a sequence of the amino terminal region of the receptor (actually 22 amino acids);

- Synthesize an oligonucleotide corresponding to seven of the 22 amino acids having the least DNA degeneracy;

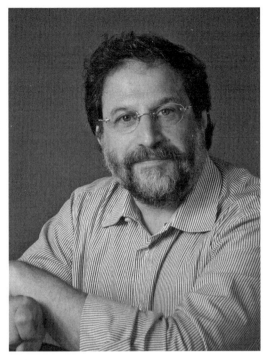

Fig. 9.5 Jeffrey Ravetch.
Reproduced courtesy of Jeffrey Ravetch.

- Use the oligonucleotide to screen a cDNA library of 50 000 'clones' from a mouse macrophage cell line;
- Sequence the positive hits found and attempt to explain the receptor organization from the sequence;
- Put the gene(s) back into receptor negative cells and measure the functional integrity of the putative receptor.

In this study Ravetch and Unkeless found two Fcγ receptor genes that were differentially expressed.[59] The first which they called Fcγα was expressed in macrophage cell lines as well as normal peritoneal macrophages. The second gene, Fcγβ, was expressed in macrophages, as well as bone marrow- (B) and thymus- (T) derived lymphocytes. Furthermore, both genes contained transmembrane regions but different intracellular portions suggesting that they may communicate different signals to the interior of the cell in response to antibody binding. The extracellular organization of both receptors consisted of two separate homologous domains that presumably were important for the IgG binding interaction. The crucial evidential step the group took was to put these genes back into cells lacking FcR and measure whether the recipient cells bound immune complexes. The cells they used were melanoma cells that after 'transfection' were able to rosette red blood cells just like the lymphocyte and macrophage. Here then was the real lift-off for the FcR field.

Notwithstanding this advance, the receptor genes that Ravetch and Unkeless identified corresponded to the 'low affinity' IgG binding class. The gene or genes for the receptor species that could bind IgG with high affinity on macrophages was still elusive. In 1989, Allen and Seed, working at the Massachusetts General Hospital in Boston, uncovered the missing DNA, this time for a human FcR.[60] The genes identified were similarly tested for function by introduction into receptor negative cells. The receptor sequence in this instance revealed an organization that was somewhat different to that seen by Ravetch and Unkeless for the low-affinity receptors, in that an additional extracellular domain was seen that was dissimilar to either of the low-affinity receptor domains.

By 1994, Ravetch was in a position to review the known functions of Fc receptors, stating in his introductory paragraph and referring to the studies of his own and other research groups:

> These studies demonstrated that FcRs have a central role in initiating immunocomplex-triggered inflammation and are likely to be major contributors to the process of lymphocyte regulation of antibody production.[61]

The immunocomplex inflammatory response referred to had just been redefined by Ravetch in a study of the Arthus reaction which until 1994 had presumed that antibody-antigen complex activation of complement via the classical pathway was responsible for this type of inflammatory response, described by Arthus in 1903. Maurice Arthus had injected rabbits intradermally with horse serum a number of times and observed that after the fourth and subsequent injections a severe inflammatory response began to build characterized by oedema, leucocyte infiltration, and after the seventh injection hemorrhage and tissue necrosis.[62] Arthus adopted the name 'anaphyllaxie' for this phenomenon from Richet and Portier who had observed a similar clinical reaction to jelly-fish toxins in dogs (Richet was awarded the Nobel Prize in 1913 for his work on anaphylaxis). In the introduction to their study Diana Sylvestre and Jeff Ravetch drew attention to the fact that hitherto the role of Fc receptors in mediating the immune complex inflammatory responses had not been considered. Using an animal model in which the key accessory γ-subunit necessary for expression of the Fc receptor at the membrane surface was genetically deleted (−/− for the γ subunit) Ravetch observed during a modified Arthus procedure, in which the antigen was injected intravenously and the antibody intradermally, a significant reduction in inflammatory responses at the intradermal site. In contrast, the expected inflammatory responses were seen in +/+ and the heterozygous +/− animals. Since deletion of the Fc receptor γ-subunit deletion also results in loss of cell surface expression of the IgE receptor which could have been responsible for the anaphylactic reactions, Ravetch carried out experiments in mice that lacked the α-subunit of the IgE receptor preventing its surface expression but which retained the normal Fcγ receptors, FcγRI and FcγRIII. In a repeat of the antigen followed by antibody challenge procedure a vigorous Arthus reaction was observed discounting any involvement of the IgE receptor.[63] Since the likely mechanism was induction of effector cell receptor cross-linking by the immune complexes formed, this suggested to Ravetch a possible therapeutic approach in which extensive tissue injury due to Fc receptor-mediated inflammatory response might be reduced by inhibition of the receptor cross-linking.

From now on researchers, using the techniques of monoclonal antibodies, DNA cloning, and cellular functional assays, would be able to unravel the structure and function of Fc receptors in all their guises and locations. The inflammatory responses Ravetch referred to were well known but were now known not to be restricted to the behaviour of the IgE isotype. Both IgG and IgE constant region interactions with specialized cells containing inflammatory mediators were possible.

The special functional behaviour of IgE

As we have seen in Chapter 8, the specific role of IgE in inflammatory responses resulting from allergen insult and subsequent triggering of mast cell and basophil histamine release were beginning to be understood by the end of the 1960s. In a key study in 1970, Ishizaka showed that IgE binds selectively to basophils and not neutrophils or monocytes which experienced only IgG binding. He further demonstrated that the IgE-basophil interaction in the presence of an allergen leads to basophil histamine release (basophils had already been shown to contain as much as 85% of the total histamine in blood). Of significance in these results was not just the isotype-target cell clarification but also that not all subjects became passively sensitized even when proven to display IgE-basophil interactions in the presence of allergen, something incidentally that had been seen[64] long before 1970.

The requirement for aggregation of receptors was teased out by Metzger and Ishizaka using slightly different approaches. Ishizaka as early as 1969 had shown in collaboration with Johansson and Bennich that anti-IgE sera, prepared by immunizing rabbits with antibodies of various isotypes, caused release of histamine from leucocytes of atopic individuals and further that the sensitivity of the leucocytes paralleled the sensitivity of the donor's skin in erythema-wheal reactions.[65] Eight years later Metzger employed chemical cross-linking of IgE molecules to form multimers and assayed the ability of monomers, dimers, and trimers to trigger histamine release (degranulation) in mast cells.[66] Ishizaka, in a development of his earlier studies, raised rabbit antibodies to cell surface proteins from a basophilic leukemia cell line and fractionated those antibodies that were specific for mast cells and whose binding to the cells was inhibited by IgE. Using purified rabbit antibody he prepared Fab' and $F(ab')_2$ fragments by pepsin digestion and assayed their ability to trigger histamine release in the mast cell assay.[67] Both groups saw the same result. Metzger's monomeric IgE against bound IgE was inactive while dimers and trimers were highly active; Ishizaka's $F(ab')_2$ against (putatively) the IgE receptor was active while Fab' was not. It was clear. Histamine release appeared to be related solely to the aggregation of IgE receptors in the membrane of target cells, dispelling other current ideas that IgG may also be involved as a 'reagin' through its Fc receptor.

As with the Fcγ receptor, DNA cloning methods would eventually shed light on the IgE receptor structural organization. During 1986 to 1988 a number of research groups, including Metzger's team, Phil Leder, and others, were cloning the DNA from rodents corresponding to two of the three elements (the alpha and beta proteins) of the receptor.[68,69,70] In 1989 Metzger produced the third element, a γ-chain, that unlocked the assembly requirements for a complete receptor model.[71] What hit the bull's eye was Metzger's reproduction of the exact IgE effects on introducing the cloned α, β, and γ genes into recipient cells lacking an IgE receptor, much as Ravetch and Unkeless had done for the Fcγ receptor. Metzger's model of the receptor would now become the paradigm for exploring the therapeutic potential of human receptor blockade in situations where activation of this receptor leads to life-threatening allergic responses.

An evolutionary relationship unfolds

With the analysis of different types of membrane receptors for antibodies and the availability of tools enabling relationships among amino acid sequences to be identified, a picture began to emerge that would explain at least in qualitative terms how antibody constant domains from different isotypes might form binding partnerships with so many different membrane bound receptors. Alan Williams (sadly taken from this world so prematurely) and his colleague Neil Barclay, working in Oxford, opened the door to a new immunological world, the 'immunoglobulin superfamily'. By cloning, sequencing of certain lymphocyte receptors, and analyzing the data of other groups Williams and Barclay began in 1988 to assemble a genealogical family relationship among proteins with key immunological functions.[72] The immunological 'domains', defined on structural principles fell into three classes, V-set, C1-set, and C2-set (there was also a truncated C2-set). The V-set were defined by their similarity to antibody variable domains, the C1-set were found in constant regions of immunoglobulins and other immune cell proteins, while the C2-set were on cells from non-lymphoid lineages. These similarities were based both on common amino acid sequence motifs and topological features since by this time a number of immune molecule structures were known, including antibodies (see Chapter 11). By 1994 the consensus was that the FcR extracellular domains were of the C2 type although the methods used at this time for establishing membership of one or another topological family were crude at best.[73] Further analysis by Raghavan and Bjorkman showed that in fact the FcR extracellular domains of the IgA (polyIg), IgG, and IgG receptors were of the V-type.[74] These types of analysis also suggested an explanation for the observed binding affinity differences between those FcR containing two versus three extracellular domains. By the time of Bjorkman's review in 1996, a clearer picture was emerging of the molecular organization of FcRs. The domain organization illustrated by Bjorkman is shown in Fig. 9.6.

Here then was the consensus view of Fc receptor molecules. Some appeared to be composed of single polypeptide chain types (e.g. pIgR, FcγRII) while others required multiple polypeptide chains for their activity. The intracellular chain segments were likely to be involved in signal transduction within the cell on antibody or immune complex binding, a detailed understanding of which is still being studied and which in any case is beyond the scope of this book.

The role of the antibody constant regions and the precise locations of receptor binding sites required even more sophisticated methods to establish. Today, this knowledge has allowed engineering of antibody constant regions to modify, remove, or

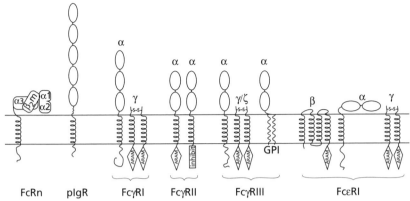

Fig. 9.6 Schematic representation of the Fc receptor family. Key: FcRn binds monomeric IgG and is the transport receptor (see Chapter 10). pIgR is the poly-immunoglobulin A receptor (see Chapter 8). FcγR1, II, and III are the Fc receptors found on macrophages, monocytes, lymphocytes, and other cells of the immune system. FcγR1 binds monomeric IgG with high affinity while FcγRII and FcγRIII bind immune complexes with lower affinity. FcεRI is the high affinity IgE receptor.

Reproduced with permission from Raghavan, M. and Bjorkman, P.J., Fc Receptors and their interactions with immunoglobulins, *Annual Review of Cell and Developmental Biology*, Volume 12, pp.181–120, Copyright ©1996 Annual Reviews Inc. Originally adapted from *Cell*, Volume 78, Issue 4, Ravetch, J.V., Fc Receptors: Robor Redux, pp. 553–560, Copyright © 1994 Elsevier, with permission from Elsevier, http://www.sciencedirect.com/science/journal/00928674

otherwise regulate interactions with the cognate Fc receptors, with significant clinical impact. An early indication that the two IgG constant domains (CH2 and CH3) were not functionally identical came from the work of Ratcliffe and Stanworth in 1983, repeating, extending, and removing some of the uncertainty from previous studies by other groups. In a study of human IgG1 binding these authors measured the relative importance of these two domains for binding to Fc receptors on heterologous (mouse) macrophages and homologous peripheral blood monocytes. Using a radiolabelled IgG1 inhibition protocol and various proteolytically-modified Fc regions, Stanworth showed that for macrophage FcR binding, the IgG CH3 domain was important while for monocyte binding the CH2 domains only were implicated.[75] Further details of the exact location on the CH2 domain important for the high-affinity receptor FcγRI were provided by the groups at the University of Sheffield (Burton and Partridge) and Greg Winter at the MRC Cambridge in 1988 exploiting the newly developed method of 'site-directed mutagenesis' in which individual amino acids could be altered at the DNA level, allowing the generation of specifically mutated proteins. Winter and colleagues showed that a single amino acid change in the CH2 domain of the murine IgG2b which normally does not bind the FcγRI receptor, endowed it with the same high affinity for the human receptor as murine IgG2a, the mouse equivalent of human IgG1. The location of this site was within the CH2 domain and close to the Fab-Fc hinge region.[76] In a follow-on study in 1991, the same groups, working this time with the University of Tokyo, further clarified the location of the binding site and showed that the binding site for the second of the three classes of Fcγ receptors, FcγRII, bound in a region on the CH2 domain overlapping with that of the FcγRI binding site.[77] It would be another nine years before it would be shown, this time by x-ray crystallography, that the third member of the FcgR family would also bind to the CH2 regions, this time not just binding but actually deforming the twin CH2 domains in the Fc region in forming the complex.[78]

For all three Fcγ receptors on cells of the immune system the CH2 domain of the Fc region supplies the binding site on IgG molecules. The role of the CH3 domain in these interactions is obscure but likely provides the structural anchor that allows the large conformational changes in the CH2 domain that accompany binding to its cellular partners without complete destabilization of the antibody. The picture with IgE recapitulates the structural hypothesis that if a domain is to be conformationally disturbed, it must also have a conformationally stable anchoring domain. With the IgE-FcεRI interaction this is precisely what was seen in the x-ray complex published in 2000 by Robert Huber and colleagues at the Max-Planck institute in Martinsried, Germany. Confirming some and contradicting other data previously published on the site of the FcεRI interaction with IgE, Huber and colleagues showed a clear interaction site at the N-terminal region of the CH3 domain with non-participation of the CH4 domain. This CH3 region was notionally equivalent to the CH2 binding region in the IgG-FcγR interactions. The controversy over the earlier binding-site studies of many laboratories had already been carefully explored in the rigorously executed site-directed mutagenesis studies of Gould, Sutton, and colleagues in 1997, whose binding model was beautifully confirmed by the Huber structure.

Some regulatory aspects of Fc receptors

During the late 1990s and into this century the story of the Fc receptor and its antibody interactions continued to unfold, generating questions as well as answers. As late as the mid-1990s the role of the low affinity type II Fc receptor, FcγRII was still not fully understood. The sister type I and type III receptors, FcγRI and FcγRIII, were known to be largely confined to cells of the myeloid lineage (granulocytes, monocytes, megakaryocytes, dendritic cells, and others) and were involved in effector functions such as phagocytosis, ADCC, and inflammatory mediator release. By contrast, FcγRII receptors are found both on myeloid and lymphoid lineages. After the earlier observations by Phillips and Parker in 1984 that Fc-bearing antibodies blocked antibody-producing cells from entering the plasma cell stage while F(ab')₂ fragments were stimulatory,[79] the concept of regulation of antibody production by a particular Fc receptor type was born. Subsequent research showed that this receptor was FcγRII. However, the complexity of interpretation of multiple inhibitory and stimulatory pathways operating with multiple Fc receptor species made absolute confirmation of this important role for the type II receptor problematic. In 1996, Ravetch, working together with the group of Toshiyuki Takai in Okayama University, probed the mechanism further using a mouse knock-out generated by Takai in which the FcγRII gene was disrupted yielding –/– mice after heterozygous inter-crossing. The results were clear-cut. As Ravetch and Takai concluded after showing that the –/– were deficient in their control of antibody production:

Our results indicate that FcγRII functions as an inhibitory receptor for both B cells and mast cells in vivo. Inactivation of this receptor results in a defect in the ability to regulate antibody levels… Defects in FcγRII function may therefore contribute to the development of autoimmunity.[80]

Four years later, Bolland and Ravetch would produce evidence that the FcγRII receptor was indeed a susceptibility factor for the development of autoimmune disease.[81]

The importance of protein–protein interactions in immunological systems has been recognized for more than 80 years. Proteins are composed of amino acids but if they operate as extracellular proteins they are often glycosylated. Antibodies are no exception. But is the carbohydrate in the Fc region just there to provide water solubility and Fc-stabilizing assistance or might it have a more important role? In 2001 and again in 2003 Astrid Samuelsson and Jeffrey Ravetch took the first steps towards understanding how FcγRII induction might regulate an IgG-induced inflammatory response. The question they addressed was why high dose immunoglobulin therapy (intravenous IgG or IVIG), used to treat a number of autoimmune conditions, does not induce inflammatory responses in patients receiving the therapy. Samuelsson and Ravetch identified a subset of macrophages that seemed to respond to Fc activation resulting in up-regulation of FcγRII and thereby increasing the threshold for inflammatory-linked FcγRIII responses.[82,83] However the model, while attractive, still lacked the sort of specific molecular control elements that typify immune response control systems. After all, Fc regions can interact with all Fc receptors and with high dose IVIG most of the Fc receptors might be equally occupied. In 2006 Kaneko and Ravetch established an absolute requirement for a particular modification to the normal Fc-linked carbohydrate, known as sialylation (the addition of sialic acid sugar molecules to the existing Fc carbohydrate) for the inhibitory effects of IgG.[84] The story was beginning to make sense. A specific macrophage subset somehow interacted with Fc regions in IgG molecules that had been differently sialylated compared with the normal IgG population. The final pieces of this particular puzzle were placed in 2008 when the Ravetch group first established the requirement for a particular modification of the Fc carbohydrate to elicit the inhibitory effect. This activity required that Fc regions contained sialic-acid sugar molecules attached in a specific chemical linkage orientation. This was determined using a recombinant antibody preparation in which specific enzymes were used to control the various linkages possible during sialic acid additions to the Fc carbohydrate. In the event, the linkage known as α2,6-sialic acid was found to be the active form. Within the IgG prepared from donors in the IVIG therapy only a small proportion (1–3%) of the IgG molecules have this particular sialic acid linkage. Here was an explanation for the IVIG effects.[85]

But what did these modified Fc regions interact with on the macrophage?

In the same year, the joint groups of Ravetch at the Rockefeller and Mikael Karlsson at the Karolinska Institute in Stockholm further rocked the inflammation boat by identifying an atypical Fc receptor on macrophages that interacts with the sialic acid modified Fc regions. These modified IgG molecules are able to bind to specific lectin (sugar-binding) receptors (known as SIGN-R1) on macrophages located in the splenic margin. Ravetch and Karlsson showed that interaction of the sialyated IgG with SIGN-R1 was responsible for suppressing the IgG induced inflammatory responses that would normally be expected to occur.[86] The excitement of these findings is perhaps modulated only by the conclusion that Fc-mediated immunological responses may be so complex that only a 'systems biology' approach to the study of humoral immunology may yield a fully comprehensible set of answers. After all, when an antigen arrives, somehow the switch from inhibition to activation needs to occur.

Despite these complexities, at the time of writing our understanding of antibody-mediated cellular activation is extensive thanks to the interplay of cell and molecular biology and its physics soulmate x-ray crystallography. Today immunologists can explain those bacterial 'killing' observations from the end of the nineteenth century and a great deal of the downstream biology to boot that accompanies foreign antigen or microorganism invasion. Were they alive today the early cell biologists and mechanistic chemists—Metchnikoff, Bordet, Ehrlich, and especially George Henry Falkiner Nuttal among them, would have gasped at the complexity. That is the beauty of science—like the universe it seems to be unbounded.

A note on nomenclature

In November 1982 the WHO convened a meeting in Paris at which data from 55 research groups in 14 countries relating to leucocyte antigens defined and differentiated by different antibodies were presented.[87] As a result a proposal was made to designate particular cell surface proteins with a CD number (CD for *clusters of differentiation*). During the fifth International Congress of Immunology at Kyoto in 1983 a nomenclature subcommittee considered and adopted suggestions arising from the Paris meeting and defined the first eleven clusters. Following this nomenclature system the leucocyte Fc receptors were given the following CD designations:

> $Fc\gamma RI$ or CD64
> $Fc\gamma RII$ or CD32
> $Fc\gamma RIII$ or CD16
> $Fc\varepsilon RII$ or CD23
> $Fc\alpha RI$ or CD89

Acknowledgements

Text extract reproduced from Metchnikoff, E. *Immunity in Infective Diseases*, translated from the French by Francis G Binnie, Cambridge University Press, Cambridge, UK, Copyright © 1907, by permission of Cambridge University Press.

References

1. **Nuttall, G. H. F.** (1888). 'Experimente über die bacterienfeindlichen einflüsse des thierischen körpers.' *Z. Hyg. Infec. Ionskir.*, **4**: 353–94.
2. **Buchner, H.** (1899). 'Über die nähere Natur der bakterientötenden Substanz im Blutserum.' *Zbl. Bakt.*, **6**: 561–5.

3. **Metchnikoff, E.** (1905). *Immunity in Infective Diseases*, F. G. Binnie (transl.). Cambridge: Cambridge University Press, p. 184.

4. **Pfeiffer, R., and Issaeff, V. I.** (1894). 'Über die Specificität der Choleraimmunisirung.' *Deutsch. Med. Wschr.*, **20**: 305–6.

5. **Metchnikoff, E.** (1895). 'Etudes sur l'immunité.' *Ann. Institut Pasteur*, **9**(6): 433–58.

6. **Metchnikoff, E.** (1905). *Immunity in Infective Diseases*,F. G. Binnie (transl.). Cambridge: Cambridge University Press, p. 186.

7. **Bordet, J.** (1895). 'Les leucocytes et les propriétés actives du serum chez les vaccinés.' *Ann. Institut Pasteur*, **9**(6): 462–506. Extract translated by Michel Kaczorek (2013), Montpellier.

8. **Bordet, J.** (1898). 'Sur l'agglutination et la dissolution des globules rouges par le serum d'animaux injectés de sang.' *Ann. Institut Pasteur*, **12**: 688–95.

9. **Metchnikoff, E.** (1905). *Immunity in Infective Diseases*, F. G. Binnie (transl.). Cambridge: Cambrige University Press, p. 196.

10. **Brooks, S. C.** (1920). 'The mechanism of complement action.' *J. Gen Physiol.*, **3**(2): 185–201.

11. **Wormall, A., Whitehead, H. R., and Gordon, J.** (1925). 'The Action of Pancreatic Extracts on Complement.' *J. Immunol.*, **10**: 587.

12. **Whitehead, H. R., Gordon, J., and Wormall, A.** (1925). 'The "Third Component" or Heat-Stable Factor of Complement.' *Biochem. J.*, **19**: 618–25.

13. **Gordon, J., Whitehead, H. R., and Wormall, A.** (1926). 'The Action of Ammonia on Complement. The Fourth Component.' *Biochem. J.*, **20**: 1028–35.

14. **Liebermann, L.** (1921). 'Über künstliches Komplement.' *Deutsch. Med. Woch.*, **43**: 1283.

15. **Eagle, H., and Brewer, G.** (1929). 'Mechanism of hemolysis by complement I. Complement fixation as an essential preliminary to hemolysis.' *J. Gen. Physiol.*, **12**: 845–62.

16. **Pillemer, L., and Ecker, E. E.** (1941). 'The terminology of the components of complement.' *Science*, **94**: 437.

17. **Pillemer, L., Ecker, E. E., Oncley, J. L., and Cohn, E. J.** (1941). 'The preparation and physicochemical characterization of the serum protein components of complement.' *J. Exp. Med.*, **74**: 297–308.

18. **Pillemer, L., Seifter, S., Chu, F., and Ecker, E. E.** (1942). 'Function of components of complement in immune hemolysis.' *J. Exp. Med.*, **76**: 93–101.

19. **Pillemer, L., Seifter, S., Chu, F., and Ecker, E. E.** (1942). 'The role of the components of complement in specific immune fixation.' *J. Exp. Med.*, **74**: 421–35.

20. **Heidelberger, M.** (1951). 'National Academy of Sciences Conference on Complement.' *Proc. Natl. Acad. Sci.*, **37**: 185–9.

21. **Rowley, D., and Wardlaw, A. C.** (1958). 'Lysis of gram-negative bacteria by serum.' *J. Gen. Microbiol.*, **18**: 529–83.

22. **Müller-Eberhard, H. J., and Kunkel, H. G.** (1961). 'Tsolation of a Thermolabile Serum Protein which Precipitates γ-Globulin Aggregates and Participates in Immune Hemolysis.' *Proc. Exptl. Biol. Med.*, **106**: 291–5.

23. **Müller-Eberhard, H. J.** (1961). 'Dynamic and Biochemical Properties of Plasma Proteins: Two proteins of human serum related to the complement system.' *Ann. NY. Acad. Sci.*, **94**: 4–13.

24. **Lepow, I. H., Naff, G. B., Todd, E. W. Pensky, J., and Hinz, C. F.** (1963). 'Chromatographic resolution of the first component of human complement into three activities.' *J. Exp. Med.*, **117**: 983–1008.

25. **Augener, W., Grey, H. M., Cooper, N. R., and Müller-Eberhard, H. J.** (1971). 'The reaction of monomeric and aggregated immunoglobulins with C1.' *Immunochemistry*, **8**: 1011–20.

26. **Calcott, M. A., and Müller-Ebergard, H. J.** (1972). 'C1q protein of human complement.' *Biochemistry*, **11**: 3443–50.

27. **Svehag, S. E., and Bloth, B.** (1970). 'The ultrastructure of human C1q.' *Acta. Path. Microbiol. Scand.*, **78**: 260.

28. **Shelton, E., Yonemasu, K., and Stroud, R. M.** (1972). 'Ultrastructure of the Human Complement Component, Clq.' *Proc. Natl. Acad. Sci.*, **69**: 65–8.

29. **Reid, K. B. M., Lowe, D. M., and Porter, R. R.** (1972). 'Isolation and Characterization of Clq, a Subcomponent of the First Component of Complement, from Human and Rabbit Sera.' *Biochem. J.*, **130**: 749–63.

30. **Reid, K. B. M., Sim, R. B., and Faeirs, A. P.** (1977). 'Inhibition of the reconstitution of the haemolytic activity of the first component of human complement by a pepsin-derived fragment of subcomponent C1q.' *Biochem. J.*, **161**: 239–45.

31. **Knobel, H. R., Villiger W., and Isliker H.** (1975). 'Chemical analysis and electron microscopy studies of human C1q prepared by different methods.' *Eur. J. Immunol.*, **5**: 78–82.

32. **Porter, R. R.** (1980). 'The complex proteases of the complement system.' Croonian Lecture. *Proc. Roy. Soc. B.*, **210**: 477–98.

33. **Goers, J. W., Schumaker, V. N., Glovsky, M. M., Rebek, J., and Müller-Eberhard, H. J.** (1975). 'Complement Activation by a Univalent Hapten-Antibody Complex.' *J. Biol. Chem.*, **250**: 4918–25.

34. **Hughes-Jones, N. C., and Gorick, B. D.** (1982). 'The binding and activation of the Clr-Cls subunit of the first component of human complement.' *Mol. Immunol.*, **19**: 1105.

35. **Ziccardi, R. J.** (1984). 'The role of immune complexes in the activation of the first component of human complement.' *J. Immunol.*, **132**: 283–8.

36. **Lu, J., Tehy, B. K., Wamg, L., Wang, Y., Tan, Y. S., Lai, M. C., and Reid, K. B. M.** (2008). 'The classical and regulatory functions of C1q in immunity and autoimmunity.' *Cellular & Molec. Immunol.*, **5**: 9–21.

37. **Ehrnthaller, C., Ignatius, A., Gebhard, F., and Huber-Lang, M.** (2011). 'New Insights of an Old Defense System: Structure, Function, and Clinical Relevance of the Complement System.' *Molec. Med.*, **17**: 317–29.

38. **Male, D., Brostoff, J., Roth, D. B., and Roitt, I. M.** (2013). *Immunology*, 8e. Philadelphia: Elsevier, Saunders.

39. **Brüggemann, M., Williams, G. T., Bindon, C. I., Clark, M. R., Walker, M. R., Jefferis, R., Waldmann, H., and Neuberger, M. S.** (1987). 'Comparison of the effector functions of human immunoglobulins using a matched set of chimeric antibodies.' *J. Exp. Med.*, **166**: 1351–61.

40. **Binden, C. I., Hale, G., Brüggemann, M., and Waldmann, H.** (1988). 'Human monoclonal IgG isotypes differ in complement activating function at the level of C4 as well as C1q.' *J. Exp. Med.*, **168**: 127–42.

41. **Coons, A. H., Creech, H. J., Jones, R. N., and Berliner, E.** (1942). 'Localization of Antigen in Tissue cells.' *J. Immunol.*, **45**: 159–70.

42. **Coons, A. H., Leduc, E. H., and Connolly, J. M.** (1955). 'Studies on antibody production.' *J. Exp. Med.*, **102**: 49–60.

43. **Boyden, S. V., and Sorkin, E.** (1960). 'The adsorption of antigen by spleen cells previously treated with antiserum in vitro.' *Immunology*, **3**: 272–83.

44. **Boyden, S. V.** (1964). 'Cytophilic antibody in guinea-pigs with delayed-type hypersensitiv-ity.' *Immunology*, **7**: 474–83.

45. **Uhr, J. W.** (1965). 'Passive sensitization of lymphocytes and macrophages by antigen-antibody complexes.' *Proc. Natl. Acad. Sci.*, **54**: 1599–1606.

46. **Uhr, J. W., and Phillips, J. M.** (1966). 'In vitro sensitization of phagocytes and lymphocytes by antigen-antibody complexes.' *Ann. N.Y. Acad. Sci.*, **129**: 793–8.

47. **Berken, A., and Benacerraf, B.** (1966). 'Properties of antibodies cytophilic for macrophages.' *J. Exp. Med.*, **123**: 119–42.

48. **Dukor, P., Bianco, C., and Nussenzweig, V.** (1970). 'Tissue Localization of Lymphocytes Bearing a Membrane Receptor for Antigen-Antibody-Complement Complexes.' *Proc. Nat. Acad. Sci.*, **67**: 991–7.

49. **Brown, J. C., de Jesus, D. G., Holborow, E. J., and Harris, G.** (1970). 'Lymphocyte-mediated transport of aggregated human g-globulin into germinal centre areas of normal mouse spleen.' *Nature*, **228**: 367–9.

50. **Paraskevas, F., Lee, S-T., and Israels, L. G.** (1971). 'Cell surface associated gamma globulins in lymphocytes: Reverse immune adherence: A technique for their detection in mouse and human lymphocytes.' *J. Immunol.*, **106**: 160–70.

51. **Hunt, S. V., and Williams, A. F.** 'The origins of cell surface immunoglobulin of marrow-derived and thymus-derived lymphocytes of the rat.' *J. Exp. Med.*, **139**: 479–96.

52. **Paraskevas, F., Lee, S-T., Orr, K. B., and Israels, L. G.** (1972). 'A receptor for Fc on mouse B-lymphocytes.' *J. Immunol.*, **108**: 1319–27.

53. **Unkeless, J. C., Fleit, H., and Mellman, I. S.** (1981). 'Structural aspects and heterogeneity of immunoglobulin Fc receptors.' *Adv. Immunol.*, **31**: 247–70.

54. **Huber, H., and Fudenberg, H. H.** (1968). 'Receptor sites of human monocytes for IgG.' *Int. Arch. Allergy Appl. Immunol.*, **34**: 18–31.

55. **Messner, R. P., and Jelinek, J.** (1970). 'Receptors for human gamma G globulin on human neutrophils.' *J. Clin. Invest.*, **49**: 2165–71.

56. **Anderson, C. L., and Abraham, G. N.** (1980). 'Characterization of the Fc receptor for IgG on a human macrophage cell line, U937.' *J. Immunol.*, **125**: 2735–41.

57. **Mcnabb, T., Koh, T. Y., Dorrington, K. J., and Painter, R. H.** (1976). 'Structure and function of immunoglobulin domains. V. Binding of immunoglobulin G and fragments to placental membrane preparations.' *J. Immunol.*, **117**: 882–8.

58. **Crabtree, G. R.** (1980). 'Fc receptors of a human promyelocytic leukemic cell line: evidence for two types of receptors defined by binding of the staphylococcal protein A-IgG1 complex.' *J. Immunol.*, **125**: 448–53.

59. **Ravetch, J. V., Luster, A. D., Weinshank, R., Kochan, J., Pavlovec, A., Portnoy, D. A., Hulmes, J., Pan, Y-C.E., and Unkeless, J. C.** (1986). 'Structural Heterogeneity and Functional Domains of Murine Immunoglobulin G Fc Receptors.' *Science*, **234**: 718–25.

60. **Allen, J. M., and Seed, B.** (1989). 'Isolation and Expression of Functional High-Affinity Fc Receptor Complementary DNAs.' *Science*, **243**: 378–81.

61. **Ravetch, J. V.** (1994). 'Fc Receptors: Robor Redux.' *Cell*, **78**: 553–60.

62. **Arthus, M.** (1903). 'Injections répétées de serum de cheval chez le lapin.' Comptes rendus des séances de la Société de biologie et ses filiales, **55**: 817–20.

63. **Sylvestre, D. L., and Ravetch, J. V.** (1994). 'Fc receptors initiate the Arthus reac-tion: Redefining the inflammatory cascade.' *Science*, **265**: 1095–8.

64. Cola, A. F., and Grove, E. F. (1925). 'Studies in hypersentitiveness XIII. A study of the atopic reagins.' *J. Immunol.*, **10**: 445–64.

65. Ishizaka, T., Ishizaka, K., Johansson, S. G. O., and Bennich, H. K. (1969). 'Histamine release from human leukocytes by anti-γE antibodies.' *J. Immunol.*, **102**: 884–92.

66. Segal, D. M., Taurog, J. D., and Metzger, H. (1977). 'Dimeric immunoglobulin E serves as a unit signal for mast cell degranulation.' *Proc. Natl. Acad. Sci.*, **74**: 2993–7.

67. Ishizaka, T., and Ishizaka, K. (1978). 'Triggering of histamine release from rat mast cells by divalent antibodies against IgE-receptors.' *J. Immunol.*, **120**: 800–5.

68. Kinet, J. P., Metzger, H., Hakimi, J., and Kochan, J. L. (1987). 'A cDNA presumptively coding for the alpha subunit of the receptor with high affinity for immunoglobulin E.' *Biochemistry*, **26**: 4605–10.

69. Shimizu, A., Tepler, I., Benfey, P. N., Berenstein, E. H., Siraganian, R. P., Leder, P. (1988). 'Human and rat mast cell high-affinity immunoglobulin E receptors: characterization of putative alpha-chain gene products.' *Proc. Natl. Acad. Sci.*, **85**: 1907–11.

70. Kinet, J. P., Blank, U., Ra, C., White, K., Metzger, H., Kochan, J. (1988). 'Isolation and characterization of cDNAs coding for the beta subunit of the high-affinity receptor for immunoglobulin E.' *Proc. Natl. Acad. Sci. U S A.*, **85**: 6483–7.

71. Blank, U., Ra, C., Miller, L., White, K., Metzger, H., and Kinet, J.P. (1989). 'Complete structure and expression in transfected cells of high affinity IgE receptor.' *Nature*, **337**: 187–9.

72. Williams, A. F., and Barclay, A. N. (1988). 'The immunoglobulin superfamily-domains for cell surface recognition.' *Ann. Rev. Immunol.*, **6**: 381–405.

73. Ravetch, J. V. (1994). 'Fc Receptors: Rubor Redux.' *Cell*, **78**: 553–60.

74. Raghavan, M., and Bjorkman, P. J. (1996). 'Fc receptors and their interactions with immunoglobulins.' *Ann. Rev. Cell Dev. Biol.*, **12**: 181–220.

75. Ratcliffe, A., and Stanworth, D. R. (1983). 'The localization of the binding site(s) on human IgG1 for the Fc receptors on homologous monocytes and heterologous mouse macrophages.' *Immunology*, **50**: 93–100.

76. Duncan, A. R., Woof, J. M., Partridge, L. J., Burton, D. R., and Winter, G. (1988). 'Localization of the binding site for the human high affinity Fc receptor on IgG.' *Nature*, **332**: 563–4.

77. Lund, J., Winter, G., Jones, P. T., Pound, J. D., Tanaka, T., Walker, M. R., Artymiuk, P. J., Arata, Y., Burton, D. R., Jefferis, R., and Woof, J. M. (1991). 'Human FcgRI and FcgRII interact with distinct but overlapping sites on human IgG.' *J. Immunol.*, **147**: 2657–62.

78. Sondermann, P., Huber, R., Oosthulzen, V., and Jacob, U. (2000). 'The 3.2 Å crystal structure of the human IgG1 fragment-FcgRIII complex.' *Nature*, **406**: 267–73.

79. Phillips, D. C., and Parker, N. E. (1984). 'Cross-linking of B lymphocyte Fcγ receptors and membrane immunoglobulin inhibits anti-immunoglobulin-induced blastogenesis.' *J. Immunol.*, **132**: 627–32.

80. Takai, T., Ono, M., Hikida, M., Ohmori, H., and Ravetch, J. V. (1996). 'Augmented humoral and anaphylactic responses in FcγRII-deficient mice.' *Nature*, **379**: 346–9.

81. Bolland, S., and Ravetch, J. V. (2000). 'Spontaneous autoimmune disease in FcγRII-deficient mice results from strain-specific epistasis.' *Immunity*, **13**: 277–85.

82. Samuelsson, A., Towers, T. L., and Ravetch, J. V. (2001). 'Anti-inflammatory activity of IVIG mediated through the inhibitory Fc receptor.' *Science*, **291**: 484–6.

83. Bruhns, P., Samuelsson, A., Pollard, J. W., and Ravetch, J. V. (2003). 'Colony-stimulating factor-1-dependent macrophages are responsible for IVIG protection in antibody-induced autoimmune disease.' *Immunity*, **18**: 573–81.

84. Kaneko, Y., **Nimmerjahn, F., and Ravetch, J. V.** (2006). 'Anti-inflammatory activity of immunoglobulin G resulting from Fc sialylation.' *Science*, **313**: 670–3.

85. **Anthony, R. M., Nimmerjahn, F., Ashline, D. J., Reinhold, V. N., Paulson, J. C., and Ravetch, J. V.** (2008). 'Anti-Inflammatory Activity with a Recombinant IgG Fc.' *Science*, **320**: 373–6.

86. **Anthony, R. M., Wermeling, F., Karlsson, M. C., and Ravetch, J. V.** (2008). 'Identification of a receptor required for the anti-inflammatory activity of IVIG.' *Proc. Natl. Acad. Sci.*, **105**: 19571–8.

87. **WHO** (1984). IUIS-WHO Nomenclature Subcommittee. 'Nomenclature for clusters of differentiation (CD) of antigens on human leucocyte populations.' *Bulletin of the World Health Organization*, **62**: 809–11.

88. **Ferrata, A.** (1907). 'Die Unwirksamkeit der Komplexen Hämolysine in salzfreien Lösungen und ihre Ursache.' *Berliner Klinische Wochenschrift*, *XLIV*: 366–9.

89. **Sachs, H., and Altmann, K.** (1909). *Handbuch der Technik und Methodik der Immunitätsforschung*, Vol. 2, p. 969. Jena: Fischer.

90. **Liefmann, H.** (1909). 'Über den Mechanismus der Seroreaktion der Lues.' *München Med Wochenschr.*, **56**: 2097.

Chapter 10

Transmission and catabolism of IgG

Protection of the unborn: a critical new function for antibodies

Unravelling the mechanism by which passive immunity is passed to the unborn child, allowing it to arrive into the world with a more or less full antibody armory, would require adding the skills of zoologists and embryologists to those of the conventional immunologists. The discovery that during evolution of the immune system a common solution to antibody protection that would be exploited in both passive transfer of immunity from mother to young and in control of the circulating lifetime of IgG molecules would yet again demonstrate the benefits of parsimony in biological mechanism. These findings would later have major implications for the use of antibodies as therapeutic agents but also expose the compromises inherent in multi-functional molecular systems.

Perinatal transmission of immunity

The question of how a neonatal child can exhibit immunity to infections to which only the mother has been exposed has been a topic of debate and investigation since the end of the nineteenth century. The first indications of some sort of passive transmission from mother to young were brought to attention by Ehrlich who after immunizing female mice to the phytotoxins ricin, abrin, and robin observed that the young mice had resistance to the toxins but only for a period of two months after birth.[1] As well as demonstrating that the second generation offspring showed no immunity, Ehrlich dismissed the theories of some others that this immune effect was transmitted by the male and suggested that in mice the lactating mother's milk containing anti-toxins would confer immunity on the young. Working with Hübener, Ehrlich followed up this study by demonstrating that a similar short-lived immunity to tetanus could be transmitted by mothers in guinea pigs and mice but not by fathers.[2] In a series of cleverly controlled experiments, Ehrlich then exposed non-immunized neonatal mice to the mother's milk of immunized mice and showed that both groups of neonatal mice exhibited the same toxin resistance. Commenting on Ehrlich's work in this area in his scintillating 1901 review of immunology, Metchnikoff observes:

> This observation proved... that the antitoxins are absorbed by the alimentary canal... researches have shown that only very young mice are capable of assimilating antitoxin through the intestinal wall. Adult mice, fed by Ehrlich with quantities of antitoxic milk, acquired neither immunity nor any antitoxic property of the blood.[3]

The observation that only neonatal mice are able to engage in passive transfer of antibodies from mother's milk (similar experiments on neonatal guinea pigs and rabbits were negative) would lie dormant for some decades, probably because of the failure to demonstrate a similar effect in humans, as Metchnikoff observed in reviewing the attempts in a number of studies to extend the paradigm,[4] but also because not all the great immunologists of the time were in agreement with the passive transfer idea. For example, Theobold Smith, in his study of transfer of immunity to diphtheria toxin from female guinea pigs to their young *in utero* draws attention to the fact that Emil von Behring himself was totally sceptical of maternally transmitted immunity, citing von Behring's comment:[5]

> … observed again and again in my countless toxin tests, that guinea pigs and mice which are descended from immune parents possess the same sensitiveness to toxins as the offspring of non-immune individuals.[6]

Ehrlich would eventually prove to be correct but it would take some time and a considerable number of contradictory studies before the true picture of antibody transmission to the foetus would become clear. It would also turn out to be very different in different animal species. In 1934, Agustin Rodolfo, an embryologist working at a Philippine government laboratory, would begin to clarify the situation in the much studied rabbit. Using carefully controlled experiments Rodolfo showed that the arrival of agglutinating antibodies from mother to foetus, generated in the mother by injection of the proteobacterium *Brucella abortus*, followed the rabbit gestation period in a sigmoidal fashion from which he concluded:

> … that the permeability of the placenta to agglutinins to Br.abortus and to hemolysins to sheep red blood cells… changes during the course of gestation. This ratio… takes the form of a sigmoid curve. The permeability of the placenta is probably a function of its histologic structure.[7]

Rodolfo's work appeared to clarify a number of discrepancies in the field and drew attention to the fact that placental anatomy may determine whether antibody transmission occurs. Confirmation of transmission of antibody via the placenta was suggested by the work of Percival Hartley, working at the Lister Institute in London, who in 1951 published results of materno-foetal transmission of anti-diphtheria toxin antibodies in guinea pigs.[8] Hartley's work was interesting for another reason. When his antibody preparation was treated with pepsin the transmission was abolished as measured by foetal anti-toxin activity. Had Porter and Edelman's work been just a little more advanced at this time Hartley might have deduced that the transfer was Fc-mediated. The fact that the pepsin treated material, which he observed 'split the antitoxin into two approximately equal halves' was not transferred more readily than the intact IgG suggested that the prevailing view of 'the smaller the fragment the more easily passage through the placenta would be', was flawed.

In another part of Britain another embryologist would enter the field and begin to provide the basic groundwork for our current understanding of materno-foetal transmission of immunity. Francis William Rogers Brambell (see Fig. 10.1), better known as Rogers Brambell, an Irish zoologist working in Bangor, North Wales with his close

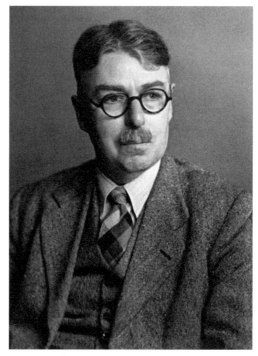

Fig. 10.1 Francis W R Brambell.

Image IM/GA/WRS/4648, Copyright © Godfrey Argent Studio. Reproduced by permission of The Royal Society, London, UK.

colleague William (Bill) Hemmings, demonstrated that transmission of immunity in the rabbit is via the yolk sac and not the placenta.[9]

Brambell would go on to study and explain the variability in the mode of passive transmission of immunity in different animal species, summarizing the known facts in his landmark publication in 1958[10] (Table 10.1).

While he was uncertain from his own experimentation about the route of transmission in man, suggesting it may be via the amniotic fluid across the foetal endoderm rather than directly from maternal to foetal blood, Brambell was certain the mechanism of transfer was 'selective' and thus likely to involve some sort of cellular receptor. His belief in a receptor-mediated transfer arose from his own experiments published later in the same year on neonatal rats in which he demonstrated dose-dependent inhibition of antibody transfer across the rat intestine by heterologous (e.g. human) gamma globulin. Unequivocal clarification of the route of transfer in man came in the same year from the MRC tropical diseases group of Terry who demonstrated that iodinated antibody in the blood of female rhesus monkeys passed from the mother to foetus[11] and must therefore have been transmitted trans-placentally. As Brambell observed in an addendum to his 1958 review, referring to Terry's publication:

Table 10.1 Time of transmission of passive immunity in mammals.

Species	Transmission of passive immunity	
	Prenatal	**Postnatal**
Ox, goat, sheep	0	+++ (36h)
Pig	0	+++ (36h)
Horse	0	+++ (36h)
Dog	+	++ (10 days)
Mouse	+	++ (16 days)
Rat	+	++ (20 days)
Guinea pig	+++	0
Rabbit	+++	0
Man	+++	0

Thus the problem of the route of transmission of immunity in primates has been solved at last by direct experiment and it must be concluded that the route in man is transplacental, as in the rhesus monkey, and not via the foetal alimentary tract. Evidently the primate placenta can transmit globulin, as does the endoderm of the yolk-sac or the gut in other groups, and displays a selectivity in transmission comparable to that of the endoderm.[12]

Brambell was obviously well aware of Hartley's work with pepsin (referring to it a number of times in his publications) and when Porter described the fragmentation of antibody by papain into Fab (Porter thought at this time the two fractions I and II were different) and Fc (or fraction III) fragments, a possible solution to the puzzle began to emerge. In collaboration with Porter, Brambell demonstrated that the passage of rabbit antibody from mother to foetus was equivalent for intact antibody and fraction III but neither fraction I nor II were transported.[13] In his short *Nature* article in 1963 Brambell proposed that the same region of 'γ-globulin' may be involved in both transmission of passive immunity and anaphylactic sensitization. It would be some years later that IgE would be discovered (see Chapter 8) as a separate isotype and the special role of the Fc region Brambell speculated on would be confirmed. He also suggested that the surviving fragment of the pepsin-treated antibody of Hartley was likely to be a fragment I+II combination with the degradation of fragment III as an explanation for the loss of transmission, supporting the notion that the Fc region played a key role in what he now believed to be a receptor-mediated antibody transfer. The search for this 'Brambell receptor' would now become a holy grail-like quest for the cell and molecular biologists of the 1970s and 1980s.

The more recent developmental history of the Brambell receptor has been described in vivid detail by Richard Junghans in his expansive review published in 1997.[14] The tracking of the location, path of absorption, and likely location of the receptor in neonatal rodents during the first three post-natal weeks were elegantly explored by Jones and Waldmann working at the NIH, Bethesda in quantitative transport studies of the rat small intestine using radiolabelled IgG and published in 1972.[15] This was in many ways a landmark study since it demonstrated that the transport machinery was saturable, that all IgG subclasses were equally well transported, and provided a plausible location for the receptor in the intestinal brush-border membranes. Waldmann further proved that the receptor was specific for the Fc region of IgG, that no other Ig class was transported, and that the interaction was pH specific, with binding at pH 6 and release at pH 7.4. In discussing the results, Jones and Waldmann drew attention to the theoretical model of Brambell published some eight years earlier in which Brambell speculated that the transport receptor within intracellular vesicles (typically a pH of ~6) might be involved in a protective recycling of circulating IgG by decreasing its catabolism.[16] It was well known that by increasing the IgG concentration in serum the observed half-life could drop by as much as 50%. Brambell proposed that when the recirculating receptor system became saturated by higher than normal levels of IgG, no protection of the artificially increased IgG would occur, leading to the apparent increased catabolism. The combination of the rigorous experimentation by Jones and Waldmann and the extraordinary insight of Brambell would now propel the field forward rapidly.

Richard Rodewald, working at the University of Virginia in Charlottesville and aware of all the published work in the area, carried out elegant cell biology studies on the rodent neonate exploring with ultrastructural (electron microscopy) methods the intracellular trafficking pathway from intestinal lumen to the neonatal blood. In his early analysis of the neonatal rat intestine Rodewald demonstrated quite clearly that binding of IgG to the surface of intestinal villi in the rat proximal jejunem was receptor mediated, satisfying the criteria of pH dependence and specificity for IgG and confirming the results of Jones and Waldmann (see Fig. 10.2). His suggestion that IgG receptor complexes transit the epithelium within 'tubular vesicles' and are associated with coated pits and coated vesicles[17] would be confirmed much later, although the precise intracellular vesicle picture would in fact become much more complicated. Electron microscopy studies on the rat proximal jejunem clearly showed the location of the receptor on the surface of the villi[18] and receptor-IgG complexes were seen to be associated with coated pits and distributed throughout the cytoplasm of the villous epithelial cells. Rodwald speculated that the pH gradient between apical and basolateral boundaries may drive this vectorial transport.[19]

In 1980 Wallace and Rees[20] provided the first quantitative characterization of the receptor-IgG interaction and three years later Simister and Rees produced evidence that the functional size of the receptor *in situ* was around 100 000 daltons using radiation target theory on neonatal rodent intestinal cells and that *ipso facto* the receptor must be a protein or protein complex.[21] Within the following two years Rodewald and colleagues[19] and independently Simister and Rees[22] isolated the receptor as a multi-subunit protein consisting of an alpha subunit of ~50 000 daltons and a smaller ~18 000 dalton beta subunit. Rees and Simister speculated that this smaller subunit may be beta2-microglobulin. This was subsequently confirmed by Simister after cloning the murine receptor in which the alpha subunit was shown to be related to the major histocompatibility complex protein, MHC type I, while the smaller beta subunit

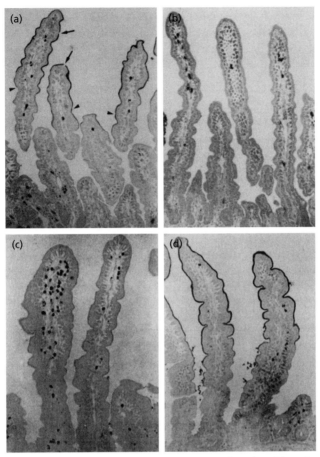

Fig. 10.2 Thick sections of villi from the proximal jejunum of 10 day old rats incubated with rat IgG-HRP (horse radish peroxidase) under various conditions. Plate a) shows staining with rat IgG-HRP at pH 6; Plate b) shows rat IgG-HRP at pH 7.4. Plate c) shows villi pre-incubated with unconjugated IgG at pH 6 and then exposed to IgG-HRP. Plate d) shows exposure to unconjugated IgG, rinsing at pH 7.4, and then exposure to IgG-HRP conjugate.

was in fact beta2-microglobulin. The crystal structure of the receptor (now referred to as the FcRn receptor for *Fc Receptor neonatal*) obtained in 1994[23] by Pamela Bjorkman in collaboration with Simister verified the structural similarity to MHC while the structure of the FcRn-Fc complex obtained in the same year[24] by Bjorkman spontaneously formed the dimer $(FcRn)_2$-Fc in the crystal (see Fig. 10.3). Bjorkman speculated that the dimerization may reflect the situation *in vivo*, consistent with the earlier results of Simister and Rees.[21]

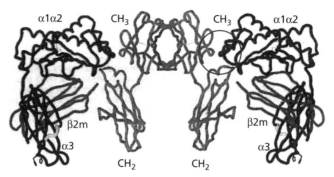

Fig. 10.3 Possible FcRn dimer bound to a single Fc region, derived from the x-ray crystal structure of the FcRn-Fc complex. The Fc region is shown in the centre with the two FcRn receptors bound on either side, proposed to interact with FcRn within the boundary region between the CH2 and CH3 domain of Fc (this author's circle).

Reprinted from Macmillan Publishers Ltd: Nature, Burmeister, W.P. et al., Crystal structure of the complex of rat neonatal Fc receptor with F., *Nature*, Volume 372, pp. 379–383, Copyright © 1994 Nature Publishing Group.

In this structural analysis by Bjorkman, the binding site for FcRn in the Fc region, which lay between the CH2 and CH3 domains, contained a number of histidine amino acids whose pK behaviour would explain the pH sensitivity of the FcRn-Fc binding (at pH 6 the histidine would be positively charged while at pH 7.4 it would be uncharged).

Antibody transfer in humans

While a large body of information existed to explain the trans-intestinal transport of IgG in neonatal rodents this did not explain the preterm transfer of passive immunity in the human. In birds and rabbits the route was also well established as occurring via the yolk sac. In human development the yolk sac is a more primitive organ providing nourishment to the embryo only while development of the foetal circulatory system is in progress. After around three weeks of foetal development it is gradually incorporated into the primitive gut and by seven weeks usually completely obliterated. Numerous studies had established the presence of receptors for IgG on cells of the placenta. In 1976 McNabb described binding to membrane preparations with binding affinities for IgG isotypes in the order IgG1= IgG3 > IgG4 >> IgG2[25] while between 1978 and 1991 Matre,[26] Kristoffersen,[27] and Kameda[28] demonstrated different types of Fc receptors on various cell types including trophoblast cells, endothelium, stroma, and Hofbauer cells. The unifying feature of all these studies however was that the binding occurred at ~pH 7 which would place their involvement outside the window for binding of IgG to the FcRn receptor, always supposing humans used the identical transfer receptor system to the rodent. In reviewing the state of the art in 1994, Colin Ockleford and colleagues noted:

> We are not able to define the precise functional role(s) of the 3 Fcγ receptors expressed by cells of the placenta. Members of the Fcγ receptor family are expressed by almost all cells of the immune system and exhibit a variety of functions. FcγRI (CD64) is the only receptor

that binds monomeric IgG with high affinity; FcγRIII (CD 16) is expressed by a variety of leucocytes but binds monomeric and aggregated IgG with low affinity and, similarly, FcγRII (CDw32) binds multivalent or aggregated IgG.[29]

In drawing attention to the unsuitability of the leucocyte receptor types (FcγI,II, and III) and the fact that in placental histology, cells bearing these receptor types did not contain IgG, Ockleford speculated that there may be a:

> … structurally distinct receptor, perhaps similar to the MHC class I-like molecule of neonatal rat jejunum.[29]

Eight months after Ockleford's comments, Simister published the cloning of an MHC Class 1-like Fc receptor from a human placental cDNA library, the sequence of which showed 69% identity in nucleotide sequence to the rat intestinal FcRn receptor.[30] Was this the answer to the human version of passive transfer of immunity to the foetus? There was still the conundrum of how IgG can bind to an FcRn-like transport receptor at the syncytial membrane surface when it is bathed by maternal blood at pH 7.4. Simister speculated that the role of the other Fc receptor types plus non-specific uptake (fluid phase endocytosis) may be to deliver IgG to the acidic endosomes within the syncytiotrophoblast which do contain the human FcRn. After arrival at the endosomal compartment, the FcRn would hold the IgG in a bound, protected state while transfer to the foetal circulation proceeded.[31]

Surprisingly, to this day, the precise mechanism by which this transport system works is still not fully understood. Of course, experimental intervention in this process is both unethical and refractory to direct placental observation during pregnancy. Until non-invasive techniques are developed to allow visualization of the trans-placental pathway, the exact mechanism operating in humans will have to rely on indirect analysis. What is clear is that a human placental FcRn receptor mediates materno-foetal transfer to the foetus providing it with a fully made up repertoire of antibodies by full term. This apparently non-discriminating physiological process would also transfer maternal IgG bearing undesirable activities (e.g. autoantibodies), potentially giving rise to pathological conditions in the unsuspecting newborn. A further particularly unfortunate consequence is that since the receptor-mediated transfer is poorly active before the third trimester, babies born preterm will have a significantly impaired passive antibody repertoire making them dangerously susceptible to infection. Evolution of the materno-foetal preparation for the outside world was in the end a compromise that depended for its maximum effectiveness on a healthy mother.

Control of antibody catabolism

Brambell's speculation in 1964 that the IgG transport receptor might play a role in regulation of IgG catabolism was almost biblically prophetic. Five years after Brambell's theory, Tom Waldmann and colleagues measured the catabolic rates of IgG isotypes in normal and multiple myeloma patients. They determined that IgG3 had the highest metabolic turnover with the other three subclasses showing similar circulating lifetimes to each other that were around three times that of IgG3. More revealing was the fact than in 12 myeloma cases with different subclass over-expression, the fractional half-lives of the myeloma and all normal IgG subclasses present were significantly shortened. As Waldmann concluded when commenting on the Brambell IgG catabolism theory and subscribing to the 'protective receptor' idea:

> The concentration-catabolism relationship demonstrated for a majority of the patients in the present study is consistent with this [Brambell] hypothesis and expands it by indicating that there are no subclass specific protective receptor sites. All four subclasses compete for the same receptors.[32]

Results from Sally Ward's laboratory in 1994 showed that if Fc fragments, whose lifetime in the blood had already been shown to be similar to that of intact IgG,[33] were mutated at certain amino acids in the CH2-CH3 region, the altered Fc fragments cleared much more rapidly from the circulation[69]. The evidence for Brambell's hypothesis was accumulating rapidly and inexorably. Two years later the final confirmation was provided through the results of Ward,[34] Junghans,[35] and Simister[36] using the new technology of 'genetic knockouts' in which the gene for β_2-microglobulin (the B chain of the FcRn receptor) had been specifically deleted from the mouse genome. Simister had already shown in 1995 that in the genetically modified mouse lacking β_2-microglobulin, intestinal transport of IgG from maternal milk in neonatal mice was completely obliterated.[37] Ward, Junghans, and Simister independently demonstrated that in the same knockout model IgG survival in the adult-mouse circulation was severely impaired (see Fig. 10.4).

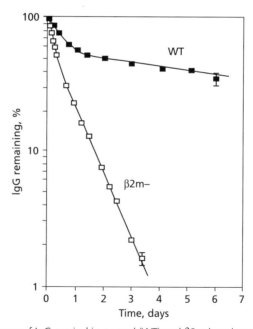

Fig. 10.4 Time course of IgG survival in normal (WT) and β2m knockout mice.

Reproduced with permission from Junghans, R.P. and Anderson, C.L., The protection receptor for IgG catabolism is the b$_2$-microglobulin-containing neonatal intestinal transport receptor, *Proceedings of the National Academy of Sciences*, Volume 93, pp. 5512–5516, Copyright © 1996 National Academy of Sciences, USA.

In passing it is pertinent to comment on the legitimacy of the term 'independent' to describe discoveries with different publication dates. If such dates are taken at face value they may mask differences in journal publication behaviour, a fact that authors often forget when claiming priority via the 'first in print' measure. These three research groups were well aware of Brambell's hypothesis although the tools for testing it were only just beginning to emerge. The first knockout mouse was produced in 1989 but specific gene 'knockouts' took a number of years to be developed. Ward, using β2m knockout mice from the Jackson Laboratory submitted her results in November 1995 and they were published in April 1996; Junghans and Anderson, also using mice from the Jackson Laboratory, submitted their work in March 1996 with publication in May of the same year; Simister, using mice from Jaenisch's laboratory at the Whitehead Institute, submitted his results in early May 1996 but they were not published until December 1996. The animal experiments described in each of these laboratories would have taken many months to perform, suggesting that the work of the three groups must have been overlapping in time. *Quod erat demonstrandum.*

In the experiments of Ward, Junghans, and Simister, the notion arose that the FcRn receptor-mediated IgG survival in adults was based on the knockout of a critical gene, β2microglobulin, which was also known to be involved in many different physiological functions. In fact β2m-deficient mice were prone to perinatal lethality, suggesting that the earlier knockout models may not have presented an ideal physiological background on which to assess critical FcRn functions. It was formally possible that the change in IgG catabolic rate was only indirectly related to the FcRn receptor. It would take another seven years before this uncertainty would be resolved. Clark Anderson at Ohio State University, who had earlier worked with Richard Junghans at Harvard on the β2m knockout, collaborated this time with Derry Roopenian at the Jackson Laboratories in targeting the alpha (heavy) chain of FcRn to produce mice defective in FcRn. Roopenian and Anderson decided that knocking out the alpha chain of the FcRn would allow functional analysis of this putative protective receptor without impacting the multitude of other functions of β2m. The FcRn$^{-/-}$ mice were normal in all tissues looked at, displayed normal weight, and were otherwise healthy. The clever experiment was then to mate a female FcRn$^{-/-}$ mouse with a male FcRn$^{+/-}$ mouse. The progeny would then be either $-/-$ or wild type ($+/-$) with respect to FcRn. The results were unequivocal. The $+/-$ neonates showed normal serum levels of IgG while the $-/-$ littermates had levels ~200 times lower, proving beyond reasonable doubt that FcRn mediates perinatal transfer of IgG. To establish the additional role of the same FcRn receptor in control of IgG catabolism, Anderson and colleagues then measured the half-lives ($t_{1/2}$) of IgG isotypes in normal and FcRn-deficient animals. As with the previous β2m-knockout experiments they observed a significant $t_{1/2}$ reduction from around nine days to one day, although in Anderson's model no difference in $t_{1/2}$ of different IgG isotypes was seen in contrast to the earlier β2m-knockout experiments. Taking this further, Anderson used a transgenic model in which the human FcRn was introduced into the genome of FcRn$^{-/-}$ mice. The same behaviour was seen. In FcRn$^{-/-}$ mice injected human IgG was cleared rapidly while in the transgene containing the human FcRn the half-life of injected human IgG was identical to that of murine IgG in the wild type.[38]

The hunt for mechanistic answers to IgG transport

By the early part of this century definitive proof was obtained that FcRn, consisting of a heavy chain protein with high similarity to class I MHC molecules and associated with a β2m light chain in a dimeric structure, was the mediator of passive transfer of IgG from mother to young and the receptor responsible for control of IgG catabolism. The presence of the receptor in yolk sac membranes, intestinal epithelial cells, or the placenta explained in full the transfer behaviour observed by many researchers and consolidated by Brambell for different animal species more than 40 years earlier. By 2003 the story seemed to be neatly rounded out, at least at the level of the molecules involved. However, there was an additional feature of this IgG protection system to explain. Exactly how were IgG molecules vectorially transferred from an apical surface, located either in the intestinal lumen or the materno-foetal placenta, to a basolateral region that emptied IgG directly into the foetal circulation? Further, what intracellular signals operated to enable IgG recycling via endocytosis and exocytosis at the same apical membrane in endothelial cells lining blood vessels without degradation?

A survey of the intensive efforts in the past 15 years to establish the mechanistic detail of IgG transport is beyond the scope of this book but a brief summary follows:

♦ Simister's molecular biology techniques identified specific amino-acid motifs in the FcRn that influenced intracellular trafficking, moving the apical ⇌ basolateral equilibrium towards an apical→ basolateral preference on IgG binding;[39]

♦ Ward's sophisticated microscopy methods have enabled visualization of the endosome pathways in polarized cells, but while providing intriguing visual information, have not yet enabled identification of the 'triggering' mechanisms for fusion with the exocytosing membranes;[40]

♦ The presence of specific N-glycan (oligosaccharides attached to proteins via the side chain of asparagine) motifs present in FcRn, described by Blumberg, may contribute to the steady state distribution and direction of IgG transport in polarized epithelia;[41]

♦ Bjorkman's electron-tomography technique enabled 3-D reconstruction of cells and was used to observe endosomes containing IgG-FcRn complexes trafficking to exit regions of the basolateral membrane in rodent intestine that are rich in a particular type of membrane-associated protein known as clathrin.[42] This had resonance with the earlier observations of Rodewald,[43] Ockleford,[44] Pearce,[45] Lin,[46] and others.

So, do we yet completely understand the molecular mechanism by which extracellular IgG is transported across an apical cell barrier to its basolateral target location? In attempting to understand the complex sorting process within cells that sends some proteins towards degradation and protects other (e.g. IgG) from the same fate, Sally Ward might perhaps be given the last word at the time of writing:

… we have characterized individual components constituting the recycling pathway of the receptor, FcRn. Specifically, several different pathways followed by TCs that intersect with larger, relatively static sorting endosomes have been defined. These pathways include a novel 'looping' process in which TCs leave and return to the same endosome. Significantly,

TCs with different itineraries can be identified by associations with distinct complements of Rab GTPases, APPL1 and SNX4. These studies provide a framework for further analyses of the recycling pathway.[47]

[Abbreviations: TC = tubulovesicular transport carrier (c.f. the tubular bodies observed by Rodewald?; Rab = family of G proteins (GTPases) involved in controlling trafficking; APPL1 = phosphatase involved in cellular cytoskeleton and lipid metabolism; SNX4 = intracellular protein involved in endosome sorting and carrying a phosphoinositide (PI) binding domain.]

We await the 'further analysis' with interest.

Some clinical sequelae of FcRn receptor activity

During passive transfer the FcRn receptor is largely promiscuous with respect to the IgG-bearing antigen specificities it donates to the human foetus. This is, of course, highly beneficial to the foetus since many millions of antigenic specificities may be present. In particular, the foetus will acquire a more or less complete repertoire of anti-infectious disease antibodies, delivering the perinatal protection essential for survival. However, deleterious antibodies produced in the mother as a result of particular autoimmune conditions, or by maternal responses to foetal antigens as a result of genetic mismatching, will also be passed to the foetus with little or no discrimination, depending on the particular IgG isotype carrying the antigen specificity. Some well recognized problems caused by reverse foetal antigen transfer to the mother are particularly dangerous for the foetus. Historical aspects of some of these pathologies are briefly described below.

Rhesus antigen incompatibility was first described and published in 1940 by Landsteiner and Wiener.[48] By injecting blood from Rhesus monkeys into rabbits, Landsteiner obtained an agglutinating antibody that was shown to have identity with immune isoagglutinins produced in humans after repeated blood transfusion or with isoagglutinins produced by pregnant mothers. In both instances those lacking the Rh factor in their red cells were immunized by the donor blood cells while in the pregnancy cases the leakage of foetal blood into the mother's circulation would be required. The following year Levine and colleagues followed up some of their earlier work with a study of the case histories of five mothers with atypical agglutinins, three of whom gave birth to infants suffering from what was then called *erythroblastosis fetalis*[49] and later renamed haemolytic disease of the newborn (HDNB) after its confirmed aetiology. The hypothesis required that the foetus inherits the Rh antigen from the father while the mother is Rh negative. Mixing of foetal and maternal blood during birth then leads to maternal anti-rhesus antibodies which, when passed to the second child via placental FcRn, can cause HDNB. The association was not proven but tantalizing. The following year Levine produced statistical evidence to prove the hypothesis[50] (see Table 10.2). In discussion of this analysis Levine states:

> The results in Table 1 [in original publication] which conform to the theoretical expectation provide striking evidence to support the importance of the Rh factor in the etiology of erythroblastosis fetalis.[49]

Table 10.2 Evidence to support the importance of the Rh factor in the etiology of *erythroblastosis fetalis.*

	Rh positive %	Rh negative %
Random population		
Male 829	86.2	13.8
Female 206	88.4	11.6
111 mothers with infants having HDNB	9	91
66 husbands of Rh negative mothers	100	
58 affected infants	100	

Table reproduced with permission © Copyright 1941 Rockefeller University Press. Originally published in Levine, P. et al., Pathogenesis of Erythroblastosis Fetalis: Statistical Evidence, *Science*, Volume 94, pp. 371–372.

Firm evidence that Rh+ cells could be removed from the circulation by antibody-driven ablation of red cells bearing the antigen was first observed in 1961[51] in a study by Clarke and colleagues at the Department of Medicine in Liverpool and in a follow-up study in 1963.[52] In these studies, Rh- male volunteers were injected with Rh+ blood followed by anti-Rh(anti-D) serum intravenously at various times. In the first of these studies, males receiving the anti-D serum had eliminated >50% of the injected cells while the controls showed full cell survival. In the follow-on study, greater amounts of anti-D serum were administered resulting in a greater percentage of elimination, even after multiple injections of Rh+ blood. In the same publication, Clarke et al also report an anecdotal result in which intramuscular anti-D γ-globulin (rather than serum) was much more effective in elimination and speculate that before clinical trials on pregnant women can be initiated 'additional experiments are indicated'.

Parallel studies in the USA, referred to by Clarke and colleagues in their letter to *The Lancet* in 1964,[53] were being carried out in New York by Freda, Gorman, and Pollack and were published in 1964. In this study nine unsensitized Rh- males were challenged with Rh+ blood over a five-month period. In four of the volunteers anti-Rh IgG was administered intramuscularly 24 hours before each antigenic challenge. In the four protected subjects no anti-Rh antibodies were detected even six months after the last passive IgG injection while in the controls four of the five volunteers were all strongly sensitized.[53] What was also observed was that if the injection of the anti-D globulin was delayed for 72 hours after injection of the Rh+ cells, the same protection was afforded as the 24-hour delay. This was not a trivial observation since it brought the timing within the likely time window for normal hospital practice. The first experiment on a pregnant woman seems to have taken place in Australia in 1964 but was not part of a formal clinical trial. The case is referred to by Clarke and colleagues[54] whose Liverpool (UK) laboratory tested the patient's blood immediately after the birth, finding about 5mL of foetal blood present. Forty-eight hours after anti-D was administered no foetal blood cells were detectable.

The results in the male volunteers gave enormous impetus to the field resulting in the initiation of clinical trials in several centres between 1964 and 1968. The results of these trials were unequivocal and ground-breaking. In the British,[55] American,[56] and Dutch[57] trials prevention of immunization in Rh⁻ women by foetal Rh⁺ cells provided irrefutable evidence of the efficacy of post-natal anti-D treatment in the prevention of HDNB. By 1972 Clarke, in summarizing the state of anti-D treatment and drawing attention to the key evidence of protection by reducing HDNB in the second child of susceptible mothers, stated:

> Reports from all parts of the world where haemolytic disease of the newborn is a problem continue to show the value of giving anti-D gamma globulin to previously-immunized Rh-negative women after the delivery of an Rh-positive baby… The final results of two Liverpool trials show a protection rate of 95% six months after delivery, and 86% at the end of the second Rh-positive pregnancy…[58]

In 1980, Clarke (Sir Cyril), Ronald Finn, Vincent Freda, John Gorman, and William Pollack were awarded the Albert Lasker Clinical Medical Research Award for their contributions towards the prevention of haemolytic disease of the newborn.

In alloimmune thrombocytopenia (ITP) where the foetal platelet antigen 1a is inherited from the father with the mother being negative for this antigen, maternal anti-1a antibodies produced by the mother traverse the placenta and cause platelet destruction in the foetus. The involvement of antibody in this pathology was first reported by Zucker et al[59] in 1959 while in the same year van Loghem and colleagues associated the condition with a heritable antigen which they named Zw.[60] The direct relationship between this platelet antigen and the presence of antibodies to the platelets after blood transfusion was established in an exhaustive study by Shulman at the NIH (USA), who identified a similar complement-fixing platelet antigen naming it P1A1. In collaboration with van Loghem, Shulman provided anti- P1A1 antibodies to van Loghem who showed that Shulman's antibodies reacted with Zw⁺ but not Zw⁻ platelets, proving that Zw and P1A1 were identical. Summarizing his observations, Shulman concluded:

> An isoantibody provoked by a mismatched platelet antigen destroyed platelets in the individuals. It is proposed, as a mechanism of thrombocytopenia, that foreign antigen survives in vivo longer than the period of antibody induction and that antibody, complexed with foreign antigen, is adsorbed by autologous platelets.[61]

Although Shulman examined parent and children families he did not at this time make the connection between maternal transport of anti-1a antibodies and the paediatric platelet pathology. He did however go on to become a major scientific force in platelet disease.

In mothers with systemic lupus erythematosus (NLE), auto-antibodies against the nuclear antigens Ro/SSA and/or La/SSB are transferred to the unborn foetus. Their auto-reactivity with these antigens, which are involved in critical RNA control functions, can give rise to cutaneous rash, liver and blood damage, but more seriously, can interfere with proper development of the heart (inducing fibrosis) leading to congenital heart block (CHB). Palmeira[62] has recently reviewed the contemporary issues relating to placental transfer of IgG whereas Capone[63] and colleagues review the cardiac manifestations of neonatal lupus.

The second and third examples above illustrate two differing clinical consequences of the materno-foetal antibody transfer process and the important interplay of developmental factors. The first case concerns the treatment of thrombocytopenia by administration of high levels of exogenous IgG (produced by extensive pooling of blood donors' IgG fractions), pioneered by Imbach and colleagues at the University Children's Hospital in Bern, Switzerland. In 1979 Imbach observed that a child with Wiskott-Aldrich Syndrome when treated with intravenous immunoglobulin (IVIG) showed an increase in platelet count.[64] When the procedure was repeated during 1980 on a child with severe, refractory ITP, a similar increase in platelets was observed.[65] These results triggered a massive series of clinical trials and mechanistic studies in other laboratories so that by 2012 Imbach notes that more than 34 000 articles on IVIG could be found in PUBMED. While for thrombocytopenia the exact mechanism of action for amelioration of the condition is not fully understood, it has been proposed that saturation of the FcRn receptor by the exogenous IgG establishes a 'recycling blockade', shortening the lifetime of endogenous antibodies which include the anti-platelet specificities. Of course, high levels of IgG can bind to all Fc receptor types and by fortuitous antigen specificities form antibody-antigen complexes which could impact many other cells of the immune system. The importance of FcRn in the protective effect of IVIG was explored in 2002 by Hansen and Balthasar in an animal model of immune thrombocytopenia. FcRn⁻ mice showed no clearance of an anti-platelet antibody after IVIG treatment compared with controls while FcRn⁺ mice cleared the antibody five times more rapidly. Today, IVIG is either a first or second line recommendation for treatment of neonatal alloimmune thrombocytopenia, reviewed by Imbach.[66]

In the ITP example, the effectiveness of post-natal treatment relies on the presence of a reversible pathology in the neonate. The regenerative process for platelets which are actually cell fragments deriving from megakaryocytes in the bone marrow, producing ~10^{11} new platelets per day, provides an avoidance mechanism for the life-threatening consequences of anti-platelet antibodies. This is not the case in neonatal lupus where anti-lupus antibodies may appear in the foetus as early as 11 weeks and immediately begin to affect normal tissue development. In the heart where tissue regeneration is absent, Capone et al note that 'the permanent reversal of third degree CHB [congenital heart block] has never been observed[67]'.

Predicting the future of FcRn as a potential therapeutic target, Ellinger and Fuchs make some interesting observations:

> In adults, hFcRn is assumed to represent a promising therapeutic target... Due to hFcRn expression and function in the placenta, such therapies will also affect the fetus. **Alternatively, specific therapeutic molecules transported by hFcRn might be designed for the fetus only.** (The author's bold).[68]

Acknowledgements

Text extract reproduced from Metchnikoff, E. *Immunity in Infective Diseases*, translated from the French by Francis G Binnie, Cambridge University Press, Cambridge, UK, Copyright © 1907, by permission of Cambridge University Press.

Text extract reproduced with permission from Gan, Z et al., Using Multifocal Plane Microscopy to Reveal Novel Trafficking Processes on the Recycling Pathway, *Journal of Cell Science*, Volume 126, pp. 1176–88, Copyright © 2013 The Company of Biologists, Ltd.

Text extract reproduced with permission from Clarke, C.A., Prevention of Rh Haemolytic Disease: the Present Position [Summary], *Proceedings of the Royal Society of Medicine*, 1972, Volume 65, p.169, Copyright © 1972 Sage Publications Ltd.

Text extract reproduced with permission from Brambell, F.W.R., The passive immunity of the young mammal, *Biological Reviews*, Volume 33, Issue 4, pp. 488–531, Copyright © 1958 Wiley and Sons, Ltd.

References

1. Ehrlich, P. (1892). 'Über Immunität durch Vererbung und Säugung.' *Zeitschr. f. Hygeine*, **12**: 183–203.

2. Ehrlich, P., and Hübener, F. Z. (1894). 'Über die Vererbung der Immunität bei Tetanus.' *Hyg. Infekt.-kr.*, **18**: 51–64

3. Metchnikoff, E. (1907). *Immunity in Infective Diseases*, F. G. Binnie (transl.). Cambridge: Cambridge University Press, pp. 449–50.

4. Metchnikoff, E. (1907). *Immunity in Infective Diseases*, F. G. Binnie (transl.). Cambridge: Cambridge University Press, pp. 450–3.

5. Smith, T. J. (1907). 'The degree and duration of passive immunity to diphtheria toxin transmitted by immunized female guinea-pigs to their immediate offspring.' *Med. Res.*, **16**: 359–79.

6. von Behring, E. (1899). In A. Eulenberg and S. Samuel (eds.), *Lehrbuch der allgemeinen Therapie und der Therapeutischen methodik*, Vol. 3, p. 998. Vienna and Leipzig: Urban and Swarzenberg.

7. Rodolfo, A. (1934). 'A Study of the Permeability of the Placenta of the Rabbit to Antibodies.' *J. Exp. Zool.*, **68**: 215–35.

8. Hartley, P. (1951). 'The effect of peptic digestion on the properties of diphtheria antitoxin.' *Proc. Roy. Soc. B.*, **138**: 499–513.

9. Brambell, F. W. R., Hemmings, W. A., Henderson, M., Parry, H. J., and Rowlands, W. T. (1949). 'The route of antibodies passing from the maternal to the foetal circulation in rabbits.' *Proc. Roy. Soc. Lond. B*, **136**: 131–144.

10. Brambell, F. W. R. (1958). 'The passive immunity of the young mammal.' *Biol. Reviews*, **33**: 488–531.

11. Bangham, D. R., Hobbs, K. R., and Terry, R. J. (1958). 'Selective placental transfer of serum-proteins in the rhesus.' *The Lancet*, **272**: 351–4.

12. Brambell, F. W. R. (1958). 'The passive immunity of the young mammal.' *Biol. Reviews*, **33**: 531.

13. Brambell, F. W. R., Hemmings, W. A., Oakley, C. L., and Porter, R. R. (1960). 'The relative transmissions of the fractions of papain of homologous γ-globulin from the uterine cavity to the foetal circulation in the rabbit.' *Proc. Roy. Soc. B.*, **151**: 478–82.

14. Junghans, R. P. (1997). 'Finally! The Brambell Receptor (FcRB).' *Immunologic Res.*, **16**: 29–57.

15. Jones, E. A., and Waldmann, T. A. (1972). 'The Mechanism of Intestinal Uptake and Transcellular Transport of IgG in the Neonatal Rat.' *J. Clin. Invest.*, **51**: 2916–27.

16. **Brambell, F. W. R., Hemmings, W. A., and Morris, I. G.** (1964). 'A Theoretical Model of γ-Globulin Catabolism.' *Nature*, **203**: 1352–5.

17. **Rodewald, R. J.** (1973). 'Intestinal transport of antibodies in the newborn rat.' *Cell. Biol.*, **58**: 189–214.

18. **Rodewald, R. J.** (1980). 'Distribution of immunoglobulin G receptors in the small intestine of the young rat.' *Cell. Biol.,*, **85**: 18–32.

19. **Rodewald, R. J., and Kraehenbuhl, J.-P.** (1984). 'Receptor-mediated transport of IgG.' *J. Cell Biol.*, **99**: 159s–164s.

20. **Wallace, K. H., and Rees, A. R.** (1980). 'Studies on the Immunoglobulin-G Fc-Fragment Receptor from Neonatal Rat Small Intestine.' *Biochem. J.*, **188**: 9–16.

21. **Simister, N. E., and Rees, A. R.** (1983). 'Properties of immunoglobulin G-Fc receptors from neonatal rat intestinal brush borders.' *Ciba Found Symp.*, **95**: 273–86.

22. **Simister, N. E., and Rees, A. R.** (1985). 'Properties of immunoglobulin G-Fc receptors from neonatal rat intestinal brush borders.' *Eur. J. Immunol.*, **15**: 733–8.

23. **Burmeister, W. P., Gastinel, L. N., Simister, N. E., Blum, M. L., and Bjorkman, P. J.** (1994). 'Crystal structure at 2.2 A resolution of the MHC-related neonatal Fc receptor.' *Nature*, **372**: 336–43.

24. **Burmeister, W. P., Huber, A. H., and Bjorkman, P. J.** (1994). 'Crystal structure of the complex of rat neonatal Fc receptor with Fc.' *Nature*, **372**: 379–83.

25. **McNabb, T., Koh, T. Y., Dorrington, K. J., and Painter, R. H.** (1976). 'Structure and function of immunoglobulin domains. V. Binding of immunoglobulin G and fragments to placental membrane preparations.' *J. Immunol.*, **117**: 882–8.

26. **Matre, R., Kleppe, G., and Tonder, O.** (1981). 'Isolation of characterization of Fcγ receptors from human placenta.' *Acta Path. Microbiol. Scand.*, Section C, **89**: 209–13.

27. **Kristoffersen, E. K., Ulvestad, E., Vedeler, C. A., and Matre, R.** (1990). 'Fc gamma receptor heterogeneity in the human placenta.' *Scand. J. Immunol.*, **31**: 561–4.

28. **Kameda, T., Koyama, M., Matsuzaki, N., Taniguchi, T., Saji, F., and Tanizawa, O.** (1991). 'Localization of three subtypes of Fc gamma receptors in human placenta by immunohistochemical analysis.' *Placenta*, **12**: 15–26.

29. **Bright, N. A., Ockleford, C. D., and Anwar, M.** (1994). 'Ontogeny and distribution of Fcγ receptors in the human placenta. Transport or immune surveillance?' *J. Anat.*, **184**: 297–308.

30. **Story, C. M., Mikulska, J. E., and Simister, N. E.** (1994). 'A major histocompatibility complex class I-like Fc receptor cloned from human placenta: possible role in transfer of immunoglobulin G from mother to fetus.' *J. Exp. Med.*, **180**: 2377–81.

31. **Simister, N. E., Israel, E. J., Ahouse, J. C., and Story, C. M.** (1997). 'New functions of the MHC class I-related Fc receptor, FcRn.' *Biochem. Soc. Transac.*, **25**: 481–6.

32. **Morrel, A., Terry, W. D., and Waldmann, T. A.** (1970). 'Metabolic Properties of IgG Subclasses in Man.' *J. Clin. Invest.*, **49**: 673–80.

33. **Spiegelberg, H. L., and Weigle, W. O.** (1965). 'The catabolism of homologous and heterologous 7S gamma globulin fragments.' *J. Exp. Med.*, **121**: 323–38.

34. **Ghetie, V., Hubbard, J. G., Jin-Kyoo, K., May-Fang, T., Yukfung, L., and Ward, E. S.** (1996). 'Abnormally short serum half-lives of IgG in β2-microglobulin-deficient mice.' *Eur. J. Immunol.*, **26**: 690–6.

35. **Junghans, R. P., and Anderson, C. L.** (1996). 'The protection receptor for IgG catabolism is the β2-microglobulin-containing neonatal intestinal transport receptor.' *Proc. Natl. Acad. Sci.*, **93**: 5512–16.

36. **Israel, E. J., Wilsker, D. F., Hayes, K. I. C., Schoenfeld, D., and Simister, N. E.** (1996). 'Increased clearance of IgG in mice that lack β2-microglobulin: possible protective role of FcRn.' *Immunology*, **89**: 573–8.

37. **Israel, E. J., Patel, V. K., Taylor, S. F., Marshak-Rothstein, A., and Simister, N. E.** (1995). 'Requirement for a beta 2-microglobulin-associated Fc receptor for acquisition of maternal IgG by fetal and neonatal mice.' *J. Immunol.*, **154**: 6246–51.

38. **Roopenian, D. C., Christianson, G. J., Sproule, T. L., Brown, A. C., Akilesh, S., Jung, N., Petkova, S., Avanessian, L., Choi, Y., Shaffer, D.J., Eden, P. A., and Anderson, C. A.** (2003). 'The MHC Class I-Like IgG Receptor Controls Perinatal IgG Transport, IgG Homeostasis, and Fate of IgG-Fc-Coupled Drugs.' *J. Immunol.*, **170**: 3528–33.

39. **Newton, E. E., and Simister, N. E.** (2005). 'Characterization of basolateral-targeting signals in the neonatal Fc receptor.' *J. Cell Science*, **118**: 2461–9.

40. **Prahbat, P., Gan, Z., Chao, J., Ram, S., Vaccaro, C., Gibbons, S., Ober, R. J., and Ward, E. S.** (2007). 'Elucidation of intracellular recycling pathways leading to exocytosis of the Fc receptor, FcRn, by using multifocal plane microscopy.' *Proc. Natl. Acad. Sci.*, **104**: 5889–94.

41. **Kuo, T. T., de Muinck, E. J., Claypool, S. M., Yoshida, M., Nagaishi, T., Aveson, V. G., Lencer, W. I., and Blumberg, R. S.** (2009). 'N-Glycan Moieties in Neonatal Fc Receptor Determine Steady-state Membrane Distribution and Directional Transport of IgG.' *J. Biol. Chem.*, **284**: 8293–300.

42. **Ladinsky, M. S., Huey-Tubman, K. E., and Bjorkman, P. J.** (2012). 'Electron tomography of late stages of FcRn-mediated antibody transcytosis in neonatal rat small intestine.' *Mol. Biol. Cell.*, **23**: 2537–45.

43. **Rodewald, R.** (1976). 'Intestinal transport of peroxidase-conjugated IgG fragments in the neonatal rat.' In W. A. Hemmings (ed.), *Maternofoetal Transmission of Immunoglobulins*, pp. 137–49. New York: Cambridge University Press.

44. **Ockleford, C. D., and Clint, J. M.** (1980). 'The uptake of IgG by human placental chorionic villi: a correlated autoradiographic and wide aperture counting study.' *Placenta*, **1**: 91–111.

45. **Pearce, B. M. F.** (1982). 'Coated vesicles from human placenta carry ferritin, transferrin, and immunoglobulin.' *G. Proc. Natl. Acad. Sci.*, **79**: 451–5.

46. **Lin, C. T.** (1980). 'Immunoelectron microscopy localization of immunoglobulin G in human placenta.' *J. Histochem. Cytochem.*, **28**: 339–46.

47. **Gan, Z., Ram, S., Ober, R. J., and Ward, E. S.** (2013). 'Using Multifocal Plane Microscopy to Reveal Novel Trafficking Processes on the Recycling Pathway.' *J. Cell Science*, **126**: 1176–88.

48. **Landsteiner, K., and Wiener, A. S.** (1940). 'An agglutinable factor in human blood recognized by immune sera for Rhesus blood.' *Proc. Soc. Exper. Biol. Med.*, **43**: 223–4.

49. **Levine, P., Katzin, E. M., and Burnham, L.** (1941). 'Isoimmunization in pregnancy: its possible bearing on the etiology of erythroblastosis foetalis.' *J. Amer. Med. Assoc.*, **116**: 825–7.

50. **Levine, P., Vogel, P., Katzin, E. M., and Burnham, L.** (1941). 'Pathogenesis of Erythroblastosis Fetalis: Statistical Evidence.' *Science*, **94**: 371–2.

51. **Finn, R., Clarke, C. A., Donohoe, E. W. T. A., McConnell, R. B., Sheppard, P. M., Lehane, D., and Kulke, W.** (1961). 'Experimental studies on the prevention of Rh haemolytic disease.' *Brit. Med. J.*, **1**: 1486–90.

52. **Clarke, C. A., Donohoe, W. T. A., McConnell, R. B., Finn, R., Krevans, J. R., Kulke, W., Lehane, D., and Sheppard, P. M.** (1963). 'Further experimental studies on the prevention of Rh haemolytic disease.' *Brit. Med. J.*, **2**: 979–84.

53. Freda, V. J., Gorman, J. G., and Pollack, W. (1964). 'Successful prevention of experimental RH sensitization in a man with an anti-RH gamma2-globulin preparation: A preliminary report.' *Transfusion*, **4**: 26–32.

54. Clarke, C. A., Finn, R., McConnell, R. B., Woodrow, J. C., Lehane, D., and Sheppard, P. M. (1964). 'Prevention of haemolytic disease.' *Br. Med. J.*, **1**(5390): 1110.

55. Liverpool Group: Clarke, C. A., Donohoe, W. T. A., Durkin, C. M., Finn, R., Lehane, D., McConnell, R. B., Sheppard, P. M., Towers, S. H., and Woodrow, J. C.; Sheffield Group: Bowley, C. C.; Leeds and Bradford Group: Shaw, J., Speight, R. B., and Tovey, A. D.; Baltimore Group: Bias, W. B., Krevans, J. R., Light-Orr, J. K., and Montague, A. C. W. (1966). 'Prevention of Rh-Haemolytic Disease: Results of the Clinical Trial: A Combined Study from Centres in England and Baltimore.' *Br. Med. J.*, **2**: 907–14.

56. Freda, V. J., Gorman, J. G., and Pollack, W. (1966). 'Rh factor: prevention of isoimmunization and clinical trial on mothers.' *Science*, **151**: 828–30.

57. de Wit, C. D., Borst-Eilers, E., van der Weerdt, M., and Kloosterman, G. J. (1968). 'Preventie van rhesus-immunisatie met behulp van anti-rhesus (D)-immunoglobuline.' *Ned. T. Geneesk*, **112**: 2345–51.

58. Clarke, C. A., (1972). 'Prevention of Rh Haemolytic Disease: the Present Position [Summary].' *Proc. Roy. Soc. Med.*, **65**: 169.

59. Zucker, M. B., Ley, A. B., Borrelli, J., Mayer, K., and Firmat, J. (1959). '13. Thrombocytopenia with a circulating platelet agglutinin, platelet agglutinin, platelet lysin and clot retraction inhibitor.' *Blood*, **14**: 148–61.

60. van Loghem, J. J., Jr., Dorfmeijer, H., van der Hart, M., and Schreuder, F. (1959). 'Serological and genetical studies on a platelet antigen.' *Vox Sang.* (Basel), **4**: 161–9.

61. Shulman, R., Aster, R. H., Leitner, A., and Hiller, M.-C. (1961). 'Immunoreactions involving platelets V. Post-transfusion purpura due to a complement-fixing antibody against a genetically-controlled platelet antigen: A proposed mechanism for thrombocytopenia and its relevance in "autoimmunity".' *J. Clin. Invest.*, **40**: 1597–620.

62. Palmeira, P., Quinello, C., Silveira-Lessa, A. L., Zago, C. A., and Carneiro-Sampaio, M. (2012). 'IgG placental transfer in healthy and pathological pregnancies.' *Clin. Dev. Immunol.*, Vol. 2012: 1–13.

63. Capone, C., Buyon, J. P., Friedman, D. M., and Frishman, W. H. (2012). 'Cardiac manifestations of neonatal lupus: a review of autoantibody-associated congenital heart block and its impact in an adult population.' *Cardiol. Rev.*, 20(2): 72–6.

64. Imbach, P., Barandun, S., Baumgartner, C., Hirt, A., Hofer, F., and Wagner, H. P. (1981). 'High-dose intravenous gammaglobulin therapy of refractory, in particular idiopathic thrombocytopenia in childhood.' *Helv. Paediat. Acta*, **46**: 81–6.

65. Imbach, P., Barandun, S., d'Apuzzo, V., Baumgartner, C., Hirt, A., and Morell, A. (1981). 'High-dose intravenous gammaglobulin for idiopathic thrombocytopenic purpura in childhood.' *The Lancet*, **1**: 1228–31.

66. Imbach, P. (2012). 'Treatment of immune thrombocytopenia with intravenous immunoglobulin and insights for other diseases.' *Swiss Med. Weekly*, **142**: w13593, pp. 1–10.

67. Capone, C., Buyon, J. P., Friedman, D. M., and Frishman, W. H. (2012). 'Cardiac manifestations of neonatal lupus: a review of autoantibody-associated congenital heart block and its impact in an adult population.' *Cardiol. Rev.*, **20**(2): 73.

68. **Ellinger, I., and Fuchs, R.** (2012). 'hFcRn-mediated transplacental immunoglobulin G transport: Protection of and threat to the human fetus and newborn.' *Wien. Med. Wochenschr.*, **162**: 207–13.

69. **Kim, J. K., Tsen, M. F., Ghetie, V., and Ward, E. S.** (1994). 'Localization of the site of the murine IgG1 molecule that is involved in binding to the murine intestinal Fc receptor.' *Eur J. Immunol.*, **24**(10): 2429–34.

Chapter 11

The structural context of antibody diversity

Antibody-antigen recognition revealed through structural analysis

We have seen in Chapters 6 and 7 that the antibody, as revealed by the protein chemists Porter and Edelman in the late 1960s and the molecular biologists Tonegawa, Hood, Leder, Talmage, and many others in the early 1980s, was beginning to be understood in terms of its polypeptide chain topology and genetic organization. There were light and heavy chain constant regions that were linked with any one of a number of variable regions interspersed with shorter joining (J) and diversity (D) segments to generate full length chains that would then assemble into tetra-chain molecules. As suggested by Burnet, Talmage, Nossal, and others, each individual B cell would synthesize only one antibody type with a defined specificity determined by the variable region gene segment selected for the assembly. This was all well and good. However, the question of how variation in antibody structure gave rise to changes in antigen specificity and further, how the affinity for an antigen could change over time with the same V-gene represented in the antibody was not understood at this time. Several contemporary advances would begin to provide answers. Analysis of light and heavy chain sequences would generate important clues on the variability segments in the N-terminal regions of the chains while x-ray crystallography on Fab fragments would provide the structural framework on which the sequence variation could be interpreted. The development of monoclonal antibodies would enable analysis of the antibody sequence changes during primary and secondary antigen challenges and spark the search for selective mutational mechanisms, thereby putting somatic theories on a more solid, mechanistic foundation. As a result, the homologous recombination (Smithies), DNA repair (Brenner and Milstein), insertional (Dreyer and Bennet), and episomal (Kabat) theories, brilliantly conceived as they were, would be soundly debunked.

Antibody sequences and the antigen binding site

The first indications of 'focused' sequence variability in the antibody N-terminal variable domain were beginning to be picked up in the late 1960s. Cesar Milstein commented on regions of greater than average variability, stating:

> There are … positions that are extremely variable, and the best examples are found in two clusters. The first occurs around residue 30/32 where several extra residues have been observed… and the second is in residues 92, 93, 94 and 96… other clusters may still appear…[1]

A year later, Elvin Kabat, whose precocious antibody career had started in 1933 in Michael Heidelberger's laboratory at Columbia University when he was only 19, began to unravel the variable and conserved features in a small number of antibody sequences and partial sequences from Bence-Jones proteins and other light chains from mouse and rabbit. At this time his view was that there was a clear indication that two sub-portions of the variable domain sequence were important for antibody recognition and that since these elements were common to mouse and human antibodies, there must have been a selection process during evolution to retain them:

> … a set of variable regions, or more precisely a set of those portions of the variable regions whose primary sequences may determine antibody complementarity, are present in man and mouse, having been preserved throughout the period in which they were evolving from a common ancestor.[2]

In a symposium in Slapy, Prague in 1969, Franĕk identified a third region within the variable domain (in porcine antibodies) which appeared to be hypervariable at sequence positions 50–55,[3] adding to Kabat's two regions around positions 30 and 92–96. What was now required was some sort of statistical analysis of the burgeoning antibody-sequence database to see if these hypervariable sequences were common to different antibodies. In 1970 Kabat, working with Tai Te Wu, carried out an extensive analysis of 77 different Bence-Jones and other light chain sequences and presented the positional variation in amino acid between different chains in the now famous 'variability plot'.[4] In attempting to explain the results Kabat was somewhat preoccupied, as were others, with the genetic origin of this excessive variability (see Chapter 7) but he was also interested in the reasons for the many conserved positions in the light chain variable domain. Of particular interest to Kabat was the frequency of conserved glycine residues, which as a good protein chemist he deduced should give rise to chain flexibility. Still obviously influenced by the Pauling 'flexible configuration' model (see Chapter 4) since no x-ray structures were yet available, Wu and Kabat commented:

> The data now available… amply support the earlier suggestions for the role of the invariant glycines of the variable region both in conferring flexibility… to permit substitutions at the variable positions, and… in functioning as a pivot to permit optimal fitting around the antigenic determinant…[4]

> Text extract reproduced with permission ©1970 Rockefeller University Press. Originally published in The Journal of Experimental Medicine, Volume 132, pp. 211–250.

Despite their scientific predilections, Wu and Kabat's analysis of antibody sequences was a major advance from which a specific set of ideas about antigen complementarity emerged. As Leroy Hood commented in a short retrospective in 2008:

> The Wu and Kabat paper in 1970 was a classic that gave us our first real view of Ab diversity.[5]

Their analysis provided a clear picture of the light chain variable domain geography although without at this time being able to establish exactly how an elevated diversity in short discontinuous stretches of sequence could arise.

In Fig. 11.1 the original variability analysis from the 1970 paper is shown.

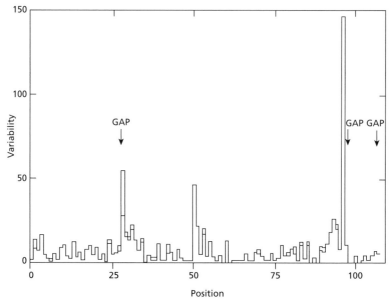

Fig. 11.1 Variability at different amino acid positions for the variable region of the light chains. GAP indicates positions at which insertions were proposed.

The analysis preceding the graphical output went as follows. A quantity is defined for each amino acid position in the light chain variable domain sequence such that: variability, $V = N/F$; where N = Number of different amino acids at a given position and F = Frequency of the most common amino acid at that position.

F is calculated by measuring the number of times the most common amino acid occurs divided by the total number of proteins examined. Kabat (see Fig. 11.2) gives an example:

> Thus at position 7, 63 proteins were studied, serine occurred 41 times and 4 different amino acids, Pro, Thr, Ser, and Asp, have been reported. The frequency of the most common is $41/63 = 0.65$ and the variability is then $4/0.65 = 6.15$.[4]

From the graph it would be obvious to the reader that positions having a variability value of 40 or 50 in 77 proteins studied would be 'hypervariable'. By examining the plot it was immediately clear that light chain variable domains contained three 'hypervariable' regions of sequence, although Kabat took the position that only two of these were involved in antigen interaction, residue positions 24–34 and 89–97. However, the fact was that even one hypervariable sequence was difficult to explain—how could somatic mutation target short, specific sequence regions and leave others alone, except via any

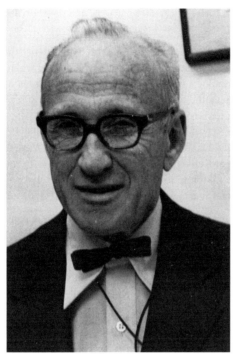

Fig. 11.2 Elvin Kabat.

one of the prevailing but complicated mechanisms of gene mutation. The genetic puzzle fostered a rich tapestry of speculative notions, no less so than for Wu and Kabat in a discussion of their results where they concluded that the two important high variability sequence regions (24–34 and 89–97) are 'inserted' as episomes.

Confirmation of Kabat's variability distribution seen in the human Bence-Jones proteins came shortly afterwards from Martin Weigert's group at the Salk Institute. Weigert sequenced ten mouse lambda chains and superimposed the observed sequence variation onto the variability plot. The lambda chain sequence hot spots were identical in position to Kabat's hypervariable regions.[6] The 'how' was to some extent also dodged by Weigert, commenting that the problem with the germ line model was how to target mutation to only a subset of sequences (*vide supra*) but then concluding that for the somatic mutation model:

> … the six identical λ chains are coded by one germ line Vλ gene which is diversified somatically by spontaneous mutation to yield the four variants.[6]

A spontaneous and high mutation frequency at some parts of the sequence but not others was proposed as a selection process operating to distinguish structurally important and less important positions:

> Invariant residues are preserved because mutations affecting them destroy antibody struc-
> ture. The replacements in specificity regions are strongly selected for antigen.[6]

This was a nice idea but there was not a single shred of evidence that such a mechanism existed in the mammalian genome. That would emerge later when the powerful mono-clonal antibody technology would allow multiple generations of the same antibody to be followed to determine what somatic events occurred and where and how in the sequence they were generated.

The search for the answers took one further step forward in 1971 from Kabat at the Rockefeller and Donald Capra at Mount Sinai School of Medicine. Capra, who had been a PhD student of Kunkel and was an up-and-coming immunology star, carried out sequencing of human immunoglobulin heavy chains and when referring back to the light chain data of Kabat concluded:

> We have shown a similar area of hypervariability is present in human immunoglobulin
> heavy chains...[7]

In addressing how such hypervariability arose Capra further speculated that:

> This suggests that a separate mechanism may generate the diversity within the hypervari-
> able region while simple point mutations probably explain the diversity elsewhere.[7]

In a follow-on study later the same year Capra confirmed the presence of three CDRs within the heavy chain, at the same time suggesting that these three regions might be in close steric contact in the antibody providing a recognition area for antigen binding.[8]

By the close of 1971 Kabat and Wu had analysed yet more light chain but also some heavy chain sequences from multiple species. The same picture emerged as for the light chains. This time however, Kabat recognized the presence of Franěk's third hypervari-ability sequence and noted that the three regions were more or less identical in human and mouse light chains. In comparing heavy chain sequences, a similar set of hyper-variable regions stuck out from the background of sequence variation, recapitulated in human, mouse, rabbit, horse, and shark antibodies. In summarizing the data it is worth recalling Kabat's conclusions:

> The symmetry in the location of hypervariable regions in the light and heavy chains which
> are brought into relatively close proximity by the respective intrachain disulfide bonds can
> provide a three-dimensional site which could contain the complementarity determining
> residues, e.g., those which make contact with the antigenic determinant. As with the light
> chains, deletions or insertions occur in these two hypervariable regions. The role of the
> other hypervariable region is not clear. It is possible that it too is involved in site comple-
> mentarity or, alternatively, it could contribute to the specificity of recognition of heavy and
> light chains. Its role will be more clearly established when some idea of its relation to the
> other hypervariable regions in three dimensions emerges. More sequence data on heavy
> chains are obviously needed. The hypervariability at positions 81 and 83–85, if substantial
> when more sequences are available, might also be related to site complementarity.[9]

A number of important messages were embedded in these words. Firstly, Kabat was still convinced that the hypervariability of amino acids around chain positions 30 and 90 originated from small pieces of DNA (episomes) inserted into existing V-region genes. (By the way, the work of Hood, Tonegawa, and others on antibody gene organi-zation had not yet appeared.) Secondly, the third region (around position 50) was not confirmed as an antigen-contacting region but was certainly 'hypervariable'. Thirdly, a possible fourth region (positions 81–85) was identified that might also be involved in antigen contact. Finally, the descriptive term, 'Complementarity-determining residues' solidified the notion that these sequence positions were critical for antigen specificity and became the permanent terminology for the hypervariable regions in antibodies, now more commonly known as complementarity-determining regions, or CDRs. What Kabat realized was that the sequence information needed to be placed in a three-dimensional context, a crude two-dimensional attempt for which had already been suggested by Capra.[8] In 1972 Kabat published a three-dimensional model of the variable region he and Wu had constructed based on the sequence analysis in the litera-ture and the presumption that the hypervariable regions must somehow come together in space to make an antigen combining site.[10] His model was a crude first attempt using 'nearest neighbour' methods that were somewhat biased toward alpha helical struc-tures, but it was a start. In the absence of any experimental structure by x-ray crystal-lography it was actually the only method available for exploring his hypothesis.

Even when a low-resolution structure of a Fab' fragment (VH+Vλ) appeared from Robert Poljak's laboratory at Johns Hopkins School of Medicine while Kabat's paper was in the proof stage, allowing Kabat to add a claim of 'striking resemblance' to his model, a proper comparison was not really possible since the x-ray structure at this low resolution (6Å) could say little more than that the variable and constant regions in the Fab' fragment were 'globular'.[11] The beginnings of a breakthrough came during 1973 when Roberto Poljak and colleagues published a follow-up study to their low-resolution Fab' *New* structure with a much higher resolution structure (2.8Å) of the same human Fab' fragment,[12] and at exactly the same time Allen Edmundson's group at the Argonne National Laboratory revealed a 3.5Å structure of the lambda light chain dimer, Mcg.[13]

For the reader's information, the Research Collaboratory for Structural Bioinformatics (RCSB) defines *resolution* as:

> Resolution is a measure of the level of detail present in the diffraction pattern and the level of detail that will be seen when the electron density map is calculated. High-resolution struc-tures, with resolution values of 1 Å or so, are highly ordered and it is easy to see every atom in the electron density map. Lower resolution structures, with resolution of 3 Å or higher, show only the basic contours of the protein chain, and the atomic structure must be inferred.[14]

What Poljak's and Edmundson's x-ray diffraction studies showed was that the polypep-tide sequences in the constant domains of the Fab fragment were in close proximity to each other (C_L-C_H) as were the light chain dimer constant domains (C_L- C_L) and that each domain assumed a folded conformation, referred to by Poljak as the 'immuno-globulin fold' (see Fig. 11.3).

The two variable domains (V_L or V_H) assumed the same folded conformation but in addition they possessed two extra strands of sequence. These strands were extremely important because they allowed the folded domain to present three exposed loops as each piece of sequence turned back on itself. As Poljak showed in a wire model of the Fab', generated by tracing the amino acid polypeptide chain within the electron density

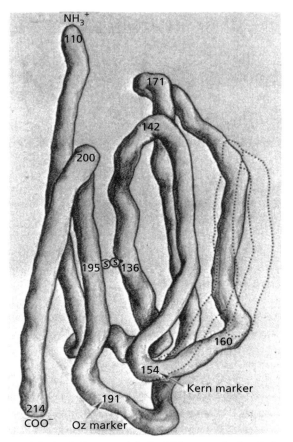

Fig. 11.3 Diagram of the basic 'immunoglobulin fold' as seen in the CL domain. The numbers follow the normal light chain numbering system in which the CL domain begins after the VL domain at residue 110. The dotted line indicates where the additional strand and loop in the variable domain occurs. The labels Oz and Kern refer to the non-allelic serological markers Oz⁺ and Kern⁻ in the λ-chain.

Reproduced from Poljak, R.J. et al., Three-dimensional structure of the Fab' fragment of a human immunoglobulin at 2.8Å resolution, *Proceedings of the National Academy of Sciences,* Volume 70, Number 12, Part 1, pp.3305–10, Copyright © 1974, with permission of the author.

generated from the x-ray crystallographic data (by the way, well before the advent of computer modelling) and then building a wire model based on the trace, this immunoglobulin fold of the two variable domains as they paired with each other presented Kabat's hypervariable sequences 'at one end of the molecule in close spatial proximity'. While clearly seeing a beta sheet structure, oddly Poljak makes no mention of Pauling's original proposal for beta sheets in the antibody 'core'. He also only 'presumes' that the layer structure is stabilized by hydrogen bonds—at this resolution their presence could only be inferred. A further observation from Poljak's structure, in line with practical immunology, was the surface accessibility of the known human lambda chain allotypic markers (Kern and Oz) while the kappa chain *inv* markers occupied the same surface region and would also have been accessible to allotypic anti-antibodies (positions 154 and 191 in λ and 153 and 191 in κ).

Edmundson was much more explicit about the core structure of the light chain domains. Despite his structure being a low resolution light chain dimer with the added requirement that the second light chain was a reliable mimic of the normal heavy chain partner, he stated:

> The appearance of the layers in the C regions is reminiscent of the 'twisted sheet' of β structure noted in carboxypeptidase A … In the Bence-Jones dimer there are many examples in which the chains are separated by distances appropriate for hydrogen bonding…[13]

He also commented that the layers in the V region were more irregular than in the C region. Here then was the first indication of a Pauling-type beta structure in the antibody domains, its ubiquity suggesting an evolutionary relationship between these domains and allowing Poljak to postulate:

> … that κ and λ chains have the same overall three-dimensional structure, and that the VH and CH regions of different classes of H chains (α, γ, μ etc) also have the same overall pattern of polypeptide folding.[12]

Poljak extended the analysis of Fab New a year later (1974) to a resolution of 2Å.[15] This now allowed him to say much more about the folded properties of the variable domains. The constant domain consisted of two layers of twisted anti-parallel beta sheets, one with four strands and one with three and a dense hydrophobic core, while the variable domain had a similar structure but with two extra strands generating three inter-strand 'hairpin-bend' regions at one end of the domain corresponding to the hypervariable sequences. The higher resolution structure also explained the role of the conserved glycine residues, identified by Kabat through sequence comparisons and located without exception at the hairpin-turn regions. Rather than allowing 'flexibility' to facilitate molding of the antibody around the antigen, as contemplated by Pauling and resurrected by Kabat, the glycine residues served an essential structural role enabling tight hairpin-turn formation (glycine has no side chain to spatially block a tight turning of the polypeptide chain) and were held rigidly in place by the hydrogen-bonded anti-parallel beta strands on either side.

Confirmation of the family relatedness of all immunoglobulin domains, regardless of isotype, was obtained from two different structural studies in 1973 and 1974. Robert Huber and colleagues at the Max-Planck Institute in Martinsried, described the structure of a kappa chain dimer REI[16] which showed many of the structural properties of the lambda chain dimer of Edmundson and the Fab of Poljak in having two beta sheets in a 'sandwich' arrangement (held together by a disulphide bond between the sheets), whose individual strands were punctuated by hairpin bends requiring the conserved glycine residues. Presentation of the hypervariable regions was again seen to be via loops at one end of the V-domain coming together in space to form a 'cavity' for potential antigen binding. The team of David Davies at the NIH took the story one chapter further. They determined the three-dimensional structure of a murine Fab first at 4.5Å[17] and then at 3.1Å[18] resolution, but this time from an antibody able to bind a small molecule antigen, phosphorylcholine (PC), despite being derived from a myeloma IgA (known as McPC 603). The Fab fragment showed the same immunoglobulin fold and location of the hypervariable regions. A further important observation made by Davies was enabled by having an x-ray structure of the Fab fragment complexed with the PC ligand, clearly showing the ligand location within a pocket surrounded by amino acids from the hypervariable sequences, or CDRs. Here for the first time was definitive structural evidence for the functional role of the hypervariable sequences in binding antigen. The observations of Milstein, Franĕk, Weigert, and others and the conclusions from the extensive analyses of Kabat and Wu would from now on become established immunological dogma (see Fig. 11.4).

The variable domain and antigen recognition

By the end of the 1970s structural information on proteins was accumulating at a high rate. Many different proteins with a large variety of folded motifs called for the type of analysis that would enable structural family relatedness to be understood. This might explain evolutionary structural relatedness (divergence from common ancestors) to be established but also might give clues to common mechanisms or functions that might have originated by structural 'convergence' from structurally unrelated ancestors. A significant advance in our understanding of core protein structural principles was made by Michael Levitt and Cyrus Chothia in 1976 who analysed 31 different protein structures and proposed a classification of different topology 'classes'.[19] Among Class II was the immunoglobulin variable region for which the topology and connectivity of the repeated beta strands in the V_H and V_L domains were defined in a more rigorous manner than previously. In 1981 Jane Richardson at Duke University, North Carolina published what was without doubt the most comprehensive analysis of protein structural motifs yet undertaken,[20] a *tour de force* of comparative protein analysis.

In describing the variable region of antibodies, Richardson drew attention to the fact that the formation of beta sheets coming together from two different protein domains (V_L and V_H) to form a core structure was uncommon. The path of the beta strands in the individual V_L or V_H variable domains corresponded to a 'Greek key' (after the Greek art motif) as shown in Fig. 11.5. In this diagrammatic representation of the beta structure the extra two strands in the variable domain (nine strands) compared with the constant domain (seven strands) provided the third hypervariable loop or CDR, giving three CDRs per chain.

Richardson uses simple geometric images to describe the two variable domains. As Levitt and Chothia had already indicated, in three-dimensions the V motif in Fig. 11.5 actually forms a cylindrical barrel for each of the V_H and V_L domains as a result of the beta strands twisting as they progress. When the two barrels come together to form a V_L-V_H pair they each contribute a four-stranded wall (a half barrel), creating a third barrel forming the interfacial region between the domains, as Richardson explains:

> Back-to-back β barrels that share one wall occur in the variable half of immunoglobulin Fab structures (except for Rhe …) where V_L and V_H are each antiparallel β barrels and the contact between them forms an even more regular eight-stranded barrel with four strands contributed from each domain.[20]

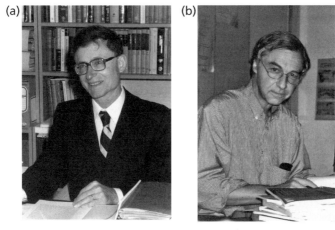

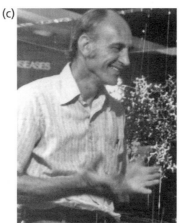

Fig. 11.4 (a) Robert J. Poljak; (b) Robert Huber; and (c) David Davies.

(a) Reproduced courtesy of Roberto J. Poljak; (b) reproduced courtesy of Robert Huber; and (c) reproduced courtesy of David Davies.

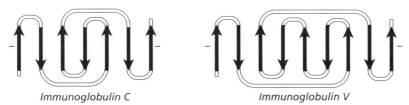

Immunoglobulin C   *Immunoglobulin V*

Fig. 11.5 The Greek key beta sheet motif found in antibody variable (V) and constant (C) domains (left).

Reprinted from *Advances in Protein Chemistry,* Volume 34, Richardson, J., The anatomy and taxonomy of protein structure, pp. 167–339, Copyright © 1981, with permission from Elsevier: http://www.sciencedirect.com/science/bookseries/00653233

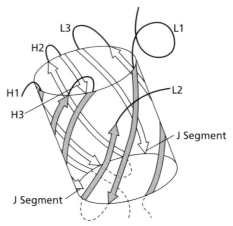

Fig. 11.6 Topology of the binding site barrel from the antibody variable region showing the eight beta strands (four contributed by each of the VL and VH barrels) forming the surface of a new barrel whose central axis bisects the VL-VH interface.

Reproduced from Novotný J. et al., Molecular anatomy of the antibody binding site, *Journal of Biological Chemistry*, Volume 258, Number 23, pp.14433–37, Copyright © 1983 The American Society for Biochemistry and Molecular Biology.

Two years after Richardson's broad-ranging analysis, Novotný, Bruccoleri, Haber, Karplus, and colleagues dissected the antibody binding site in even more detail, extending Richardson, Levitt, and Chothia's analyses but focusing on the antibody variable region. In their 1983 'molecular anatomy' study the Harvard group sought to define the boundaries between the core beta structure of the variable region and its antigen-binding hypervariable sequences, its CDRs.[21] The barrel of Novotný et al (see Fig. 11.6) now made clear the relationship between the beta sheet 'framework' and the terminal loops (CDRs) that formed an antigen-binding region.

A number of important observations were made following this analysis. Firstly, by positioning the two variable domains together as required from the x-ray structures and then examining the locations of the hypervariable residues, Novotný found that some of these amino acid side-chains were buried, away from the solvent (water) exterior. Amino acids that were known to be critical for the PC-antibody interaction in McPC603 were mapped to inaccessible regions at the bottom of the binding site, close to or part of the interface between the VL and VH beta sheets and sitting on the buried top of the barrel. The obvious conclusion was that if any of these residues were changed (mutated) the impact on the binding site could be large since, as buried residues, they could influence the local conformation by disrupting the packing at the interface. Was this a mechanism for antigen-induced conformational change? The importance of the VL-VH interface was reinforced by a more extensive study by Chothia in 1985. In this packing analysis Chothia showed that as much as 25% of this interface derives from the hypervariable sequences. In addition, Chothia's analysis identified a peculiar packing motif, different to all other beta sheet interactions, in which certain strands fold over against their own beta sheet at two opposite corners of the interface forming an atypical third sheet of hydrophobic side-chains and acting as a 'glue' holding together the VL and VH domains.[22]

The second observation of Novotný was that certain of the hypervariable regions were not close to the central binding-site 'cavity' at all and in fact some were part of the outlying beta sheet structure, restricting their conformational freedom to form antigen contacts. Novotný speculated that of the 80 amino acids in the hypervariable sequences 'only 47 are intimately involved in the binding site'. This observation would spark studies by the structural biologists that would draw different conclusions about Kabat's CDRs: their definitions, their sequence boundaries, and their structural context.

These were early days in developing models for how antigens would interact with the antibody. So far, only small molecule haptens had been studied and by analogy with enzymes, their binding requirement would require only a small number of antibody amino acid side-chains to form suitable cavities. Novotný's second observation was laid to rest in 1985 by two sets of data. The first was an x-ray structure of a Fab fragment complexed with the protein antigen, hen's egg lysozyme. Although only at 6Å resolution at this stage a clear picture of the antibody-antigen interface was revealed. In an unambiguous statement Poljak, now at the Institut Pasteur in Paris with his team that included Roy Mariuzza and Simon Phillips, observed:

> The interactions between Fab and lysozyme extend over a large area... and involve all six complementarity-determining regions (CDRs) of the antibody.[23]

So, when antibodies interact with a protein antigen, all six CDRs may be required, but did that mean 80 hypervariable amino acids had to be available for mutation to create the specificity repertoire?

One of the reasons Poljak chose hen lysozyme was that the sequence of this protein in different avian species showed small sequence differences, mainly on the protein surface. In particular, a single amino acid replacement in several different lysozymes whose binding to the Fab was measured by Poljak, influenced the binding to the Fab fragment in a manner that allowed him to deduce that this amino acid occupied a central part of the antigenic contact area, exactly as predicted from the x-ray structure. His conclusion was:

> Thus, the effect of a single amino acid substitution on antigenic specificity and antigen recognition by the antibody are explained readily in terms of our three-dimensional model.[23]

This was in some ways a very important observation. A single change within a large protein surface could have an impact on binding but would it always abolish it altogether, as in Poljak's study? It would be a nice explanation of known anti-allotypic antibody behaviour but did the concept stretch as far as permitting absolute specificity?

There was however a further important result that emerged from this structure. The antigenic region of lysozyme that interacted with the Fab was a topographical rather than a sequential determinant. This meant that the multiple protein segments recognized by the antibody on lysozyme (the antigenic determinant) were discontinuous in sequence but spatially contiguous. In a landmark paper in 1984, Richard Lerner's group at the Scripps Clinic and Wayne Hendrickson at Columbia University carried out an analysis of antibodies that recognized peptides and looked at which of those antibodies cross-reacted with the protein from which the peptide was taken. To their surprise they found that when the peptide came from a region of the protein that was highly mobile (as measured by its 'temperature factor' in the crystal structure) it was more likely to react with the native protein than if it came from a well-ordered region. This suggested that simple linear peptides might not always be good antigen candidates for protein recognition, a concept that would keep immunologists busy in the debating chambers for some time. Poljak may not have been particularly impressed by this notion, as he comments in the last sentence of the 1985 paper, perhaps in a moment of disguised irony:

> Recent reports show the importance of segmental mobility in antigenic recognition;… the residues of lysozyme recognized by antibody D1.3 are not in regions of above-average mobility.[23]

From an improved resolution (2.8Å) of this same antibody-lysozyme complex published in 1986, Poljak was able to draw a number of conclusions about the exact positioning and involvement of amino acids in the V-J joining region of the light chain and V-D-J joining region of the heavy chain in the antigen combining site.[24] In this particular complex, all four amino acid side-chains in CDR3 of the heavy chain that interact with lysozyme are encoded by the D segment. By contrast, none of the V-J junctional amino acids forming CDR3 of the light chain or CDR3 of the heavy chain contribute to the antigen binding. Of course in this one example it was not possible to be sure this would always be the case.

On the subject of antibodies that were reactive with other antibodies where the respective hypervariable regions interact with each, as in 'idiotypic antibodies', Poljak had some further debunking in store for the conformational change-ists. It was known that small molecule haptens could inhibit this anti-idiotypic interaction and this was supposed to occur by the hapten changing the conformation of the antibody so that its idiotypic partner could no longer bind. Poljak's explanation was rather simpler:

> … given the area of antigen-antibody interactions and the location of the antibody interacting residues, antigen binding should sterically hinder the reaction between combining site idiotypes and antibodies against them. No conformational change is involved.[24]

On the question of whether Poljak's anti-lysozyme was 'optimized' for its antigen, the three-dimensional structure offered up a tantalizing suggestion. On inspection of the antigen-antibody interface Poljak noticed that the surface contained 'holes'. Some of these were filled by water molecules but others were not. He speculated that these were prime targets for somatic mutation, new 'fitter' amino acids providing greater interaction and thereby higher affinity binding. Here was a *raison d'etre* for the somatic machinery but just how did it work? A further decade would pass before the answer arrived.

As a follow-up to this x-ray structure, Chothia, Lesk, and Levitt along with the x-ray team of Poljak carried out a comparative modelling study of the variable region of this antibody (we shall look at the development of modelling methods in Chapter 13). In the manner typical of the rigour with which Chothia and Lesk approached structure analysis, they observed that only parts of the Kabat CDR sequences were actually located within the accessible 'loops' at the junctions of the beta strand pairs while other parts were either part of the beta sheet structure itself or buried.[25] Table 11.1 compares the Kabat and Chothia CDRs as first presented in the comparative-modelling paper.

An example of a 'Chothia CDR', as they became known, is shown in Fig. 11.7. The numbering scheme is not of great interest per se unless antibody variable domains are being analysed structurally or residue positions that might be antigen contact positions are targeted for mutation. The main difference between the Kabat number-ing scheme and that of Chothia and Lesk was that the former is based on sequence variability alone while the latter takes into account the position of the amino acids in the structure. If they are not in a loop that is accessible to antigen but part of the beta sheet structure then *strictu sensu* they should not be called complementarity-deter-mining residues. This rather strict classification was to change several times over the years and would also fall foul of the observations that amino acids *outside* the CDRs even as defined by Kabat could engage in antigen binding. Nevertheless, it was more correct from a protein structural point of view. The particular importance of the altered numbering scheme to the antibody community was that when a CDR had an insertion—for example CDR L1 in the antibody McPC603 has 13 amino acids—those extra amino acids would be accommodated in the Kabat scheme (inserted into residue number 24–34) without respecting the structural context while in the Chothia scheme the additional amino acids would be inserted as a 'bulge' at the top of the loop, maintaining the conformation of the parent core loop structure[26] (see Fig. 11.7).

While this may seem an esoteric aspect of antibody structural symbolism, it would become highly important for immunologists attempting to model and then modify or improve antibodies by artificially introducing mutations into CDRs. By respecting the Chothia structures they would be reasonably confident that the change would not drastically change the CDR shape or, more importantly, would not disrupt the core beta sheet structure of the variable domain.

Table 11.1 Comparison of Kabat and Chothia numbering for CDR regions[25]

CDR	Kabat numbering	Chothia (1986) numbering
L1	24–34	26–32
L2	50–56	50–52
L3	89–97	91–96
H1	31–35B	26–32
H2	50–65	53–55
H3	95–102	96–101

Source: data from Chothia, C. et al., The Predicted Structure of Immunoglobulin D1.3 and its Comparison with the Crystal Structure, *Science*, Volume 233, Number 4765, pp.755–758, Copyright © 1986 American Association for the Advancement of Science. All Rights Reserved.

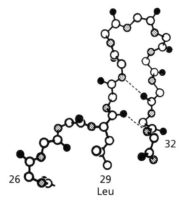

Fig. 11.7 The conformation of the L1 (kappa) CDR from antibody McPC603. In antibodies with shorter L1 sequences the positions of amino acids 26, 29, and 32 are identical to those shown here.

Reprinted from *Journal of Molecular Biology*, Volume 196, Issue 4, Chothia, C. and Lesk, A.M., Canonical Structures for the Hypervariable Regions of Immunoglobulins, pp. 901–917,Copyright © 1987, with permission from Elsevier: http://www.sciencedirect.com/science/journal/00222836

Allosteric signalling by antigen to the Fc region: fact or fiction

An aspect of antibodies that was still unresolved was how binding of antigen could affect the Fc region via an allosteric mechanism to activate or trigger Fc-mediated complement or Fc receptor binding. During the Fab and light chain dimer studies the temptation by the structural crystallographers to comment on this was understandably difficult to resist. Davies observes in his 4.5Å phosphorylcholine antibody study that no drastic conformational changes occurred on ligand binding although subtle changes could not be ruled out.[17] Poljak's comments on the unliganded New structure at 2Å in 1974 were:

> The possibility of a conformational change as a biological signal triggered by antigen binding is an important question to be considered in discussing immunoglobulin structure… These observations suggest that a conformational change could take place by a hinge-like movement at one or both switch regions.[15]

The switch regions that Poljak refers to are the intervening pieces of polypeptide chain joining the globular variable to the globular constant domain in both the light and heavy chains. In the same year Poljak, working with Fred Richards at Yale, determined the structure of Fab New complexed with the adventitious hapten vitamin K (actually a hydroxylated form) and concluded that hapten binding, which involved hypervariable residues lining a groove between the light and heavy chain CDRs, showed no evidence of any conformational change in the Fab.[27] Structures were being searched diligently for any evidence of change on antigen binding but so far the antibody was not giving up its secrets while the Fc theorists were watching with anticipation. But these were studies of the Fab fragment only and what was needed to answer the question of Fab to Fc signalling was a structure of the complete antibody.

The first structural study on a complete IgG actually took place using electron microscopy before any of the crystallographic structures were published. In 1967 Valentine and Green, working at the National Institute for Medical Research in London took an anti-dinitrophenyl (DNP) rabbit IgG and complexed it with a bivalent form of the hapten in which the DNP group was attached to either end of a short methylene (CH_2) chain.[28] This would, they supposed, drive both Fab arms to bind the same hapten molecule, thus enabling them to visualize the antibody complexes more easily. Images in the electron microscope (EM) allowed them to reconstruct a model for the intact antibody, shown as a Y-shape in Fig. 11.8 in one of the forms observed and interpreted as the anti-DNP antibody forming a trimeric complex with the divalent antigen. The observed Y-shape was remarkably consistent with the solution data produced two years earlier by Tanford (see Chapter 6, Fig. 6.5). The attribution of the different pieces in the EM pictures was proved by repeating the experiments after digesting away the Fc region with pepsin and observing the triangular forms but without the protrusions at the apices. Extraordinarily, the predicted molecular weights of the Fab and Fc arms, estimated by assuming these arms were cylinders with the dimensions shown and a partial specific volume of 0.73 (partial specific volume is the protein volume divided by its molecular weight; 0.73 was the accepted average value for many different proteins, typically derived from density or equilibrium sedimentation methods), were 50 000 daltons for each part, in full agreement with Porter's calculation from sequencing of the heavy and light chains. The images obtained with or without hapten were not resolved sufficiently to allow any conclusions about conformational changes on DNP binding (see Fig.11.8).

In 1971 David Davies and colleagues made a crystallographic study of the myeloma IgG1, Dob.[29] This IgG had a 15 amino acid deletion in the hinge region and might

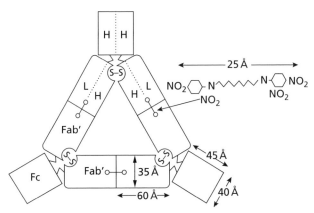

Fig. 11.8 Scale drawing of the bivalent DNP hapten associated with three anti-DNP antibodies, as modelled from electron micrographs. The labelling is according to the normal antibody chain and fragment nomenclature.

Reprinted from *Journal of Molecular Biology*, Volume 27, Issue 3, Valentine, R.C. and Green, N.M., Electron Microscopy of an Antibody-Hapten Complex, pp. 615–617, Copyright © 1967, with permission from Elsevier: http://www.sciencedirect.com/science/journal/00222836

therefore not have been typical of all IgG1 isotypes. Because it was a low-resolution structure due to the poor quality of the crystals the authors were forced to consider a number of possible models for IgG that were consistent with the experimental data. The model they selected had a T-shape which did not correspond exactly with the Y-shape of Valentine and Green but was consistent with their own EM studies on crystals of the antibody, carried out in parallel with the crystallography and showing that the IgG appeared to vary between a T- and Y-shaped molecule.[30] On the question of conformational change, Davies was circumspect, referring to the work of others such as that of Melvin Cohn at the Salk Institute who proposed a model for induction of a cell response by antibody binding. In Cohn's model, the surface-bound antibody (e.g. in a B cell) was required to change conformation in its invariant (or Fc) region on simultaneous binding of two incoming antigen molecules via a mechanism he referred to as 'stretching', a change thought necessary to enable the two Fab arms to reach two antigens.[31] As yet there was no direct evidence either way and in any case for Davies and colleagues Dob was just an itinerant antibody with no antigen partner to allow bound and unbound conformations to be assessed.

In his review in 1975, Poljak makes no further comment on the conformational change issue other than to recite the pre-existing data on McPC 603 with and without phosphorylcholine and the New/vitamin K example. In 1976, the structure of a new myeloma antibody on the block, Kol, was under investigation by Peter Colman and Robert Huber.[32] Kol had some intriguing behaviour that led the authors to indulge in yet more speculation on the conformation change story. Kol showed evidence of considerable disorder in the crystals such that the Fc region was not visible. One explanation was that this part of the molecule had 50:50 occupancy of two different positions with respect to the Fab arms, implying considerable flexibility in the hinge region ('flex point' as the authors describe it) connecting the Fab arms to Fc. Was this for or against the allostery theory? It could be argued that with such flexibility, reminiscent of the earlier electron microscopy observations, conformational signalling might be difficult given such an intrinsic disorder in the hinge. Colman and Huber took a different view, although with some caveats:

> The biological significance of the Fc flex point however, is not clear. The evidence for a conformational change in antibody structure as a prerequisite for complement fixation is not overwhelming... Nevertheless, the differences in the structures of two free Fab fragments, New... and McPC603... and Fab in complete antibody as reported here, together with the difference between the structures of the myeloma proteins Dob... and Kol, suggests a plausible starting model for the description of antibodies as allosteric proteins... We are aware of the speculative nature of the foregoing. It is unclear whether antibodies exhibit co-operative allosteric properties at all.[32]

So far, allosteric signalling by antigen binding seemed to be at an immunological *impasse*?

In 1977 Davies revisited the Dob low-resolution structure using some new crystallographic techniques. The new version of the structure had the T-structure suggested in the initial study and was the first 'close-up' view of the antibody molecule (see Fig. 11.9).[33]

More interesting was that the Fc region showed no structural differences to the structure of an isolated Fc. In addition, Davies was able to position the carbohydrate known to be present in the C_H2 domain. In doing so it became clear that direct protein-protein interaction between the C_H1 and C_H2 domains was not possible except via the carbohydrate. This would have complicated any model for signalling via polypeptide chain flexion. Davies then nails his position to the mast by taking his own crystallographic data and those of others who had seen significant segmental flexibility in antibodies (e.g. Stryer's study in solution using fluorescence techniques, although Stryer was less dogmatic about the possibility of conformational signalling[34]). Davies concluded:

> On the basis of the differences between the structures of the Fab of Kol and of the isolated Fabs of McPC 603 and New... Huber et al... proposed an allosteric Ig model in which antigen binding would cause a stiffening of the flexible antibody molecule by formation of longitudinal inter-domain contacts in the heavy chain. They suggested that the hinge deletion in Dob would also result in rigid Fab arms. The observation here that the elbow bend of Dob (147°) is intermediate between that of the fragment Fab structures and that of Kol, together with a similar intermediate set of inter-domain contact distances, would argue against a two-state allosteric model and would add support instead to the general concept of longitudinal flexibility in the Fab.[33]

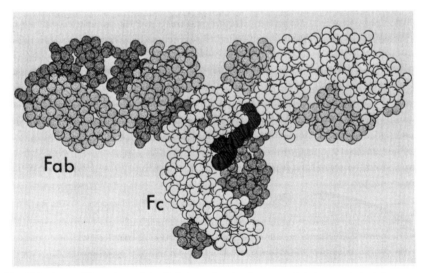

Fig. 11.9 Space-filling view of the Dob Ig molecule. One complete heavy chain is in white and the other is dark gray; the two light chains are lightly shaded. The large black spheres represent the individual hexose units of the complex carbohydrate. In this view, the two-fold axis of symmetry is vertical. A crevasse is seen between the CH2 of the white heavy chain and the CL domain of the Fab on the left.

Reproduced with permission from Silverton, E.W., Navia, M.A. and Davies, D.R. Three-dimensional structure of an intact human immunoglobulin, *Proceedings of the National Academy of Sciences*, Volume 74, pp. 5140–44, Copyright © 1977.

But others were not as convinced as Davies. At the Weizmann Institute in Rehovoth, Israel Pecht and Ruth Arnon, using a variety of experimental techniques and theoretical analysis, provided evidence that antigen-induced changes do occur within the antibody and in one example demonstrated a gain in complement activation by an anti-peptide (a hen-egg lysozyme fragment) antibody when it was complexed with the bivalent form of the peptide antigen but not when the antigen was monovalent.[35] Furthermore, the activation of complement was accompanied by domain changes in the antibody as shown by spectroscopic measurements. Since these reactions were carried out in the solution phase, Pecht and Arnon's conclusions were:

> The data… support… a unique mechanism… for activating the effector functions of antibodies of the IgG class… conformation changes induced both by antigen binding and by cross-linking the two sites of an IgG molecule are essential for the transformation into the active state.[35]

Pecht and others would continue to beat the allostery drum while the field waited for further structural information. For a second intact antibody study it would have to wait until 1983 when Edmundson and colleagues published the structure of yet another hinge-deleted IgG1 myeloma, MCG.[36] This too formed a T-structure although the relationship of the Fab arms to the Fc region was different from Dob or Kol, further obscuring any clear conclusions. At this time large protein structure determination by x-ray crystallography took many years and the 'allosterists' would have to resort to solution phase studies and theoretical arguments until, in 1992, Alexander McPherson at the University of California published the structure of a 'normal' murine IgG2a antibody.

McPherson's structure was only at 3.5Å resolution but this was sufficient to see all the major antibody features and in particular to comment on the 'flexibility of immune response proteins'.[37] This particular antibody assumed a domain relationship that was somewhat different from previous structures in that it showed an asymmetric positioning of the two Fab arms with respect to the Fc region, reflecting what McPherson refers to as an inherent structural variability. In drawing some conclusions about the role of the hinge regions that connect the Fab arms to the Fc region he comments:

> The hinge polypeptides are not really hinges, but rather they are tethers that allow the Fab components to drift from the Fc to bind antigen or potentially allow the Fc to move in such a way to trigger effector functions, such as the activation of complement. The connecting polypeptides gives the Fabs the freedom to move and twist so as to align hypervariable regions with antigenic sites… The antibody is an assembly of units possessing a high degree of flexibility…[37]

Was the jury about to deliver its verdict? A year after McPherson's study, Allen Edmundson returned to the structure of MCG which he had obtained at low resolution in 1983. MCG carried a hinge deletion but oddly was able to bind protein A (a bacterial protein able to bind with high affinity to the C_H2 region) and the high-affinity Fc receptor FcγR1 but not complement. Rather than exhorting an allosteric explanation for complement Edmundson introduced the study by stating in the abstract:

> Potential complement (Clq) binding sites on Fc are sterically shielded by the Fab arms, but putative attachment sites are accessible for docking with the FcR1 receptor on human monocytes and with protein A of Staphylococcus aureus.[38]

Edmundson went on to state in the concluding comments:

> The structure shown... is compatible with the view... that the docking of complement component Clq is obstructed by the Fab arms in IgG proteins without hinge regions.[38]

With Poljak's 1986 lysozyme-anti-lysozyme structure a further nail was put in the conformational casket. When an antigen binds to the tip of the Fab arm any conformational signalling to the Fc region must pass information through the Fab chains in some way. Commenting on the difference between the lysozyme-bound Fab structure and other known unliganded Fab structures Poljak observes:

> ... the angle observed in the lysozyme-Fab D1.3 complex corresponds to that postulated to occur in unliganded Fabs. Thus, the allosteric model of antibodies... in which antigen binding induces changes in quaternary structure resulting in closer contacts across V and C domains is not consistent with the structure of this complex.... No other change of conformation in the antibody or antigen can be established by the present analysis. The classical 'lock and key' metaphor is an adequate simplification...[24]

At this point there seemed to be a convergence of opinion, at least amongst the structural biologists. Normal antibodies (those without hinge deletions) were fully capable of eliciting all sorts of effector functions such as Fc receptor binding, complement activation, and so on. The key seemed to be that subsequent to binding, some other type of activity was required to elicit the full effector response. This might be intracellular signal activation via Fc receptor domains inside the cell, bivalent or multivalent assembly of antigen-antibody complexes on a cell surface that were able to bind complement components with higher affinity than in solution, and so on. The antibody was in fact a flexible, multicomponent vehicle for antigen-induced effector 'assembly' and may not require a complex 'through the polypeptide chain' allosteric change mechanism to accomplish its functions, what this author described as an 'immunological Swiss army knife' in an opening address to the 1990 Biochemical Society main meeting in Bath, UK.

The story does not end there however. As late as January 2013 the debate continues. A group of Italian physical chemists, after analysing different antibody Fab structures, 28 with antigen bound and 28 without antigen bound, drew the following conclusion:

> The use of a common structural reference reveals preferential changes in the dynamic coordination and intramolecular interaction networks induced by antigen binding and shared by all antibodies. Such changes propagate from the binding region through the whole immunoglobulin domains...[39]

This most intriguing aspect of antigen-induced antibody signalling continues to defy a fully acceptable explanation.

Light chain absenteeism in the Tylopoda

In 1993, the extraordinary plasticity of the immune system was further revealed with the discovery of a novel form of antibody in the *Camelids* family (sub-order Tylopoda). Hamers and his team, working at the Free University of Brussels, on fractionation of the serum of camels discovered an antibody species having a molecular weight only two-thirds that of a normal IgG. On further analysis these forms turned out to be heavy chain dimers only, completely lacking light chains.[40] In addition to these heavy chain antibodies the camel also had normal IgG molecules. The heavy chains were however different to normal heavy chains. On reduction they had a molecular weight lower than normal heavy chains. On further examination they were shown to be completely lacking the CH1 domain hitherto present in all gamma heavy chains. In some ways this was logical if there was no light chain with which to form a VL-CH1 interaction. The story did not finish there however. The missing CH1 domain was replaced either by a short or a long hinge region. The long hinge, which could extend to 70Å as the crow flies due to the presence of a particular sequence motif that generates a somewhat rigid rod-like structure, was more than enough to span the distance from the N-terminus of the CH2 domain to the C-terminus of the VH domain in a normal IgG. In the short hinge species the lack of a flexible connection could prevent the two VHH domains coming close to one another and would, Hamers speculated, have restricted their ability to engage in normal IgG functions such as complement binding or antigen cross-linking. The Hamers' graphical representation of the various iso-forms of *camelid* antibodies (known as HCAbs for heavy chain antibodies) is shown in Fig. 11.10.

A number of questions are raised by this novel discovery. The 'why' is not really possible or even profitable to try to answer. The 'what' was explored by Hamers in the initial communication in 1993 and in a series of studies leading to the germ line gene analysis in 2000. From the initial studies a partial 'how' also emerged but new questions were raised. One obvious function question the group asked was 'Does the VH-only immunoglobulin (the terminology was VHH domains) express a large repertoire of antigen-binding capabilities or might it have evolved to satisfy some particular specificity gap in the normal antibody repertoire'? Two facts seemed to provide an answer, if somewhat puzzling from a parsimonious evolution point of view. First, the VHH antibodies represented about 75% of the total protein A binding antibodies (in human IgG all isotypes except IgG3 bind the bacterial IgG-binding protein, protein A, strongly), a result that reflected what must have been an extraordinarily strong selection pressure operating in the *Tylopoda* for this species of antibody. Analysis of the binding capability of the V_HH antibodies showed a wide antigen recognition capability, dispelling the notion that this form of antibody might have evolved to meet a very specific niche role. In follow-on studies, the Belgian group began to piece together a remarkably interesting story that may have reflected the use of genetic elements from both mammalian and avian sequence diversification mechanisms. In 2000, Nguyen and the Belgian team published analysis of the dromedary immunoglobulin V-region germ line sequences and via cDNA analysis, the expressed V_HH region sequences.[41] Several surprising results emerged. Firstly, the VHH genes seemed to have evolved with the VH subgroup III, suggesting a focused gene duplication and diversification origin. Within this group

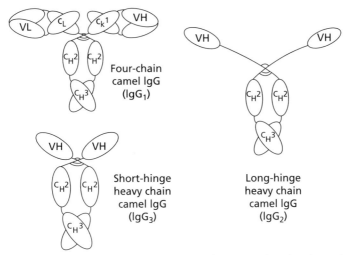

Fig. 11.10 Cartoons of the normal Camel IgG (top left), the HCab with either a short hinge (lower left) or a long hinge (right).

Reprinted by permission of Macmillan Publishers Ltd: *Nature*, Hamers-Casterman, C. et al., Naturally occurring antibodies devoid of light chains, Volume 363, Issue 6428, pp. 446–448, Copyright © 1993.

of VHH genes, representing about half the number present in the human VH gene repertoire, an additional disulphide bond was present that may stabilize the domain and diverse CDR sequences were observed. An equivalent number of normal germ line VH genes were also present in the *camelid* genome. In the cDNA sequences further CDR diversification was seen including a high frequency of somatic changes and the presence of long CDR sequences that may have arisen by a gene replacement mechanism during rearrangement (see Chapter 12). Perhaps the most extraordinary finding was suggested by performing a Kabat sequence-variability analysis of the cDNA sequences of the VHH domains (see Fig. 11.11). Subsequent x-ray structural analysis established that this new CDR does make antigen contact and extends the surface area of the VHH domain available for binding.[42,43]

The discovery of a different form of mammalian antibody (the IgH isotype?) existing in a single taxonomic group inhabiting a relatively restricted geographical area raises interesting questions about the genetic events that may have led to this divergence by the normal mammalian antibody genome. Are there, for example, specific immunological advantages to small binding domains for protection against particular forms of antigenic insult that may be endemic in tropical regions of the world? Whatever the answers, a selective advantage must have been introduced in order for this genetic variation to have been maintained so vigorously. More than ten years on, those answers must also explain the presence of similar heavy chain antibodies in cartilaginous fish, discovered in 2011 by Juarez and colleagues at the Department of Marine Biotechnology, Centro de Investigacion Cientifica y de Educacion Superior de Ensenada, Ensenada, Baja California, Mexico.[44] As Muyldermans from the *camelid* Belgian group comments in a 2013 review of the single domain antibody area:

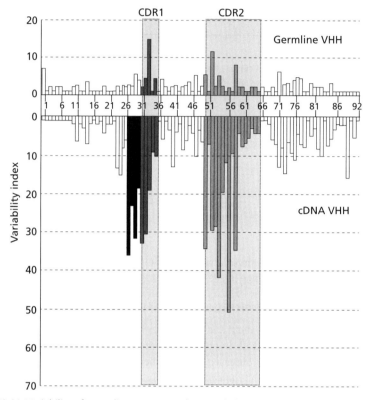

Fig. 11.11 Variability of germ line sequences (upper plot) and 103 cDNA sequences (lower plot) from the VHH regions of dromedary HCAbs. The black bars signify the additional CDR four region spanning residues 27–30.

Reprinted by permission of Macmillan Publishers Ltd: *The EMBO Journal*, Nguyen, V.K.et al., Camel heavy-chain antibodies: diverse germline VHH and specific mechanisms enlarge the antigen binding repertoire, Volume 19, Number 5, pp. 921–30, Copyright © 2000.

> The genetic elements composing HCAbs have been identified, but the in vivo generation of these antibodies from their dedicated genes into antigen-specific and affinity-matured bona fide antibodies remains largely under-investigated.[45]

Their evolutionary significance also remains to be explained. Does the genome of the mammalian immune system hold further secrets yet to be uncovered? We await the next decade with anticipation and perhaps even with some apprehension about its further complexities.

Acknowledgements

Text extracts from Kabat, E.A. and Wu, T.T., Attempts to locate complementarity determining residues in the variable positions of light and heavy chains, *Annals of the New York Academy of Sciences*, Volume 190, pp. 382–393, Copyright © 1971 The New York Academy of Sciences, with permission from John Wiley and Sons.

Text extract reproduced with permission from H.M. Berman, et al. *The Protein Data Bank Nucleic Acids Research*, Volume 28, pp. 235–242, Copyright © 2000 RCSB Protein Data Bank, www.rcsb.org

Text extract reprinted from the *Journal of Molecular Biology*, Volume 100, Issue 3, Colman, P.M. et al., Structure of the Human Antibody Molecule Kol (Immunoglobulin G1): An Electron Density Map at 5Å Resolution, pp. 257–282, Copyright © 1976 with permission from Elsevier: http://www.sciencedirect.com/science/journal/00222836

Text extracts reprinted by permission of Macmillan Publishers Ltd: *Nature*, Amit, A.G. et al., Three-dimensional structure of an antigen-antibody complex at 6Å resolution, Volume 313, pp. 156–158, Copyright © 1985.

References

1. **Milstein, C.** (1967). 'Linked groups of residues in immunoglobulin κ chains.' *Nature*, **216**: 330–2.
2. **Kabat, E. A.** (1968). 'Unique features of the variable regions of Bence Jones proteins and their possible relation to antibody complementarity.' *Proc. Natl. Acad. Sci.*, **59**: 613–19.
3. **Franěk, F.** (1970). In J. Šterzl and I. Řiha (eds), *Developmental Aspects of Antibody Formation and Structure*, pp. 311–13. New York: Academic Press.
4. **Wu, T. T., and Kabat, E. A.** (1970). 'An analysis of the sequences of the variable regions of Bence Jones proteins and myeloma light chains and their implications for antibody complementarity.' *J. Exp. Med.*, **132**: 211–50.
5. **Hood, L. E., Wu, T. T., and Kabat, E. A.** (2008). 'A Transforming View of Antibody Diversity.' *J. Immunol.*, **180**: 7055–6.
6. **Weigert, M. G., Cesari, I. M., Yonkovich, S. J., and Cohn, M.** (1970). 'Variability in the lambda light chain sequences of mouse antibody.' *Nature*, **228**: 1045–7.
7. **Capra, J. D.** (1971). 'Hypervariable region of human immunoglobulin heavy chains.' *Nature New Biol.*, **230**: 61–3.
8. **Kehoe, J. M., and Capra, J. D.** (1971). 'Localization of two additional hypervariable regions in immunoglobulin heavy chains.' *Proc. Natl. Acad. Sci.*, **68**: 2019–21.
9. **Kabat, E. A., and Wu, T. T.** (1971). 'Attempts to locate complementarity-determining residues in the variable positions of light and heavy chains.' *Ann. N.Y. Acad. Sci.*, **190**: 382–93.
10. **Kabat, E. A., and Wu, T. T.** (1972). 'Construction of a Three-Dimensional Model of the Polypeptide Backbone of the Variable Region of Kappa Immunoglobulin Light Chains.' *Proc. Natl. Acad. Sci.*, **69**: 960–4.
11. **Poljak, R. J., Amzel, L. M., Avey, H. P., Becka, L. N., and Nisonoff, A.** (1972). 'Structure of Fab NEW at 6Å Resolution.' *Nature New Biol.*, **235**: 421–5.
12. **Poljak, R. J., Amzel, H. P., Avey, H. P., Chen, R. P., Phizackerley, R. P., and Saul, F.** (1973). 'Three-dimensional structure of the Fab' fragment of a human immunoglobulin at 2.8Å resolution.' *Proc. Natl. Acad. Sci.*, **70**: 3305–10.
13. **Schiffer, M., Girling, R. L., Ely, K. R., and Edmundson, A. B.** (1973). 'Structure of a λ-Type Bence-Jones Protein at 3.5- Å Resolution.' *Biochemistry*, **12**: 4620–31.
14. **RCSB Protein Data Bank**, 'Looking at Structures: Resolution', available from http://www.rcsb.org/pdb/101/static101.do?p=education_discussion/Looking-at-Structures/resolution.html

15. **Poljak, R. J., Amzel, H. P., Chen, R. P., Phizackerley, R. P., and Saul, F.** (1974). 'Three-dimensional structure of the Fab' fragment of a human myeloma immunoglobulin at 2.0Å resolution.' *Proc. Natl. Acad. Sci.*, **71**: 3440–4.

16. **Epp, O., Colman, P., Fehlhammer, H., Bode, W., Schiffer, M., and Huber, R.** (1974). 'Crystal and Molecular Structure of a Dimer Composed of the Variable Portions of the Bence-Jones Protein RE1.' *Eur. J. Biochem.*, **45**: 513–24.

17. **Padlan, E. A., Segal, D. M., Spande, T. F., Davies, D. R., Rudikoff, S., and Potter, M.** (1973). 'Structure at 4.5Å resolution of a phosphorylcholine-binding Fab.' *Nature New Biol.*, **245**: 165–7.

18. **Segal, D. M., Padlan, E. A., Cohen, G. H., Rudikoff, S., Potter, M., and Davies, D. R.** (1974). 'The Three-Dimensional Structure of a Phosphorylcholine-Binding Mouse Immunoglobulin Fab and the Nature of the Antigen Binding Site.' *Proc. Natl. Acad. Sci.*, **71**: 4298–302.

19. **Levitt, M., and Chothia, C.** (1976). 'Structural patterns in globular proteins.' *Nature*, **261**: 552–8.

20. **Richardson, J.** (1981). 'The anatomy and taxonomy of protein structure.' *Adv. Prot. Chem.*, **34**: 167–339.

21. **Novotný. J., Bruccoleri, R., Newell, J., Murphy, D., Haber, E., and Karplus, M.** (1983). 'Molecular anatomy of the antibody binding site.' *J. Biol. Chem.*, **258**: 14433–7.

22. **Chothia, C., Novotný, J., Bruccoleri, R., and Karplus, M.** (1985). 'Domain association in immunoglobulin molecules. The packing of variable domains.' *J. Mol. Biol.*, **186**: 651–63.

23. **Amit, A. G., Mariuzza, R. A., Phillips, S. E. V., and Poljak, R. J.** (1985). 'Three-dimensional structure of an antigen-antibody complex at 6Å resolution.' *Nature*, **313**: 156–8.

24. **Amit, A. G., Mariuzza, R. A., Phillips, S. E. V., and Poljak, R. J.** (1986). 'Three-dimensional structure of an antigen-antibody complex at 2.8Å resolution.' *Science*, **233**: 747–53.

25. **Chothia, C., Lesk, A. M., Levitt, M., Amit, A. G., Mariuzza, R. A., Phillips, S. E. V., and Poljak, R. J.** (1986). 'The Predicted Structure of Immunoglobulin D1.3 and its Comparison with the Crystal Structure.' *Science*, **233**: 755–8.

26. **Chothia, C., and Lesk, A. M.** (1987). 'Canonical Structures for the Hypervariable Regions of Immunoglobulins.' *J. Mol. Biol.*, **196**: 901–17.

27. **Amzel, L. M., Poljak, R. J., Saul, F., Varga, J. M., and Richards, F. M.** (1974). 'The Three Dimensional Structure of a Combining Region-Ligand Complex of Immunoglobulin NEW at 3.5- Å Resolution.' *Proc. Natl. Acad. Sci.*, **71**: 1427–30.

28. **Valentine, R. C., and Green, N. M.** (1967). 'Electron Microscopy of an Antibody-Hapten Complex.' *J. Mol. Biol.*, **27**: 615–17.

29. **Sarma, V. R., Silverton, E. W., Davies, D. R., and Terry, W. D.** (1971). 'The three-dimensional structure at 6Å resolution of a human gG1 immunoglobulin molecule.' *J. Biol. Chem.*, **246**: 3753–9.

30. **Labaw, L. W., and Davies, D. R.** (1971). 'An electron microscopoic study of gG1 immuno-globulin crystals.' *J. Biol. Chem.*, **246**: 3760–2.

31. **Bretscher, P. A., and Cohn, M.** (1968). 'Minimal model for the mechanism of antibody induction and paralysis by antigen.' *Nature*, **220**: 444–8.

32. **Colman, P. M., Deisenhofer, J., Huber, R., and Palm, W.** (1976). 'Structure of the Human Antibody Molecule Kol (Immunoglobulin G1): An Electron Density Map at 5Å Resolution.' *J. Mol. Biol.*, **100**: 257–82.

33. **Silverton, E. W., Navia, M. A., and Davies, D. R.** (1977). 'Three-dimensional structure of an intact human immunoglobulin.' *Proc. Natl. Acad. Sci.*, **74**: 5140–4.

34. **Yguerabide, J., Epstein, H. F., and Stryer, L.** (1970). 'Segmental flexibility in an antibody molecule.' *J. Mol. Biol.*, **51**: 573–90.

35. **Pecht, I., Ehrenberg, B., Calef, E., and Arnon, R.** (1977). 'Conformation changes and complement activation induced upon antigen binding to antibodies.' *Biochem. Biophys. Res. Commun.*, **74**: 1302–19.

36. **Rajan, S. S., Ely, K. R., Abola, E. E., Wood, M. K., Colman, P. M., Athay, R. J., and Edmundson, A. B.** (1983). 'Three-dimensional structure of the Mcg IgG1 immunoglobulin.' *Mol. Immunol.*, **20**: 787–99.

37. **Harris, L. J., Larson, S. B., Hasel, K. W., Day, J., Greenwood, A., and McPherson, A.** (1992). 'The three-dimensional structure of an intact monoclonal antibody for canine lymphoma.' *Nature*, **360**: 369–72.

38. **Gudat, L. W., Herron, J. N., and Edmundson, A. B.** (1993). 'Three-dimensional structure of a human immunoglobulin with a hinge deletion.' *Proc. Natl. Acad. Sci.*, **90**: 4271–5.

39. **Corrada, D., Morra, G., and Colombo, G.** (2013). 'Investigating Allostery in Molecular Recognition: Insights from a Computational Study of Multiple Antibody–Antigen Complexes.' *J. Phys. Chem. B.*, **117**: 535–52.

40. **Hamers-Casterman, C., Atarhouch, T., Muyldermans, S., Robinson, G., Hamers, C., Songa, E. B., Bendahman, N., and Hamers, R.** (1993). 'Naturally occurring antibodies devoid of light chains.' *Nature*, **363**: 446–8.

41. **Nguyen, V. K., Hamers, R., Wyns, L., and Muyldermans, S.** (2000). 'Camel heavy-chain antibodies: diverse germline *VHH* and specific mechanisms enlarge the antigen binding repertoire.' *The EMBO Journal*, **19**: 921–30.

42. **Desmyter, A., Transue, T. R., Ghahroudi, M. A., Thi, M. H., Poortmans, F., Hamers, R., Muyldermans, S., and Wyns, L.** (1996). 'Crystal structure of a camel single-domain VH antibody fragment in complex with lysozyme.' *Nature Struct. Biol.*, **3**: 803–11.

43. **Decanniere, K., Desmyter, A., Lauwereys, M., Ghahroudi, M. A., Muyldermans, S., and Wyns, L.** (1999). 'A single-domain antibody in complex with RNase A: non-canonical loop structures and nanomolar affinity using two CDR loops.' *Structure*, **7**: 361–70.

44. **Juarez, K., Dubberke, G., Lugo, P., Koch-Nolte, F., Buck, F., Haag, F., and Licea, A.** (2011). 'Monoclonal antibodies for the identification and purification of vNAR domains and IgNAR immunoglobulins from the horn shark *Heterodontus francisci*.' *Hybridoma (Larchmt).*, **30**: 323–9.

45. **Muyldermans, S.** (2013). 'Nanobodies: natural single domain antibodies.' *Ann. Rev. Biochem.*, **82**: 775–97.

Chapter 12

Monoclonal antibodies and the mechanisms of hypermutation

The antibody gene enigma

It has been said that the 1960s was the decade that saw the biggest changes in modern history, a decade of flamboyance, inventiveness, and social revolution that saw man on the moon for the first time. For molecular immunologists it was a decade of frustration interspersed with periods of scintillating enlightenment. By 1970 the organization of antibody protein chains, the presence of immunoglobulin G isotypes and allotypes, progress in understanding the special characteristics of IgA, IgM, IgD, and IgE, models for the action of the multi-protein complement system, and concepts on how immune competence was transferred from mother to young were known or actively being worked on, and much, much more. However, one question that continued to evade explanation was how antibody diversity was generated in the adult animal. The 'large number of germ line antibody genes' versus a 'small number of genes accompanied by extensive somatic mutation' theories were still the subject of hot debate, fuelled by contradictory and puzzling observations as well as predispositions about the genetic mechanisms available to mammalian immune systems (see Chapter 7). The nub of the problem was illustrated by Milstein and Pink in a review on the structure and evolution of immunoglobulins.[1] The evolutionary conundrum pointed out by Milstein was as follows. Assuming a common ancestor model for immunoglobulins followed by Darwinian evolution it would be expected and is the case that different mammalian species would have species-specific sequences in their immunoglobulin chains (he uses λ light chains as an example). Milstein argues that this is difficult to reconcile with the existence of multiple genes:

> It is easy to see that the 'invariant residues' of the N-regions present in a large set of ancestor genes [assuming the many germ line gene model] should have been largely preserved and be common in different species, which does not seem to be the case.[1]

On the other hand, if there were only a small number of germ line genes then:

> …a simple evolutionary tree model would imply that each of them should be recognized in the different species. Such a simple evolutionary tree is unsatisfactory because although human basic sequences appear to be old in evolution corresponding basic sequences are not obvious in other species.[1]

To explain this apparent contradiction Milstein postulates a small number of germ line genes accompanied by accumulation of species differences introduced late in evolution either during speciation or via somatic mutations, or a combination of both. His illustration of this concept, with the implicit assumption that gene duplication and gene elimination are reasonably common events during evolution, is shown in Fig. 12.1.

It is never sufficient for great scientists to acknowledge problems without providing a way forward. Milstein's marker in the sand was clearly for the somatic mutation model:

> No simple model for a somatic origin of the diversity seems entirely satisfactory. One plausible model, which adds an integration mechanism to the original Brenner and Milstein proposal can be summarized as follows. There are a discrete number of genes in the germ line to code for the variable sections (say 10 for human kappa chains). Some of these genes may contain allelic forms giving rise to some of the repeated variants. Somatic point mutations give rise to low frequency variants, to the 'hot spots' and some of the repeated variants. A selective process after the somatic mutation must take place, in which the antigen plays a major role.[1]

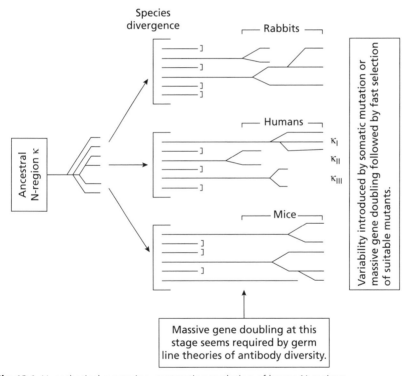

Fig. 12.1 Hypothetical expansion-contraction evolution of kappa N-regions.

This illustrates the effect of gene doubling and gene elimination (shown as]) in the evolutionary origin of the basic sequences of human kappa chains and their weak homology with possible basic sequences of other species.

The Brenner and Milstein proposal Milstein refers to was discussed in Chapter 7. What was required to answer the question was a method for reproducing antibody evolution on the timescale of 'a human scientific career', a method that would enable a single antibody's sequence changes to be followed during the lifetime of an individual anti-gen's exposure to the immune system. But IgG molecules had a relatively short lifetime (~one month in humans) and anyway how could a single molecule in a myriad of other antibodies be identified? The answer could only come from being able to follow the product of an individual antibody-producing B-cell. This presupposed of course that the generally accepted 'one cell, one antibody' clonal theory was correct which was not yet fully proven, notwithstanding the work of Nossal and Lederberg (see Chapter 5).

Driven by the feeling that protein chemistry may not yield the answers and now at the MRC in Cambridge, Milstein made a bold move along with his friend George Brownlee, triggered perhaps by his laboratory neighbour Fred Sanger who was at this time developing new methods for sequencing messenger RNA (mRNA). Yet again, a technical breakthrough opened doors to new approaches. In 1971, Stavnezer and Huang at Johns Hopkins had just published a method for translating mRNA from cells in an *in vitro* cell lysate system from reticulocytes. This allowed them to take immu-noglobulin light chain mRNA prepared from a myeloma (tumour and/or derived cell line) and produce a light chain protein encoded by the RNA 'in the test tube'.[2] A year later Brownlee and Milstein, employing the same approach but with a different cellular source of cell-free translation machinery, repeated and published the *in vitro* synthesis of a myeloma kappa chain and indicated in the last sentence of the publication that they may also have identified a 'light chain precursor'.[3] Later the same year, Milstein's team confirmed the light chain precursor identifying a protein chain modified at its N-terminus by a sequence of amino acids that was not visible in Porter or Edelman's rabbit chains. Milstein was circumspect in his interpretation of the data, perhaps apply-ing his own dictum absorbed from day-to-day association with Max Perutz, head of the MRC Cambridge laboratory and the inimitable Fred Sanger, 'Do good experiments and don't worry about the rest'.[4] While the complete sequence of the putative precursor was not fully established Milstein suggested it may allow membrane association of the precursor protein that would be required for secretion:

> Our results could throw light on the mechanism of secretion … It seems to us that a short amino acid sequence at the N-terminus of a precursor protein would be a simple way to provide such a signal.[5]

Preferring to use mRNA prepared from cells in culture rather than from solid tumours, Milstein and Brownlee prepared mRNA radiolabelled in cell-tissue culture (using high specific activity phosphorus 32 isotope labelling) and attempted to obtain RNA sequence information. RNA sequencing at this time was rather primitive. The radi-olabelled mRNA was cut into oligonucleotide segments with an RNAse enzyme that cleaved RNA at every guanine base. Further fragmentation by different ribonuclease enzymes followed by separation in two dimensions (electrophoresis then chromatog-raphy) allowed partial identification of fragments. The sequence of the intact mRNA molecule or large fragments of it produced by the first RNAse digestion could then be deduced by alignment of partially overlapping oligonucleotides.[6] Similar methods using proteases had been used by Porter, Edelman, and others for the protein sequencing of antibody chains. Phew! No methods were available at this time that enabled the complete sequence of RNA molecules to be easily determined, although Sanger was 'working on it'. The lengthy experiments Brownlee and Milstein carried out in this study laid to rest at least one of the older theories of immunoglobulin chain assembly that allowed for V and C chains to be assembled at or subsequent to protein synthesis on the ribosome, and revealed their proclivity for gene assembly occurring at a much earlier stage:

> The sequences isolated [mRNA] derive from both the V and C halves of the light chain, indicating that there is a single mRNA molecule for both variable and constant regions. Integration of V and C genes seems therefore likely to occur by rearrangement of DNA during differentiation.[5]

The search for a system by which somatic mutation could be studied led Milstein towards myeloma cells that could be cultured *in vitro* through many generations of division in the hope of identifying spontaneous somatic changes. By propagation of different myeloma 'clones' in the presence of a radiolabelled amino acid (lysine containing carbon 14, or ^{14}C) antibody protein could be isolated over time and sequenced to identify whether mutations were accumulating in the hypervariable regions. Early experiments were disappointing. Mutants were found but tended to be structurally deleterious to the antibody rather than at sites likely to be able to influence antigen specificity.[7] The hunt for a system by which antibodies could be synthesized in single clones of antibody-producing cells was sharpened by the work of Mohit published in 1971 in what would turn out to be a sort of mirror image of what Milstein would eventually discover. Mohit, working at the NIH, was able to fuse IgG-producing myeloma cells with non-antibody-producing lymphoma cells to form hybrid cells.[8] Selected clones of the resulting hybrid contained the genes for and produced both heavy chains and light chains and intact immunoglobulin. This study sought to explore why previous experiments in which myeloma cells had been fused to non-immune cells had failed to produce immunoglobulin. Mohit's results suggested that the genes for light chains and heavy chains were likely to be on different chromosomes and that chromosome loss could explain the failed previous attempts. His clones that were successfully producing antibody had higher chromosome numbers than the light chain-only-producing clones, supporting the chromosome loss argument.

In Cambridge a different approach was being taken. Richard Cotton, visiting from the University of Melbourne and working in Milstein's laboratory, fused two antibody-producing myeloma cell lines from different species, mouse and rat, with a somewhat surprising result. The hybrid myeloma exhibited co-dominant expression of both sets of antibody chains, apparently contradicting the allelic exclusion rule. Not only were the parent antibodies present but also light chain-heavy chain hybrids, as would be expected from random sorting and assembly during expression. However, there was no evidence for V-C resorting confirming earlier conclusions that V-C assembly had already taken place and could not therefore occur at the RNA or protein synthesis level.[9]

Was allelic exclusion demonstrable in normal B-cells? In 1965 Pernis, Gell, and colleagues in a collaborative study between the University of Milan and Birmingham (UK) showed that only one of two possible alleles were expressed in antibody-producing cells visualized in sections of lymph-node and spleen tissue based on the level of labelling produced by fluorescent antibodies directed against two different allotypic markers. This was contrary to previous results of Colberg and Dray who in 1964 had shown chains containing both allotypic markers within the same cell, using similar techniques.[10] In a follow-up study, reported at a 1967 Cold Spring Harbor meeting, Pernis confirmed and extended his 1965 results observing:

> … separate cells producing the 'allotype-lacking' chains, and with localization in different cells of allelic markers present in heterozygous individuals.[11] *(Author's bold.)*

While Cotton and Milstein's results might have appeared to confirm Colberg and Dray's results, their interpretation was in line with that of Pernis:

> The presence of Ig hybrid molecules indicates that… both parental genes are expressed in the same individual cell… The simplest explanation seems to be that restricted expression of V and C genes is caused by the presence in the parental cells of single already integrated V-C genes.[9]

The message was that in myelomas the antibody gene assembly was already complete. Control of antibody chains was in *cis* so that introduction of genes from another cell encoding a different set of antibody chains would receive no allelic restriction signal and both sets of antibodies would be expressed.

Despite the success of hybrid cells produced by cell-fusion techniques, the holy grail of a single antibody-producing cell whose hypermutation progression over time could be followed was still concealed. The other part of the puzzle was that in order to interpret the mutational data in terms of somatic 'improvement' an antigenic activity should be present for the antibody and measurable. So why not consider selecting and then propagating the antibody-producing plasma B-cell as a production vehicle? It was not obvious how to go about this since it was known from many published studies that spleen cells had a limited lifetime in culture.

Proving the clonal integrity of antibody-producing cells

During the 1960s the single cell clone experiment was explored in a number of places and by different approaches. One of the cleverest experimental regimes was developed in 1965 by John Playfair and Ben Pappermaster of UC Berkeley collaborating with the US Naval Radiation Defense laboratory. Playfair transferred spleen cells from normal mice to syngeneic mice whose normal lymphocyte population had been ablated by high-dose irradiation. This was then followed by injection of sheep erythrocytes into the irradiated mice. After eight days the spleens were examined and searched for the presence of specific 'active areas' producing antibodies able to lyse the erythrocytes. Not only were active areas found but two different active antibody zones could be found when pig erythrocytes were also injected, suggesting the donor spleen cells were viable for generating different antigen specificities. Playfair's interpretation of these remarkable experiments, reflecting the still uncertain question on the clonal integrity of antibody-producing cells, was:

> We conclude that if single precursor cells are in fact responsible for the areas of localized antibody formation, which are apparently of a single specificity, the progeny of each pre-cursor must be restricted to forming exclusively, or predominantly, a single type of antibody. Whether this restriction is imposed by contact with the antigen, or whether it is inherent in the pre-cursor cell itself, remains to be demonstrated.[12]

Of course, this was not an approach that would yield antibodies in any quantity. The further development of this experimental system was made by Brigitte Askonas and Alan Williamson at the National Institute for Medical Research (London) in 1970. As with Playfair, antigen reactive clones of murine B-cells were propagated through irradiated syngeneic mice but this time by sequential transfer of spleen cells (attempted by Playfair but with poor retention of spleen-cell activity) through multiple generations of irradiated mice and measurement of the retention of antigen reactivity. Survival of the transferred clone, which was antigen-dependent and presumed to be mediated by memory B-cells, was considerable (up to six months) but was more limited if the interval between transfers was too long (~65 day limit) suggesting a limited lifetime for the clones, postulated to be memory cells, carrying the specific antibody specificity.[13] While theoretically valuable as a means of measuring memory-cell longevity, a methodology that required propagation of antibody-producing cells through animals was not a particularly easy addition to the immunological toolbox.

Further evidence for the 'clonal selection' theory was obtained in 1969 by Norman Klinman, working in the University of Pennsylvania School of Medicine. Klinman's approach came closer perhaps than any other being pursued at the time to establishing the monoclonality of B-cells. Klinman immunized normal mice for four to eight months with the hapten-protein conjugate dinitrophenyl-haemocyanin before their spleen cells were introduced into irradiated mice. *In vitro* cultures of the irradiated mouse spleens, stimulated by addition of antigen, were then maintained for two to four weeks during which time antibodies were collected from various foci ('monofocal antibodies') and their binding affinities to the hapten-conjugate measured. Klinman's results still allowed the possibility that multiple antibodies were generated within a single clone, forcing him to conclude:

> Following the basic predictions of the 'clonal selection hypothesis', the immunocompetent cell is visualized as a cell that possesses genetic information for the production of one or very few... immunoglobulin primary amino acid sequences... The clonal progeny of such a cell would exhibit the same specificity.[14]

A somewhat different story unfolded with the publications in 1969 and 1970 by Joseph Sinkovics at the M.D. Anderson Hospital in Texas. Sinkovics was studying murine leukaemia virus-producing lymphoma cells and had observed that certain cell lines derived from fusion of the lymphoma with immune spleen cells produced both virus and antibody in the same cells. These cells could be grown is suspension culture allowing the possibility of antibody production. One particular cell line appeared to produce multiple antibody isotypes (IgG1 and IgG2a) in the same cell, reminiscent of the myeloma fusion results of Cotton and Milstein. This study was however directed more to understanding the underlying mechanisms of leukaemia virus infection than producing antibodies *in vitro*, despite the 'apologia' published by Sinkovics in 1981 some six years after the discovery of monoclonal antibodies.

Myelomas, spontaneous tumours for which the discovery of cognate antigens was at best down to serendipity and at worst, impossible were not ideal but they were the best tool available. In 1973 Milstein presented his results with Cotton on the myeloma-myeloma fusion experiments at a seminar in the Basel Institute of Immunology. During this visit he met Georges Köhler. Köhler was 27 years old and finishing his PhD on the immune response to the bacterial enzyme beta-galactosidase, working with Fritz Melchers while on secondment in Basel. As Melchers recollects,[15] Köhler wished to study somatic mutations in antibody-producing cells by studying single cell clonal growth over multiple generations, the exact same reason Milstein was studying myelomas. Köhler applied for and received an EMBO post-doctoral fellowship to work in Milstein's laboratory at the MRC in 1974. The story goes that Milstein invited Köhler to study the P3 myeloma cell line, developed by Horibata at the Salk Institute and derived from the MOPC-21 myeloma, to try to find its antigen. This would enable a return to the myeloma culture and screening experiments but would now be armed with a means of identifying clones that had altered antigen binding, always with the caveat that altered binding could be due to drastic changes in the antibody as well as discrete mutations within the hypervariable regions. It appears that at this point Köhler (see Fig. 12.2a) proposed an alternative strategy which Milstein (see Fig. 12.2b) had not considered. The 'strange idea' was to fuse the myeloma with an antibody-producing B-cell. The problem was not trivial since Köhler had to devise a way of selecting the hybrid cells in the presence of a proliferating myeloma producing its own antibody. By the spring of 1975 he and Milstein had solved the problem. In May they submitted the paper to *Nature* and it appeared in August after only six weeks of review.

Oddly, despite the subsequent perfectly justified fanfares, the editorial team of *Nature* in which the work appeared had not seen it as enough of a breakthrough to highlight the paper in its 'News and Views' section. Some of the opinion leaders of the time were similarly 'underwhelmed'. In a Wellcome-Trust-supported 'History of Twentieth Century Medicine Group Witness Seminar' held in 1984, Sir James Gowans, who in 1977 was Secretary to the UK Medical Research Council (and who introduced this author to the problem of antibody transport at the end of the 1970s), admitted:

> I don't remember being shattered... I remember being mightily intrigued.[16]

Brigitte Askonas (known as Ita and who sadly passed away early in 2013) observed:

> I remember the excitement, although the report of the first antigen specific hybridoma was not shattering.[15]

The failure to protect the 'invention' has been more than amply discussed elsewhere (see Milstein's short review in 2000[18]). In the mid-1970s the new age of biotechnology was only just emerging. There was not yet an Amgen while Genentech formed in 1976 was not in the antibody area. Cetus, formed much earlier (1971) did not enter the

(a)

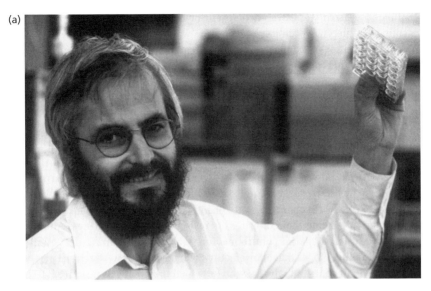

(b)

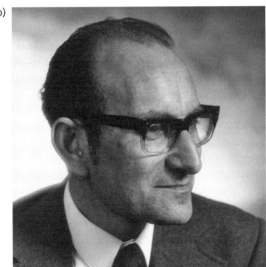

Fig. 12.2 (a) Georges Köhler and (b) Cesar Milstein.

(a) Reproduced with permission from Rolf Haid, DPA and IBL Bildbyrå, Sweden; (b) Image IM/GA/RGRS/7953, Copyright © Godfrey Argent Studio. Reproduced by permission of The Royal Society, London, UK.

antibody area until around 1981. The specialist antibody company, Hybritech, formed to exploit monoclonal antibody technology, appeared in 1978. With no UK patent and the paper published in 1975, the field was an open intellectual property-free landscape. In the UK, the seeds of the biotechnology revolution had not even been sown. Seeing the commercial potential of a single discovery is an art that the National Research and Development Corporation, the UK's central commercial exploitation body for all

UK-funded research, was naively deficient in, or as Milstein more politely puts it '... the patenting philosophy within this organization was conservative'.[18] Whatever the reasons, it has been suggested that UK plc missed out big time. The more lenient, though of course in hindsight, view might be that since only two antibodies had made it to the market (Orthoclone OKT3 for reversal of kidney transplant rejection and Reopro for prevention of blood clots in angioplasty) within the patent time period likely to have applied (assuming no continuation patents to extend the lifetime of the original discovery) there would have been a limited exploitation loss.

A key technique employed by Köhler made use of the methods described 14 years earlier by Littlefield working on cell fusion at the Massachusetts General Hospital. Prior to Littlefield's work, cell fusion had generated hybrids plus the starting cells with no easy way to deselect the non-fused cells since the fusion process was quite inefficient. Littlefield isolated mutants of his starting cell lines each of which was deficient in an enzyme that conferred its resistance to certain drugs. After carrying out the fusion a special culture medium was used containing drugs and crucial DNA building blocks that allowed only the hybrid to grow—each cell partner in the fusion would contribute the enzyme for which the other was negative.[17] Köhler's system was a little simpler since the spleen cells he was to use had only a limited life anyway so that the selection element for these cells was essentially 'time'. The first step was to develop a myeloma whose growth could be selectively inhibited. An 8-azaguanine resistant myeloma cell line was generated that lacked the enzyme hypoxanthine-guanine phosphoribosyltransferase, HPRT. *Note*: in non-resistant (i.e. normal) cells 8-azaguanine acts as an 'abnormal' substrate for HPRT leading to non-functional purine nucleotides and eventual cell death. The HPRT⁻ myeloma was then fused with spleen cells from a mouse previously immunized with sheep red blood cells (SRBC) using Sendai virus which promotes membrane fusion. By growing the fusion mixture in a medium containing hypoxanthine, aminopterin, and thymidine [known as HAT) only the fused myeloma–spleen-cell fusion cells survive. This is because in the presence of aminopterin, a folic acid inhibitor, the *de novo* pathway to nucleotide synthesis is blocked so that the myeloma cell has no mechanism remaining for syntheses of its DNA building blocks, having now lost the HPRT salvage pathway and the *de novo* pathway. The hybrid however obtains its HPRT from the spleen cells and therefore has an intact salvage pathway provided it has access to the building block hypoxanthine with which to make IMP and then on to GMP and AMP, and to thymidine. After some days the spleen cells also die, leaving fused cells only as survivors. Colonies of hybrid cells were seen after a few weeks and by exposing the cells to SRBC the presence of secreted antibody could be seen by haemolysis of the red blood cells (see Fig. 12.3). This was not however a perfectly clean experiment, great advance that it was. The myeloma partner in the hybrid still expressed its own antibody and continued to do so after fusion so that as with the myeloma-myeloma fusion of Cotton and Milstein, two sets of antibodies plus hybrid chain antibodies were also produced. The myeloma-antibody chains could be analysed and identified since the sequences were known to Köhler and Milstein. Of course, this could be simplified going forward by selecting myeloma cell lines that

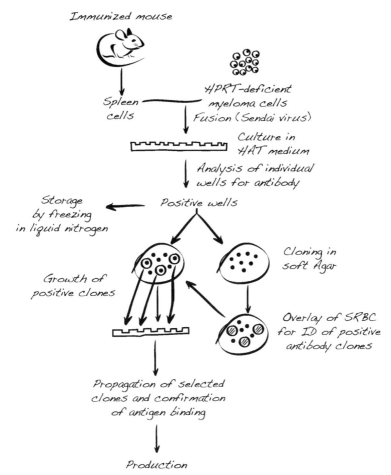

Fig. 12.3 The hybridoma method.

Source: data from Köhler, G. & Milstein, C., Continuous cultures of fused cells secreting antibody of predefined specificity. *Nature*, 1975, 256, 495–497. Copyright © 1975. Cartoon drawn by the author.

did not express any antibody, as suggested by the authors and later incorporated. In concluding this momentous development, Köhler and Milstein commented:

> It is possible to hybridise antibody-producing cells from different origins. Such cells can be grown in vitro in massive cultures to provide specific antibody. Such cultures could be valuable for medical and industrial use.[18]

The hybridoma technology development was not without its vexatious moments. A not-uncommon problem of reproducibility with a new complex set of biological techniques beset the team in Cambridge and also that of Köhler now back in Basel. It seems that a key set of reagents (the HAT medium) had been prepared by a different set of hands that failed to reproduce the exact chemical composition. The new formula resulted in hybrid cell death no doubt causing enormous consternation amongst the respective teams. Long telephone conversations between Milstein and Köhler, allegedly, were not helpful. It appears that a newcomer to the MRC laboratory, Giovanni Galfré, discovered the problem giving rise to an improved protocol, as Milstein himself recites in his Nobel lecture.[4] Writing later in a retrospective at the turn of this century, Milstein also draws attention to a disappointment with the fact that *in vitro* somatic mutation studies using the monoclonal technology were not that successful, an application that was redressed somewhat ironically by the myeloma-myeloma fusion methods that had originally proved inadequate:

> The antibody producing cells that we derived initially did not fulfill their intended purpose because we subsequently failed in our attempts to generate somatic mutants affecting binding sites.[19]

The search for models to explain affinity maturation

What Milstein had hoped was that monoclonal antibodies in culture might allow somatic changes in response to antigen challenge leading to affinity improvement to be followed over time. His early experiments with Cotton using purely myeloma fusions had generated largely deleterious mutations but it turned out this was not a *sine qua non* of the myeloma system. The experience of others working with myelomas and with the same objective of unravelling somatic mechanisms suggested this system did have something to offer. A particularly striking example of its utility was published in 1981 by Stuart Rudikoff, Matthew Scharff, and colleagues in a collaborative study between the NIH (Rudikoff) and Albert Einstein College of Medicine (Scharff). While studying a myeloma IgA with specificity for the phosphorylcholine hapten, cloning of the myeloma in soft agar generated clones for the original antibody and a variant that showed no binding. Sequencing of the variant indicated a single amino acid change in the heavy chain CDR1 (H1) in which a glutamic acid (negatively charged) was replaced by an alanine (neutral). Since the myeloma sequence was close to that of the McPC603 antibody, whose Fab structure had been determined by David Davies some seven years earlier, Scharff and colleagues generated a three-dimensional model of their variant and saw that the mutation disrupted an interaction that would almost certainly have caused a structural change in the CDR concerned. An interesting aspect of their work was that, unlike other studies, they did not use positive selection of clones by the antigen, which after all would only work if binding is retained, but relied on analysis of variants that had lost antigen binding, somewhat advantaged by the high mutation frequency of the particular myeloma cell line being used. As they concluded:

> We have shown that a single amino acid substitution is capable of completely altering antigen-binding specificity. Thus, a small number of amino acid substitutions, such as those postulated to arise by somatic mutation, can potentially be effective in generating antibody diversity in addition to that inherent in the germ-line repertoire.[20]

While Scharff's study scored a valuable point for the myeloma approach, its limitation was that a myeloma is essentially in 'immunological stasis' and further, there was no evidence that the mutation mechanism(s) operating to generate mutations in myeloma cells were the same as those in normal B-cells. The key advantage of the hybridoma method was that protocols could routinely be set up where mouse immunization followed by spleen-cell removal and hybridoma formation at different time intervals after the initial immunization, with or without further immunization, could be studied. For example, hybridomas could be produced after seven, 14, 28, 56 etc. days post-immunization and by sequencing (via the DNA) to identify the same antibody, that is an antibody using the same V-genes, J-segments, and D-regions, and individual mutations within the variable regions could be mapped and measured against their effects on antigen binding. This presumed that the sequence information would be sufficient to identify the exact same germ line V-gene and its J- and D- assembly partners through the time course of the study—not a trivial conclusion to draw since it was not entirely clear in the early 1980s exactly how many mouse V-genes there were and how close in sequence different germ line V-gene sequences were.

Notwithstanding the uncertainties, exploitation of the hybridoma method to better understand somatic diversity was reported in the period 1981 to 1984 by a number of research groups, but three examples stand out in their clarity and impact. During 1980, Lee Hood and his collaborator Patricia Gearhart at the Carnegie Institution in Baltimore carried out an analysis of 16 monoclonal antibodies generated in their own laboratory and several monoclonal antibodies and myelomas from other laboratories that bound the hapten phosphorylcholine. Of the antibodies analysed 11 were IgM, five were IgG3, four were IgG1, and nine were IgA. A number of important conclusions came from this study. Firstly, IgG light chain sequences (the first 36 amino acids, so only including the L1 CDR) contained mutations while the IgM antibodies had no mutations and only one of the nine IgAs. Sequences within the heavy chain of the IgG antibodies (again the first 36 amino acids and including only H1) were 'considerably more variable' than the IgM or IgA antibodies. Hood's interpretation of this was that the somatic mutation machinery must be activated only after class switching, a suggestion that would soon be challenged by other studies. Mutations were observed in both the framework and hypervariable regions, causing Hood and colleagues to caution:

> Therefore, either the framework variants arise from distinct germ line V_H segments or the presumptive mechanism for somatic variation is not confined to the hypervariable regions.[21]

One further important observation of Hood was that the relationship between the original germ line variable region sequences and those of the antibodies studied was unknown, precluding a rigorous evaluation of the exact level of somatic mutation activity after germ line variable gene selection.

The second example was to become a paradigm for monoclonal antibody studies on somatic variation. In a series of experiments separated by two publications just over one year apart, Milstein's team carried out an analysis of hybridomas raised against the phenyloxazolone (phOx) hapten, a Fab x-ray structure of which had been solved by Poljak. In the first study, a series of 15 anti-phOx monoclonal antibodies were produced seven days after immunization of mice and their light and heavy chain mRNAs sequenced using a modification of the new chain termination DNA sequencing method of Sanger.[22] The sequences of the light and heavy chains showed a particularly restricted germ line gene response with some initial low-level indications of somatic variants. Where there were differences they congregated in the V-J_K or V-D-J_H boundary regions. In one instance the mutation in the heavy chain could be assigned to an allotypic position leaving only a single change in the light chain that could be reasonably ascribed to an antigen-driven somatic change. The interpretation of these results was based on the premise that the small numbers of point mutations observed were indeed mutations of the same germ line V-gene, an uncertain conclusion, also noted in Hood's study, since the exact number of sequence differences between different germ line genes was unknown. The follow-up study by Milstein in 1984 clarified the response to phOx and illustrated exactly how monoclonal antibodies could be used to study the development of somatic variation over time.[23] During analysis of the primary (seven-day and 14-day) and secondary responses, significant differences were observed. In contrast to the observation of Hood, early-response antibodies showed somatic changes in the IgMs but not the IgGs while later in the response both isotypes were mutated. This appeared to contradict Hood's assertion that somatic changes are triggered by class switching. The somatic changes observed were also 'sensibly' located for the somatic theorists in that they appeared to cluster around hypervariable sequences that were known to be important for phOx binding from the x-ray structure. In addition, the binding affinities of the later-response antibodies were higher than the early responders, again providing a sound argument for linking somatic mutation and 'maturation' of the antibody response with antibody 'improvement', as Milstein concluded:

> … providing the basic structure of the antibody combining site is maintained, point mutations within the variable regions can produce antibodies with a better affinity for antigen. This increase in affinity is correlated with time, providing an explanation for the maturation effect.[23]

The third example was different. The antigen was a protein and up to this time all studies had been carried out on small haptens, albeit after conjugation to large carrier proteins. Martin Weigert and colleagues examined the mouse response to a particular antigenic determinant (named Sb) on haemagglutinin, a major coat protein of influenza virus, by sequencing and analysing the kappa light chains from seven antibodies.[24] From this study Weigert observed that around six to seven mutations per antibody occurred in the same light chain germ line gene between immunization and fusion, accumulating in a serial fashion over a period of 24 days. Using a generation time for the hybridoma cells of ~18h, Weigert calculated that this would have translated into a mutation rate of 10^{-3} per DNA base pair per generation, in accord with the observations of Scharff for the PC system—a comparative frequency for the average mutation rate of the human genome would be around 10^{-8} per base pair per generation. Clearly, something special was at work here, something that would be capable of introducing mutations and targeting them to antibody variable regions with a frequency 10^5 times that of random mutation mechanisms. Weigert further observed that his kappa chain sequences showed clustering of the changes and that they were mainly within CDRs. His concluding positioning statement was clear:

> To explain the pattern of variability in Vλ, it was proposed that antigen may act in the selection (selective expansion) of B cells expressing mutated immunoglobulin receptors that fit the

antigen. The marked clustering of replacement mutations in complementarity-determining regions of the light chains of the H36 hybridoma antibody set agrees with this proposal and further suggests that antigen selection acts on sequentially arising single-point mutations throughout the development of a B-cell lineage.[24]

Weigert also noted and elaborated something that had been commented on by Hood and that would later become of critical importance in the 'engineering' of antibodies for improvement and clinical use:

> The few mutations in framework regions also may play a role in modifying antibody specificity or else may have been coselected along with complementarity-determining region replacements.[24]

The step from framework mutation to impact on antigen specificity was not obvious at this time despite the existence of a number of three-dimensional structures of antibody Fab fragments. This was perhaps an example that antibody-antigen recognition was not a biological *gestalt* phenomenon but rather would be explained by careful identification and assembly of the individual parts eventually revealing the whole. But some parts were still missing.

The assembly of antibody genes begins to yield its secrets

By 1980 the assembly of antibody chains was well known to involve a number of complex recombination events in which light chain variable region genes would be selected and recombined with Jκ or Jλ sequences while heavy chain variable region genes would recombine with D and J_H segments. It was also known that some further junctional diversity accompanied this assembly process but the precise mechanism by which V-J and V-D-J recombination occurred was unclear.

In 1980 Hood and Tonegawa had separately observed that certain palindromic DNA sequence motifs were present in the flanking regions of V, J, and D regions which suggested a mechanism by which the relevant ends of the various segments could be brought together (see Chapter 7). However, the final variable region sequences were not precisely as they would have been if the component segments were simply attached 'end-to-end' with the palindromic sequences acting as a guidance system. Some additional diversity was also introduced either by deletion or addition of nucleotides during the joining process but how this occurred was unresolved. This extra diversification was not in itself a contributor to somatic diversity since once formed the V-J or V-D-J sequences would be fixed in time and space. Of course, formally these regions could also be targets post-assembly for somatic changes.

In 1982 Alt and Baltimore at the Whitehead Institute in Boston added further important pieces to the puzzle. From analysis of the rearranged chromosomal DNA in virally transformed foetal liver cells (development of the human immune system occurs in the foetal liver with both pre-B and B-lymphocytes already present in the human foetal liver at 12 weeks gestation) the joining events for heavy chains that bring D and J_H segments together were explored.[25] Three types of joining event were seen, two of which were considered 'irregular' and one normal. A model for the normal joining process derived by Alt and Baltimore is reproduced in Fig. 12.4.

The Alt and Baltimore model had five different stages:[25]

Stage I: The D and J DNA double strands are 'nicked' by a nuclease to present four open-ended single DNA strands ready for joining;

Stage II: the recombination signal sequences (RSS; palindromic sequences) are joined but the coding sequences remain open (Baltimore suggests they must be held in close proximity by a protein to facilitate ligation);

Stage III: deletions at the terminal ends of the D and J segments are made, (possibly) by an exonuclease activity;

Stage IV: additional nucleotides are added to the ends of the D and J segments;

Stage V: DNA polymerization to fill in any single strand 'overhangs' followed by ligation take place to form a contiguous VDJ sequence.

The most intriguing aspect of this model was its explanation for the fact that in many heavy chains amino acids had been found within CDR3 that had not originated from either the D or the J segment and must therefore have arisen from nucleotide changes introduced during formation of the junction. Baltimore suggests that a terminal transferase activity could perform just this action thereby creating additional diversity at the V_H-D junction. The candidate enzyme proposed, terminal deoxynucleotidyltransferase (TdT), was known to be present in thymus and bone marrow and furthermore showed a specificity preference for deoxyguanine (dG) nucleotides that are often found in abundance at the D-J_H junctions after assembly. Baltimore referred to this additional diversifying event in the heavy chain as 'N diversity' giving rise to the N-region. In the light chain, V_L-J junctions are not exposed to this type of additional modification, as Baltimore comments:

> N regions are not detected in light chain variable region sequences, suggesting that cells that are joining κ segments should lack terminal transferase as has been observed (unpublished data).[25]

The functional importance of TdT in creating heavy chain N-diversity would be confirmed much later using transgenic mouse technology—mice in which the TdT gene is disrupted are unable to carry out N-diversity additions.[26,27]

Adding to the complexity of V-D-J joining, Darsley and Rees sequenced five anti-peptide antibodies in 1985 and noted a possible mechanism that would further diversify the heavy chain D region. As Darsley explained when describing the gene organization of two related anti-lysozyme antibodies:

> … the junctional diversity of VH-D joining has resulted in a frame-shift in the D-segment, compensated for in the D-JH junction to regain the correct reading frame… This has… implications for… rearrangements of the germ line pools, effectively trebling the number of available D-segments.[28]

The N-region story had not ended here however. N-diversity was generated by an essentially random addition of nucleotides to the chain termini. In 1989, while

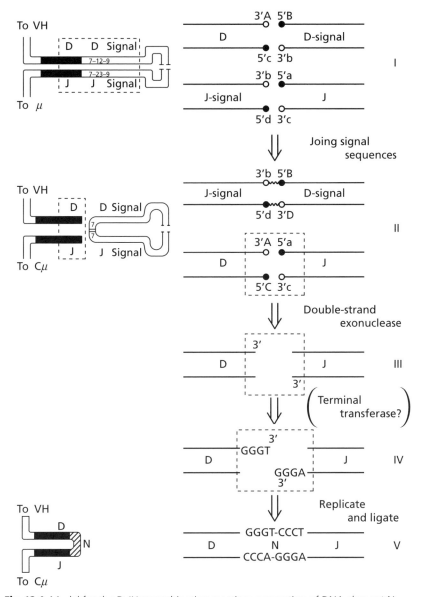

Fig. 12.4 Model for the D-JH recombination reaction: generation of DNA element N.

Reproduced from Alt, F.W. and Baltimore, D., Joining of immunoglobulin heavy chain gene segments: Implications from a chromosome with three D-JH fusions, *Proceedings of the National Academy of Sciences*, Volume 79, pp.4118–22, Copyright © 1982, with permission of the author.

dissecting the T-cell receptor, Tonegawa discovered an additional junctional diversity mechanism that also turned out to be present in antibody heavy chain V-D junctions. He named this new process P-diversity (P for palindrome).[29] Gellert illustrates this new diversity-adding mechanism of Tonegawa in his excellent review in 2002[30] (see Fig. 12.5).

As Gellert points out, this was an important new diversity mechanism and what is more, the added amino acids originate from the germ line coding sequence itself. Of course, if the hairpin nicking is exactly central there is no complementary chain overhang and no P nucleotides are added.

In short, the recombination machinery that marries V-J and V-D-J regions together brings with it elements of imprecision targeted to critical regions of the sequence, CDRs L3 or H3, that would be expected to impact antigen binding. This was not

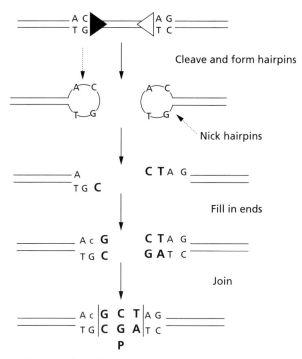

Fig. 12.5 The mechanism of templated nucleotide insertion at the junction of V-gene coding regions. During cleavage of DNA at the recombination signal sequence (RSS) coding border, the ends of coding DNA are converted to hairpins. These hairpins can be nicked a few bases off-centre (shown here as one base off-centre on the left, two bases off-centre on the right). This nicking leaves self-complementary single-strand extensions (large letters). After fill in and joining, these extensions (marked P) can be incorporated in the junction.

somatic mutation but it was a means of further diversifying the variable gene repertoire even beyond that created by the combinatorial assembly of variable genes with J and D fragments.

Despite these extraordinary advances of Tonegawa, Hood, and others, made possible by rapidly developing molecular biology tools, any specific protein involvement in the recombination and assembly steps was largely guesswork, apart from the obvious enzymatic requirements of cutting (nicking) DNA, removing or replacing nucleotides, converting single-stranded DNA to double-stranded DNA and ligating open DNA ends together. At the Whitehead Institute David Baltimore had begun to develop the tools that would eventually open the mechanistic box. In 1988, David Schatz and Baltimore reported the results of a study in which genomic DNA from a B-cell lymphoma had been introduced into fibroblast cells. Fibroblasts are normally incompetent in recombination of antibody genes, as are all non-immune system cells. After receiving the lymphoma DNA however, the fibroblasts were able to recombine a V-J antibody gene construct in the normal way.[31] They speculated this might be the result of a single gene product, encoding a recombinase protein or more likely, an enzyme. In a continuation of this approach published the following year, Schatz and Baltimore, now joined by Marjorie Oetinger, turned this speculation into reality. Using a clever DNA construction containing a V-gene and J regions in an orientation that only permitted expression of an enzyme conferring resistance to the drug mycophenolic acid if the antibody gene construction had undergone recombination, they were able to select those cells that must have expressed a recombinase. Further genomic analysis using genomic fragments tagged with an oligonucleotide that could be followed during segregation of the 'foreign' DNA allowed cloning of the protein RAG1 (recombinase active gene 1).[32] RAG1 was proposed as the VDJ recombinase enzyme system that functioned to hold the RSS sequences together, nick the DNA at relevant positions, and facilitate the subsequent joining of the V-D and D-J regions. As the team comments, having considered and then dismissed the possibility that RAG1 was merely an activator of the recombinase and not the recombinase itself:

> … evidence leads us to favor the hypothesis that RAG-1 encodes some or all of the V(D) J recombinase (where 'V(D)J recombinase' refers to the essential, lymphoid-specific component(s) of the enzymatic machinery of recombination).[32]

The scientific discovery process is like a Russian doll. When you think you have the answer and are immensely happy with it, another layer appears that makes reassessment necessary. The puzzlement in the team after the RAG1 study was how cells receiving the purified gene, the cDNA containing the recombinase RAG1, could be no more efficient at recombination than the genomic DNA and '100- to 1000-fold less active than the theoretical maximum'. In that study the fact that the clone containing RAG1 was missing a large amount of DNA from its 5'-end, which typically might contain those regulatory elements essential for correct expression, was a candidate explanation. The answer was different. The year after the RAG1 discovery, Baltimore and his team discovered a second protein, RAG2, by further examination of the genomic clone containing RAG1.[33] The sequences of the two proteins were completely unrelated and further, no similar sequences to either were found in the database of protein sequences determined to date. When the two genes were introduced into the cell system used to measure recombination, the 1000-fold theoretical recombination frequency was reached. This was undoubtedly a 'eureka' moment for the team and the fact that both RAG1 and RAG2 appeared to be highly conserved in evolution (dog, hamster, rabbit, cow, opossum, and turtle were tested) underlined the importance of the discovery. A speculative but biologically intriguing observation by Baltimore was the unusual organization of the two genes in the context of the then current understanding of evolutionary mechanism:

> More striking is the compact organization of RAG-1 and RAG-2 on the chromosome;... In mammalian cells, adjacent genes with related or identical function usually reflect the occurrence of gene duplication events... The absence of sequence similarity between RAG1 and RAG 2 suggests... this is not the case...[33]

This was an exciting time and the unravelling of recombination mechanism quite important. Baltimore himself (see Fig. 12.6), who received the Nobel Prize in 1975 for his work on retroviruses and their interaction with the mammalian genome, noted in his autobiographical addendum in 2005 that his most important contribution to immunology was the discovery of the RAG1 and RAG2 recombinase system.[34]

The somatic mutation machinery is discovered

But the Matryoshka doll of antibody maturation was not yet completely opened. Exactly how somatic changes introduced during progression of an immune response occurred

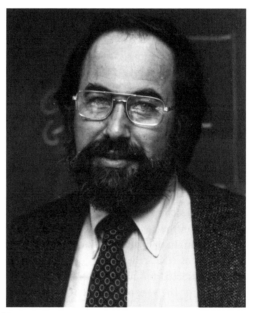

Fig. 12.6 David Baltimore.
Image reproduced courtesy of Dr Alice Huang.

and their selection and accumulation in hypervariable regions were still not understood. Brenner and Milstein's 1966 'DNA cleavage and error prone repair' hypothesis was still the main candidate mechanism, although as Neuberger points out '… without much supportive evidence'.[35]

In the hunt for mechanism a supplementary question that occupied the attention of a number of research groups focused on the origins of somatic mutation was 'How extensive is the region in and around the variable regions in which somatic changes are introduced?' As Weigert's study had suggested, antibody gene mutations appear to have a considerably higher frequency than the random mutation frequency in the rest of the genome, so would not be expected to operate too far outside the immediate vicinity of the rearranged variable genes and their constant region partners. Some differences between the findings of different groups were evident however. Two studies in 1981 suggested some uncertainty in defining the spatial limits of the somatic mutation machinery. Pech and colleagues analysed the sequences of rearranged Vκ-genes and their presumed germ line parents and concluded:

> The results reported here… because of the clustering of several sequence differences in a small region and the absence of any differences in fairly large adjoining regions, argues in favour of a localized mutation mechanism.[36]

The 'adjoining regions' Pech refers to included relatively short upstream and downstream DNA sequences that are untranslated. In these experiments six base-pair differences were observed that were considered somatic changes, giving rise to two changes in the framework region and three in the hypervariable region (L3). The second study came from Lee Hood's laboratory, this time focused on the heavy chains of two phosphorylcholine-binding IgA myeloma antibodies and a germ line VH gene common to both. In Hood's system the two somatic variants had 11 amino acid changes between them from the germ line VH sequence. Sequence sampling from regions upstream and downstream from the VH region was also carried out as well as parts of the upstream region from the alpha constant region gene. The two antibodies exhibited differences but a common factor was that the extensive mutation seen was localized in and around the VH gene. At a distance of 5 000 bases upstream and downstream of the VH region no somatic changes were visible, consistent with the view that the somatic mechanism was focused on rearranged antibody genes.

In a mini-review in the same year Baltimore describes a number of other studies that drove the immunology community to the inevitable conclusion that somatic mutations were focused on antibody variable regions but not confined to the CDRs, that single bases or two adjacent bases could be changed with some considerable contradiction on whether pyrimidine or purine bases were favoured, that changes could be silent (no amino acid change) and that the activation of the responsible somatic players follows class switching since few changes are observed in IgM antibodies. Perhaps the most prophetic observation by Baltimore was the suggestion that somatic mutation, triggered as it seemed to be by antigen interaction with the B-cell, must occur in the peripheral lymphocyte system while combinatorial rearrangement occurs in the central lymphoid organs.

In one of a series of follow-on studies Gearhart carried out a more extensive analysis of hybridoma and myeloma cells in 1983. The results were in many aspects consistent with previous results but in this study genomic rather than cDNA sequences were determined to establish the boundaries of mutation upstream and downstream of the variable and constant region genes and within untranslated intervening sequences. Four rearranged antibody genes expressed 32 point mutations throughout the DNA examined but these were present in clusters rather than randomly spread, although the clusters themselves appeared to be randomly located by statistical analysis. Gearhart's conclusion was that the likely candidate for a somatic machine was an error prone polymerase and that in order to arrive at a cluster distribution of mutations the enzyme would need to initiate several separate repair events. The 1966 model of Brenner and Milstein would not lie down!

In 1987, O'Brien, Storb, and Brinster used the now popular transgenic mouse model to introduce prearranged kappa chain genes. The question they sought to answer was whether somatic mutation occurs on an already rearranged gene. This would establish whether the recombination events and somatic mutation are somehow interdependent. Transgenic mice containing a donated myeloma kappa chain able to bind the phosphorylcholine (PC) hapten and containing marker mutations to distinguish it from endogenous kappa chains were hyperimmunized with a protein-PC conjugate and hybridomas produced. The results were clear. The transgenic mice were fully capable of introducing mutations into the donated rearranged light chain (eight mutations in four different hybridoma clones) all of which were located within the V_L region. Further, the chromosomal location of the transgene did not appear to be important, suggesting all the information for somatic mutation existed in the transgenic DNA introduced. Again, few mutations were seen in the region downstream from the V gene or around the constant domain gene. Storb and Brinster's conclusions were consistent with those of others before:

> The localization of the mutations to the V gene suggests that a special mutator exists that must recognize specific sequences in or around immunoglobulin V genes... The absence of mutations near the C gene suggests the mutator is confined to the vicinity of the V region.[37]

A more quantitative analysis by Patricia Gearhart in 1990 seemed to be homing in on the key DNA region. From an analysis of 17 light and heavy chain genomic clones containing the antibody genes, Lebeque and Gearhart constructed a mutation frequency map of the VJ and VDJ regions and their surrounding DNA (see Fig. 12.7).[38]

Some key conclusions from Gearhart's study were that the majority of mutations occurred in the V-region (between x-axis values 0 and 0 in Fig. 12.7) but not exclusively, recapitulating the observations of many other studies. The upstream promoter (directs transcription of the gene into mRNA) appeared to be the limit of the boundary suggesting to Gearhart that somatic mutation is somehow linked to the transcriptional state of the V-genes. In a somewhat wide-ranging model Gearhart goes much further. A component of the model was the possible role of the downstream 'enhancer' sequence. An enhancer is a region of DNA that typically binds transcription factors that increase (enhance) the rate of transcription of a nearby gene or gene cluster. In 1983 Tonegawa and Schaffner had independently identified (in back-to-back publications)

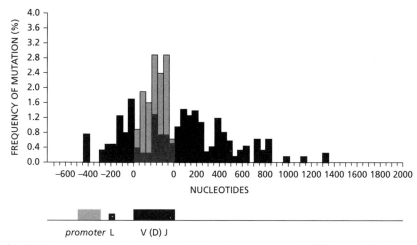

Fig. 12.7 Frequency of mutation versus distance from rearranged V(D)J genes. The bottom drawing shows the positions of the promoter, leader, and V(D)J gene sequences. Negative numbers on the abscissa correspond to 5′ flanking DNA; the coding region sits between 0 and 0 (350 nucleotides); positive numbers correspond to 3′ flanking DNA. The ordinate values give the relative frequency of mutation.

Reproduced with permission © 1990 Rockefeller University Press. Originally published in Lebeque, S.G. and Gearhart, P.J., Boundaries of somatic mutation in rearranged immunoglobulin genes: 5′ boundary is near the promotor, and 3′ boundary is ~1kb from V(D)J gene, *Journal of Experimental Medicine*, Volume 172, pp. 1717–27.

such an enhancer close to the V-region's genes and sitting between the J- and C-regions. Tonegawa's results showed that the enhancer could operate normally whether it was upstream or downstream of the V-genes and was even active when in a reverse orientation on the DNA strand. Importantly, the enhancer appeared to be tissue specific since it was inactive in fibroblast cells.[39] Schaffner's study reinforced the observations of Tonegawa but also demonstrated that the enhancer was able to increase the transcription of non-antibody genes (e.g. the rabbit β-globin gene) provided the relevant constructs were present in B-lymphocytes, confirming the tissue-specific activity of this special sequence of DNA.[40]

One more piece of the antibody gene organization puzzle was added in 1987 around the same time that Storb and Brinster reported their transgenic experiments. William Garrard's group at the University of Texas in Dallas had identified another feature of the light and heavy chain gene locus that seemed to make sense if the antibody gene cluster was to be viewed as a special genetic unit whose transcription and rearrangement activity might be switched on or off depending on the cell type. This feature was known as a 'matrix association region' or MAR. The chromosomal DNA was known to be organized into large looped domains, the anchor points of which are specific sequences of DNA that define where the ends of the looped domains interact with the nuclear matrix. Such looped domains can then be either active or inactive in transcription depending on the topological environment of the DNA and the presence or activity of transcription activating factors. Garrard had identified two such MAR sequences on either side of the V-region gene enhancer previously identified by others as sitting between the J- and constant regions. This was an alluring situation and suggested to Garrard that the MAR elements 'may act as positive or negative regulators of enhancer function'.[41] Was this a possible explanation for the tissue-specific expression of antibody gene rearrangement?

During 1993, Michael Neuberger and colleagues at the MRC in Cambridge were taking this story much further and adding complexity that had not been previously seen (Fig. 12.8). First, they showed that the immunoglobulin gene promoter could be quite happily replaced by a promoter for another gene (β-globin) suggesting it had no direct role in the somatic mutation process. But there was more. There were actually two different enhancers present, one close to the V-gene region, as described by Garrard and others, and a second enhancer 3' of the constant region gene. Using a transgenic mouse model and cloning of the DNA from B-cells in germinal centres of peripheral lymph tissue (Peyer's patches) Neuberger found that both enhancers were essential for effective hypermutation:

> The question, therefore, arises as to whether the enhancers are potentiating hypermutation by directly recruiting a factor unique to the hypermutation process or one shared by the transcriptional apparatus; alternatively, their stimulation of hypermutation might be secondary to an effect on transcription or chromatin structure. While the results demonstrate the importance of the enhancers in controlling hypermutation, we know nothing about the efficacy of these elements as regulators of transcription or chromatin structure in those very cells in which the hypermutation is taking place.[42]

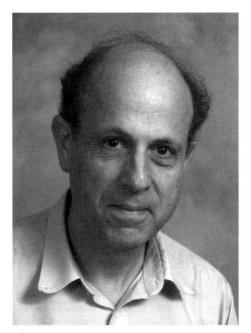

Fig. 12.8 Michael Neuberger.
Reproduced courtesy of MRC Laboratory of Molecular Biology, UK and Michael Neuberger.

Baltimore had suggested in 1981 that hypermutation activity should be confined to the peripheral immune system. The germinal centres in Peyer's patches had been shown by Butcher and colleagues in 1982 to be a plausible site for generation of plasma cell precursors and of mature memory B-cells.[43] The high antigen exposure in such secondary lymphoid tissues leading to stimulation of B-cell responses and the wealth of experimental evidence accumulated led to the notion that germinal centres are the sites where heavy chain class-switching (e.g. IgM to IgG or IgA etc.) occurs and where somatic mutations accumulate.[44]

Constant region class switching and hypermutation: mechanistic insights

Against this immense backdrop of antibody genetics the stage was set for entry of what seemed the most likely players to perform, the molecular biologists. But a relatively new player in the somatic mutation debate entered stage east! Tasuku Honjo had worked with Phil Leder at the NIH in the early 1970s and after returning to Tokyo in 1974 and later moving to Kyoto University he turned his attention to the problem of constant region class switching, not realizing at that time where it would lead. In 1978 through to 1982 Honjo had established the order of constant region genes for the various isotypes and proposed and subsequently confirmed that class switching from IgM to any other isotype occurs by deletion of the other isotype C-regions 3' to the IgM C-gene by a 'looping out' and deletion mechanism.[45,46] An expected set of results allowed Honjo to propose that the switch from IgM to IgG1 is actually triggered by an exogenous factor, the cytokine interleukin 4 (IL-4).[47] But this was not enough to fully understand what was taking place in the cell, as Honjo recollects in his 2008 memoir:

> By this time the outline of the CSR [class switch recombination] was complete... and everyone in the field was eager to discover the class-switch recombinase. Missing, however, was a cell line with efficient and specific class switching...[48]

The cell line that Honjo sought came to his attention as a result of a further visit to the NIH as a Fogarty scholar in 1991. The B-lymphoma cell line was being looked at to study IgA class switching, albeit with very low efficiency but it could be switched on and off with a combination of various protein factors. Back in Kyoto three years later Honjo's laboratory isolated a subclone of this cell line that exhibited a much higher class-switching behaviour while his graduate student, Muramatsu showed that for this class switching to occur, the cell was required to initiate new protein synthesis. This was exciting. Using a cloning technique in which cDNAs from non-induced cells were 'subtracted' from the cDNAs of the switch-induced cells leaving only (theoretically) those cDNAs that arose from the class-switching induction, a specific gene encoding an enzyme was identified. The enzyme was called *a*ctivation-*i*nduced cytidine *d*eaminase, or AID, and appeared to be closely related to a deaminase enzyme (APOBEC-1) involved in RNA-editing of another known protein by converting the base cytosine to uracil—if a base in RNA is deaminated, or 'edited' at a particular position the protein translation machinery will stop at that point and a truncated protein will result. Was this the end of the trail or just the beginning? AID was shown to be expressed in germinal centre B-cells at times coincident with the onset of class switching, it increased in splenic B-cells when mice were immunized with sheep red blood cells and was absent in many different cell types that cannot undertake class switching of immunoglobulin genes.[49] The evidence was tantalizingly close but not yet proven. After all, it was not immediately obvious how a cytidine deaminase enzyme that operated on RNA converting cytidine to uracil could be involved in class switching and rearrangement of regions of DNA. Reflecting their uncertainty, Honjo's team screened other candidates that differed between the induced and non-induced cells but all roads appeared to lead to AID in terms of its temporal and spatial appearance during B-cell class switching events. Honjo walked out on a limb and speculated:

> Furthermore, the possibility of RNA editing activity on other templates inspires us to speculate that AID may participate in regulatory steps unique to GC [germinal center] function such as somatic hypermutation and CSR [class switching recombination].[49]

In a further immensely detailed study in 2000 Honjo (see Fig. 12.9) provided the cell biology proof that AID was involved both in class switching and somatic hypermutation. By disrupting the gene in transgenic mice or by analysis of spleen cells from AID-defective mice, class switch recombination was severely impaired. Further, immunization of AID-deficient mice and analysis of the antibody genes after two antigen injections over several weeks showed hypermutation levels ten times lower than those of normal mice, with an observed mutation frequency at about the level expected of a random mutation mechanism. The message was clear: AID was the leading candidate for the recombinase by a Swedish mile and was heavily implicated in the hypermutation mechanism. But, did it work on RNA or DNA? Honjo plumped for the RNA option at the same time expressing doubt in any involvement of DNA:

> The most straightforward possibility for the function of AID is, therefore, an RNA editing enzyme with a substrate specificity determined by an additional co-factor… Obvious candidates of the AID target may be the DNA repair enzymes, DNases, and DNA polymerases… Although less likely, AID may edit DNA directly.[50]

It took another system and another research group to set the mechanistic hunt back on track. In 2002 Michael Neuberger, convinced that AID needed to be able to operate on DNA, decided to test a model for the deamination of DNA bases in a bacterial system. Fast generation times and ease of read-out made the bacterial system an efficient test vehicle. The essence of Neuberger's model was that AID deaminates cytosine (C) in a guanine:cytosine (G:C) base pair in DNA and in so doing the cytosine is converted to uracil, a non-DNA base but found in RNA. If instead of repairing this modification (known as base-excision repair) the altered base is used as a template for DNA synthesis, the result would be that the original C would become a T and its base-pairing partner an A. Thus, a G:C base pair would have become a T:A base pair, *ergo* a mutation. Other possibilities were discussed but the bacteria needed to speak. By introducing the AID gene into bacteria and analysing the mutations in a gene conferring resistance to the antibiotic rifampicin that allowed bacteria to escape the antibiotic inhibition Neuberger confirmed that in the AID-transformed bacteria

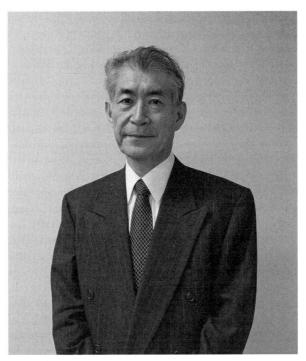

Fig. 12.9 Tasumu Honjo.
Reproduced with permission of Tasumu Honjo, Copyright © JT Biohistory Research Hall in Japan.

80% of the mutations looked at were GC=> AT changes, compared with 31% in controls. The targeting of the AID-generated mutations in the bacteria was not a random process however. Some G:C pairs were favoured over others and the frequency of mutations was greatly enhanced when the bacteria were deficient in the uracil repair pathway, strongly implicating uracil as an intermediate. Neuberger's conclusions were stark and bold:

> Our data indicate that AID triggered the deamination of dC [deoxy-C)] residues in DNA. It will be interesting to ascertain whether AID is sufficient to mediate dC deamination directly in vitro or whether it works with or through other factors. The homology of AID to Apobec-1 and cytidine deaminase... obviously argues in favour of a close involvement of AID in the DNA deamination process itself. The preferential targeting of mutation to the immunoglobulin loci in lymphocytes presumably depends on the proteins with which AID associates.[51]

While the plot was now becoming clearer, the 'preferential targeting' Neuberger referred to was still a part of the story that was missing. G:C base pairs are pretty common in the genome but hypermutation was only occurring (it was thought) within the antibody gene loci. Furthermore, AID would only deaminate cytosine in a single-stranded piece of DNA, but DNA is double-stranded. Within a further two years, Frederick Alt would provide at least a partial explanation to the targeting conundrum. In 2004, using an *in vitro* hypermutation screening method which required transcription of the target DNA during the assay, Alt identified a protein, replicating protein A (RPA), which appeared to be important as an AID cooperating factor.[52] The deamination activity of AID alone was only visible during transcription where the double-stranded DNA is opened to form single-stranded R-loops (see Chapter 7, Fig. 7.4) during copying to mRNA. When the target double-stranded DNA sequence contained a large number of RGYW sequence motifs that were known to be 'hot-spots' of AID activity (the motif RGYW was known to be preferred by AID, where R = adenine or guanine, G = guanine, Y = cytosine or thymine, and W = adenine or thymine) but that are unable to form stable single-stranded R-loops during *in vitro* transcription, no AID activity was seen. However, in the presence of RPA the deamination of double-stranded DNA during transcription was significantly enhanced. The role of RPA appeared to be to stabilize the single-stranded DNA generated during transcription progression to allow AID-catalysed deamination at the RGYW motifs. Alt demonstrated the single-strand behaviour of RPA by showing it was able to bind short stretches of DNA in the transcription 'bubbles' with a preference for RGYW sequences. After deamination by AID, this protein dissociates from the transcription complex leaving RPA bound. Alt speculates that RPA may then act as a 'guidance system' for recruitment of other enzymes in the mutator machine (e.g. DNA repair enzymes) that complete the nucleotide switch. Alt's concluding comment was a statement confirming his belief that the function of AID in somatic mutation was now clearly established. At least there now appeared to be one hand on the Grail:

> Finally, these functions strongly support the deamination model of AID function and mechanistically link the SHM requirements of transcription, AID and RGYW motifs.[52]
>
> [SHM = somatic hypermutation]

By 2008 Neuberger posed a number of still unanswered questions about the SHM mechanism. For example, how is AID targeted to the immunoglobulin loci and further what signals direct it either to the V-region for SHM or to the switch region for class switching of the immunoglobulin genes. Again why are the C=>U mutations not simply repaired as they would be by high fidelity DNA polymerases operating elsewhere in the genome?[32] By 2012 AID would have been identified in many other regions of the genome and not just in B-cells, a fact that not only brought Neuberger's question into sharp focus for the immunology community but caused some concern among the geneticists about how such a 'mutator' machine is controlled within both somatic and germ cells to avoid accumulation of frequent deleterious genomic mutation. For SHM, the key steps were beginning to be understood with a large number of associated protein and enzyme members of the somatic mutation ensemble already identified or at least as having a postulated involvement. By 2012 the mutable motifs in the V-region DNA were either known or proposed to be husbanded by a multitude of proteins and other factors. In his review of the state of the art in 2012, Matthew Scharff at the Albert Einstein College of Medicine illustrates the complexity of the process (see Fig. 12.10).[53] Scharff's stages can be summarized as follows:

1. Initiation of DNA transcription;

2. Binding of AID to single-stranded transcription-mediated loops of DNA at preferred regions of the V-gene containing RGYW motifs. The single-strand loops formed are stabilized by the RPA protein and other factors followed by AID-mediated deamination of the base cytosine creating a uracil base;

3. Excision of uracil from the single strand of DNA by the enzyme uracil-DNA glycosylase (UNG), leaving a gap; at the same time recruitment of DNA mismatch recognition proteins (MSH2–MSH6) that orchestrate specific enzymatic processes that create a single-stranded 'patch' (single-strand gap) around the original mismatch targeted at nearby A:T base pairs (Scharff's 'resection factors');

4. Recruitment of 'error prone' DNA polymerase enzymes that carry out repair of the single-strand 'patches', which may be as much as 20 base pairs on either side of the original mismatch, followed by re-creation of the double-stranded DNA but now containing mutations.

In his commentary in the same special issue of the journal, Jayanta Chaudhuri, working at the Memorial Sloan-Kettering Cancer Institute, brought the current understanding of the somatic hypermutation process centre stage, drawing attention at the same time to the dangers associated with releasing a profligate mutation machine loose on the entire genome:

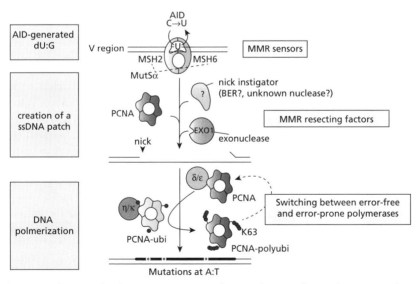

Fig. 12.10 The cascade of processes necessary for introduction of somatic mutations into the antibody variable genes. The steps shown in the figure are summarized above.

Generating mutations across two different chromosomes during SHM and inducing DSBs across several kilobases of sequence on one chromosome during CSR, AID has the unique ability to promote DNA diversification unlike any other characterized protein involved in Ig diversification… Because AID has the power to radically alter the organization of DNA as well as the coding sequences of DNA, mechanisms must exist to limit its activity specifically at the Ig loci. Significant progress has been made in identifying transcriptional, post-transcriptional, and post-translational regulatory mechanisms. In addition, several factors that influence AID binding to DNA have been identified. However, a specificity-factor, if it exists, that dictates how AID is able to precisely induce very high levels of mutations and DSBs at Ig loci remains elusive. Identifying how AID gains access to non-Ig genes, the mechanisms that promote (or restrict) this access and the process through which normal error-free repair by the general DNA repair pathways are subverted to induce mutations and DSBs in the genome during CSR and SHM will constitute the next frontier of investigation on the biology of AID.[54]

[SHM = somatic hypermutation; CSR = class switch recombination; Ig = immunoglobulin; DSB = double-stranded breaks]

Here was a truly remarkable example of the beauty of the genome organization and the complexity of its regulatory processes. An understanding of controlled diversity *in vivo* and antibody structure would give rise to 'engineered diversity' or '*in vitro* evolution' and take the antibody repertoire orders of magnitude beyond its *in vivo* counterpart. This development would make possible the effective use of antibodies in human therapy and diagnostics and make Ehrlich's 'magic bullet' concept a magical reality.

Acknowledgements

Text extracts reprinted from *Progress in Biophysics and Molecular Biology*, Volume 21, Milstein, C. and Pink, J.R.L., Structure and evolution of immunoglobulins, pp. 209–263, Copyright © 1970 with permission from Elsevier, http://www.sciencedirect.com/science/journal/00796107

Text extract reproduced from Playfair, J.H.L., Pappermaster, B.W. and Cole, L.J. Focal Antibody Production by Transferred Spleen Cells in Irradiated Mice, *Science*, Volume 149, pp. 998–1000. Copyright © 1965. Reprinted with permission from AAAS.

Text extract reproduced with permission from McKean, D., et al., Generation of antibody diversity in the immune response of BALB/c mice to influenza virus haemaglutinin, *Proceedings of the National Academy of Sciences*, Volume 81, pp. 3180–3184, Copyright © 1984.

Text extracts reprinted from *Cell*, Volume 77, Issue 2, Betz, A.G. et al., Elements regulating somatic hypermutation of an immunoglobulin κ gene: Critical role for the intron enhancer/matrix attachment region, pp. 239–248, Copyright © 1970 with permission from Elsevier, http://www.sciencedirect.com/science/journal/00928674

Text extract reprinted from *Seminars in Immunology*, Volume 24, Issue 4, Vuong, B.Q. and Chaudhuri, J., Combinatorial mechanisms regulating AID-dependent DNA deamination: Interacting proteins and post-translational modifications, pp. 264–272, Copyright © 2012 with permission from Elsevier, http://www.sciencedirect.com/science/journal/10445323

References

1. **Milstein, C., and Pink, J. R. L.** (1970). 'Structure and evolution of immunoglobulins.' *Prog. Biophys. Mol. Biol.*, **21**: 209–63.

2. **Stavnezer, J., and Huang, C. C.** (1971). 'Synthesis of a mouse immunoglobulin light chain in a rabbit reticulocyte cell free system.' *Nature*, **230**: 172–6.

3. **Brownlee, G. G., Harrison, T. M., Matthews, M. B., and Milstein, C.** (1972). 'Translation of messenger RNA for immunoglobulin light chains in a cell-free system from Krebs II ascites cells.' *FEBS Lett.*, **23**: 244–8.

4. **Milstein, C.** (1984). 'From the structure of antibodies to the diversification of the immune response.' Nobel Lecture, Nobelprize.org.

5. **Milstein, C., Brownlee, G. G., Harrison, T. M., and Matthews, M. B.** (1972). 'A possible precursor of immunoglobulin light chains.' *Nature*, **239**: 117–20.

6. **Brownlee, G. G., Cartwright, E. M., Cowan, N. J., Jarvis, J. M., and Milstein, C.** (1973). 'Purification and sequence of messenger RNA for immunoglobulin light chains.' *Nature New Biol.*, **244**: 236–40.

7. **Secher, D. S., Cotton, R. G. H., and Milstein, C.** (1973). 'Spontaneous mutation in tissue culture—chemical nature of variant immunoglobulin from mutant clones of MOPC21.' *FEBS Lett.*, **37**: 311–16.

8. **Mohit, B.** (1971). 'Immunoglobulin G and free kappa-chain synthesis in different clones of a hybrid cell line.' *Proc. Natl. Acad. Sci.*, **68**: 3045–8.

9. **Cotton, R. G. H., and Milstein, C.** (1973). 'Fusion of two immunoglobulin myeloma cells.' *Nature*, **244**: 42–3.

10. **Colberg, J. E., and Dray, S.** (1964). 'Localization by Immunofluorescence of Gamma-Globulin Allotypes in Lymph Node Cells of Homozygous and Heterozygous Rabbits.' *Immunology*, **7**: 273–90.

11. **Pernis, B.** (1967). 'Relationships between the heterogeneity of immunoglobulins and the differentiation of plasma cells.' *Cold Spring Harbor Symp. Quant. Biol.*, **32**: 333–41.

12. **Playfair, J. H. L., Pappermaster, B. W., and Cole, L. J.** (1965). 'Focal Antibody Production by Transferred Spleen Cells in Irradiated Mice.' *Science*, **149**: 998–1000.

13. **Askonas, B. A., Williamson, A. R.**, and Wright, B. E. G. (1970). 'Selection of a single antibody forming cell clone and its propagation in syngeneic mice.' *Proc. Natl. Acad. Sci.*, **67**: 1398.

14. **Klinman, N.** (1971). 'Purification and analysis of "monofocal" antibody.' *J. Immunol.*, **106**: 1345–52.

15. **Melchers, F.** (1995). 'Georges Köhler (1946–1995).' Obituary. *Nature*, **374**: 498.

16. **Tansey, E. M., and Catterall, P. P.** (1994). 'Monoclonal antibodies: A witness seminar in contemporary medical history.' *Med. Hist.*, **38**: 322–7.

17. **Littlefield, J. W.** (1964). 'Selection of hybrids from matings of fibroblasts in vitro and their presumed recombinants.' *Science*, **145**: 709–10.

18. **Köhler, G., and Milstein, C.** (1975). 'Continuous cultures of fused cells secreting antibody of predefined specificity.' *Nature*, **256**; 495–7.

19. **Milstein, C.** (2000). 'With the benefit of hindsight.' *Immunol. Today*, **21**: 359–64.

20. **Rudikoff, S., Giusti, A. M., Cook, W. D., and Scharff, M. D.** (1982). 'Single amino acid substitution altering antigen-binding specificity.' *Proc. Natl. Acad. Sci.*, **79**: 1979–83.

21. **Gearhart, P. J., Johnson, N. D., Douglas, R., and Hood, L.** (1981). 'IgG antibodies to phosphorylcholine exhibit more diversity than their IgM counterparts.' *Nature*, **291**: 29–34.

22. **Sanger, F., Nicklen, S., and Coulson, A. R.** (1977). 'DNA sequencing with chain terminating inhibitors.' *Proc. Natl. Acad. Sci. USA*, **74**: 5463–7.

23. **Griffiths, G. M., Berek, C., Kaartinen, M., and Milstein, C.** (1984). 'Somatic mutation and the maturation of immune response to 2-phenyl oxalolone.' *Nature*, **312**: 271–5.

24. **McKean, D., Huppi, K., Bell, M., Staudt, L., Gergard, W., and Weigert, M.** (1984). 'Generation of antibody diversity in the immune response of BALB/c mice to influenza virus haemagglutinin.' *Proc. Natl. Acad. Sci.*, **81**: 3180–4.

25. **Alt, F. W., and Baltimore, D.** (1982). 'Joining of immunoglobulin heavy chain gene segments: Implications from a chromosome with three D-JH fusions.' *Proc. Natl. Acad. Sci.*, **79**: 4118–22.

26. **Gilfillan, S., Dierich A., Lemeur, M., Benoist, C., and Mathis, D.** (1993). 'Mice lacking TdT: mature animals with an immature lymphocyte repertoire.' *Science*, **261**: 1175–8.

27. **Komori, T., Okada, A., Stewart, V., and Alt, F. W.** (1993). 'Lack of N regions in antigen receptor variable region genes of TdT-deficient lymphocytes.' *Science*, **261**: 1171–5.

28. **Darsley, M. J., and Rees, A. R.** (1985). 'Nucleotide sequences of five anti-lysozyme monoclonal antibodies.' *The EMBO Journal*, **4**: 393–8.

29. **Lafaille, J. J., DeCloux, A., Bonneville, M., Takagaki, Y., and Tonegawa, S.** (1989). 'Junctional Sequences of T Cell Receptor γδ Genes: Implications for γδ T Cell Lineages and for a Novel Intermediate of V-(D)-J Joining.' *Cell*, **59**: 859–70.

30. **Gellert, M.** (2002). 'V(D)J recombination: RAG proteins, repair factors, and regulation.' *Ann. Rev. Biochem.*, **71**: 101–32.

31. **Schatz, D. G., and Baltimore, D.** (1988). 'Stable expression of immunoglobulin gene V(D)J recombinase activity by gene transfer into 3T3 fibroblasts.' *Cell*, **53**: 107–15.

32. **Schatz, D. G., Oettinger, M. A., and Baltimore, D.** (1989). 'The V(D)J Recombination Activating Gene, RAG-1.' *Cell*, **59**: 1035–48.

33. **Oettinger, M. A., Schatz, D. G., Gorka, C., and Baltimore, D.** (1990). 'RAG-1 and RAG-2, Adjacent Genes That Synergistically Activate V(D)J Recombination.' *Science*, **248**: 1517–23.

34. **Baltimore, D.** (2013). *David Baltimore—Autobiography*. http://www.nobelprize.org

35. **Neuberger, M. S.** (2008). 'Antibody diversification by somatic mutation: from Burnet onwards.' *Immunol. Cell Biol.*, **86**: 124–32.

36. **Pech, M., Höchtl, J., Schnell, H., and Zachau, H. G.** (1981). 'Differences between germ line and rearranged immunoglobulin coding sequences suggest a localized mutation mechanism.' *Nature*, **291**: 668–70.

37. **O'Brien, R. L., Brinster, R. L., and Storb, U.** (1987). 'Somatic hypermutation of an immunoglobulin transgene in κ transgenic mice.' *Nature*, **326**: 405–9.

38. **Lebeque, S. G., and Gearhart, P. J.** (1990). 'Boundaries of somatic mutation in rearranged immunoglobulin genes: 5' boundary is near the promotor, and 3' boundary is ~1kb from V(D)J gene.' *J. Exp. Med.*, **172**: 1717–27.

39. **Gillies, S. D., Morrison, S. L., Oi, V. T., and Tonegawa, S.** (1983). 'A tissue-specific transcription enhancer element is located in the major intron of a rearranged heavy chain gene.' *Cell*, **33**: 717–29.

40. **Banerji, J., Olson, L., and Schaffner, W.** (1983). 'A lymphocyte-specific cellular enhancer is located downstream of the joining region in immunoglobulin heavy chain genes.' *Cell*, **33**: 729–40.

41. **Cockerill, P. N., Yuen, M.-H., and Garrard, W. T.** (1986). 'The Enhancer of the Immunoglobulin Heavy Chain Locus is Flanked by Presumptive Chromosomal Loop Anchorage Elements.' *Cell*, **44**: 273–82.

42. **Betz, A. G., Milstein, C., Gonzales-Fernandez, A., Pannell, R., Larson, T., and Neuberger, M. S.** (1994). 'Elements regulating somatic hypermutation of an immunoglobulin κ gene: Critical role for the intron enhancer/matrix attachment region.' *Cell*, **77**: 239–48.

43. **Butcher, E. C., Rouse, R. V., Coffman, R. L., Nottenburg, C. N., Hard, R. R., and Weissman, I. L.** (1982). 'Surface phenotype of Peyer's patch germinal centre cells: implications for the role of germinal centres in B cell differentiation.' *J. Immunol.*, **129**: 2698–707.

44. **Thorbecke, G. J., Amin, A. R., and Tsiagbe, V. K.** (1994). 'Biology of germinal centers in lymphoid tissue.' *FASEB J.*, **8**: 832–40.

45. **Honjo, T., and Kataoka, T.** (1978). 'Organization of immunoglobulin heavy chain genes and allelic deletion model.' *Proc. Natl. Acad. Sci.*, **75**: 2140–4.

46. **Shimitu, A., Takahashi, N., Yaoita, Y., and Honjo, T.** (1982). 'Organization of the Constant-Region Gene Family of the Mouse Immunoglobulin Heavy Chain.' *Cell*, **28**: 499–506.

47. **Noma, Y., Sideras, P., Naito, T., Bergestedt-Lindquist, S., Azuma, C., Severinson, E., Tanabe, T., Kinashi, T., Matsuda, F., Yaoita, Y., and Honjo, T.** (1986). 'Cloning of cDNA encoding the murine IgG1 induction factor by a novel strategy using SP6 promoter.' *Nature*, **319**: 640–6.

48. **Honjo, T.** (2008). 'A memoir of AID, which engraves antibody memory on DNA.' *Nature Immunology*, **9**: 335–7.

49. **Muramatsu, M., Sankaranand, V. S., Anant, S., Sugai, M., Kinoshita, K., Davidson, N. O., and Honjo, T.** (1999). 'Specific Expression of Activation-induced Cytidine Deaminase (AID), a Novel Member of the RNA-editing Deaminase Family in Germinal Center B Cells.' *J. Biol. Chem.*, **274**: 18470–6.

50. **Muramatsu, M., Kinoshita, K., Fagarasan, S., Yamada, S, Shinkai, Y., and Honjo, T.** (2000). 'Class switch recombination and hypermutation require activation-induced cytidine deaminase (AID), a potential RNA editing enzyme.' *Cell*, **102**: 553–63.

51. **Petersen-Mahrt, S. K., Harris, R. S., and Neuberger, M. S.** (2002). 'AID mutates E.coli suggesting a DNA deamination mechanism for antibody diversification.' *Nature*, **418**: 99–103.

52. **Chaudhuri, J., Khuong, C., and Alt, F. W.** (2004). 'Replication protein A interacts with AID to promote deamination of somatic hypermutation targets.' *Nature*, **430**: 992–8.

53. **Chahwan, R., Edelmann, W., Scharf, M. D., and Roa, S.** (2012). 'AIDing antibody diversity by error-prone mismatch repair.' *Sem. Immunol.*, **24**: 293–300.

54. **Vuong, B. Q., and Chaudhuri, J.** (2012). 'Combinatorial mechanisms regulating AID-dependent DNA deamination: Interacting proteins and post-translational modifications.' *Sem. Immunol.*, **24**: 264–72.

Chapter 13

Antibody structure prediction and development of humanization strategies

Early modelling ideas

The relationship between amino acid sequence and the three-dimensional structure of proteins began to exercise the minds of protein chemists after the first protein x-ray structure breakthroughs at the end of the 1950s. In 1960, the groups of Kendrew and Perutz, working on myoglobin and haemoglobin respectively, published back-to-back papers on the structures of these two proteins, both of which contained a significant proportion of helical 'rods' interrupted by non-helical disordered segments which allowed the helical 'secondary structure' elements to be packed together to form a compact 'tertiary structure'.[1,2] The haemoglobin structure was a much more complicated target since it consisted of four subunits held together in a tetrahedral array but was at a lower resolution than myoglobin. Interaction between the research groups suggested that the individual subunits in Perutz' structure resembled the myoglobin of Kendrew and the more resolved features in myoglobin were used to aid the structural interpretation of haemoglobin. Perutz was aware that there would be two forms of haemoglobin, oxidized and reduced, and made the trenchant observation that the transition between the two forms was likely due to movement of the subunits with respect to each other rather than changes within the subunits, a remarkable insight from Perutz. From that point, haemoglobin was set to become the archetypical protein system for the development of theories explaining allosteric changes in proteins.

Before these two protein structures emerged no real understanding existed of how a polypeptide chain was folded in globular proteins. In 1951 Pauling, Corey, and Branson had suggested the dimensions of alpha helices[3] based on solution studies of polyamino acids that formed long helical structures analogous to those observed by Bragg in structures of fibrous proteins such as keratin, but whether these were present in other globular proteins was unknown. The structures of myoglobin and haemoglobin not only resolved this but confirmed Pauling and Corey's alpha helix properties and dimensions (see Fig. 13.1).

Other protein structures arrived rapidly with the first enzyme x-ray structure, hen's egg lysozyme, determined in 1966 by David Phillips and co-workers. Lysozyme contained both alpha helix and beta sheet structures (now referred to as 'secondary structure' elements while the complete folded protein adopted a 'tertiary structure'),[4] the latter also described in some detail in a separate paper by Pauling and

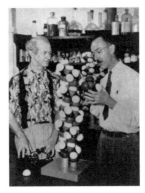

Fig. 13.1 Pauling (left) and Corey examining a wooden model of an alpha-helix (a-helix) as proposed in 1951. The scale is 1Å = 1 inch (1:~250 000 000). Despite his chemistry brilliance, Pauling in fact built a left-handed a-helix with D-amino acids, the exact mirror image of what actually occurs in natural proteins. See Eisenberg's beautifully concise recollections.[4] The a-helix proposed by Pauling had 3.7 amino acid residues per complete turn and was stabilized by longitudinal hydrogen bonds between the first and the fourth peptide bond units.

Corey in 1951,[5] one form of which (the anti-parallel) had also been anticipated by Pauling in 1940 as a possible core structural element in antibodies.[6]

The structural information was all very useful but in order to make predictions from amino acid sequence alone it required some indication of whether protein folding required a coordinated, simultaneous assembly of multiple regions of secondary structure in order to form the three-dimensional whole, or whether individual sections of sequence would form stretches of secondary structure that would be stable while the protein-folding process moved towards its native tertiary structure. A clear indication that the protein sequence 'knew' how to discover its folded conformation after being unfolded by denaturing reagents (e.g. urea) which were then removed, came from the work of Anfinsen[7] on the enzyme ribonuclease, establishing the important principle that the information for protein folding to the native structure was contained solely in the amino acid sequence. This was later confirmed by Levinthal for the enzyme alkaline phosphatase.[8] Anfinsen's observations were an exceptionally important advance since it finally laid to rest the notion that proteins acquire their folded structure by an 'instructional process', as earlier suggested for antibodies whose shape in the antigen-binding regions was thought to be templated by the antigens themselves—see Chapter 4.

Armed with this information, biophysicists began to explore the relationship between sequence and structure, a journey that would eventually lead to methods for modelling proteins of unknown structure, including antibodies. One of the earliest attempts was made by Anthony Guzzo working in the Biophysics Department at the University of Chicago. Using the rather limited data set provided by the myoglobin and haemoglobin structures and sequences from the different haemoglobin forms (α, β, and γ) plus the myoglobin sequences, Guzzo attempted to correlate amino acid type and helix 'propensity'.[9] In a simple but revealing diagram Guzzo proposed that protein chains could be generated using helix segments containing 'helix-liking' amino acids, interrupted by non-helical regions that contained helix-disrupting amino acids (see Fig. 13.2). In a flurry of predictions Guzzo used his primitive method to predict the helical regions in lysozyme with moderate success.

In a follow-up 'Letter to the Editor' in 1966 Prothero captured Guzzo's analysis in a set of rules that became known as 'Prothero's Rules'.[10] His simple algorithm stated that stretches of five amino acids in a protein chain would be helical (forming about one-and-a-half turns of an alpha helix which has 3.6–3.7 amino acid residues per full turn) if at least three of the amino acids were alanine, valine, leucine, or glutamic acid. If a sequence segment of seven amino acids contained three of those same amino acids and in addition contained one from glutamine, isoleucine, or threonine, that segment would also be helical. Further, as Guzzo had suggested, proline acts as a helix breaker (it cannot form hydrogen bonds) and is restricted to the last or last-but-one position in

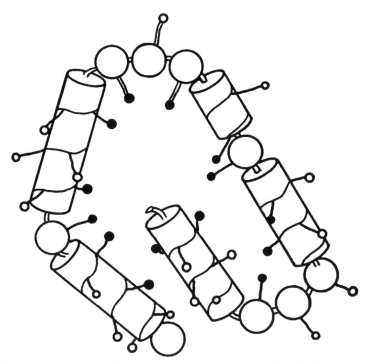

Fig. 13.2 A suggested model for use in considering the relationship of helical sub-assemblies. The lengths of the helical sections are determined by inspection of the amino acid sequence. The arrangement should presumably be such that, in general, hydrophilic groups (indicated by the open circles) are external, and hydrophobic groups (indicated by the dark circles) are internal to the molecule.

a helical segment. Indicating the embryonic state of modelling and the uncertainty of whether certain amino acids were either banned from helices or only found in helices, Prothero, in a moment of scientific humility, invited the reader to 'revise the above rules to free it from… criticism'. Guzzo and Prothero's early ideas were widely tested and as more sequence information became available, statistical techniques by Oleg Ptitsyn at the USSR Academy of Science in Puschino,[11] Barry Robson and Roger Pain[12] at the University of Newcastle (UK), and others were used to improve the classification of amino acids as helical or non-helical. In a more physical chemistry approach, Scheraga used conformational energy calculations to suggest that nearest neighbour interactions were also important,[13] highlighting the possibility that individual positions within the amino acid sequence taken in isolation without considering whether their neighbouring amino acids might negate or enhance their structural preferences could lead to false propensities.

It was probably this type of study that stimulated Wu and Kabat to look at the probability of an amino acid, n, in the centre of a tripeptide segment (n-1, n, n+1) to be in a helix or non-helix environment, a preparatory study to their investigation of antibody structure by modelling. In this approach, nearest-neighbour effects in all possible three-amino-acid segments were used to classify helix potential for a particular residue n rather than scoring individual amino acids in isolation.[14] Having built a set of helix propensities for every amino acid using a database of known crystal structures (myoglobin, lysozyme, the α and β chains of horse oxyhaemoglobin, tosyl-α-chymotrypsin, and carboxypeptidase A) Wu and Kabat then looked at antibody light and heavy chain variable sequences and predicted that light chains contain about 10% helix and heavy chains about 17%. They referenced supporting evidence for their percentage estimates from solution studies by Ross on Bence-Jones light chains using the method of 'optical rotatory dispersion' where organized structural elements such as helices and beta sheets, which contain an intrinsic asymmetry, can be observed in absorption spectra using polarized ultraviolet light.[15] Wu and Kabat's conclusions that variable regions contain helices in low amounts surprisingly did not include discussion of other possible structural elements such as beta structures, despite the comments of Ross in the discussion section of his paper:

> Examination of polymer films has shown that the β conformation can be correlated with the appearance of a positive maximum in the rotatory dispersion curves at 207 mμ… The Bence-Jones protein curves have similar maxima.[15]

Armed with a method for prediction of helices in proteins, Wu and Kabat attempted to model the three-dimensional structure of the light chain variable domain. By specifying the two rotational degrees of freedom of the peptide bond from inspection of tripeptides in the database of protein structures, they were able to assign conformations to each peptide unit in the light chain variable region sequence. After assignment of all such conformations they arrived at a three-dimensional model for the light chain variable region.[16]

Their results were understandably biased by the frequency with which helical regions dominated the known protein structures, with little or no attention paid to possible beta structure—topologically a beta strand is also a helix with two amino acids per turn

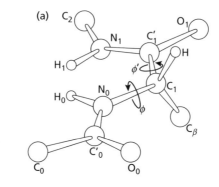

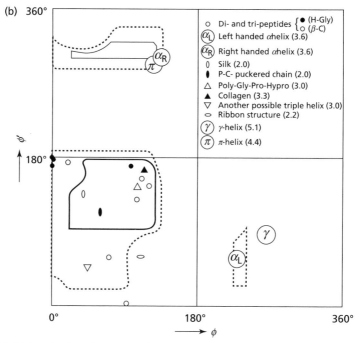

Fig. 13.3 (a) Standard configuration of two peptide residues linked at an a-carbon atom and forming two planes that can be rotated with respect to each other by changing the angles φ (phi) and φ' (later designated φ and Ψ (psi)); (b) A plot of φ versus φ' angles showing the values of these two angles that define the different regions of secondary structure (alpha helix, beta sheet etc). In 1963 Ramachandran defined these angular preferences based on very few protein x-ray structures. Since then it has been frequently refined but is still known as the Ramachandran plot.[17]

Reprinted from *The Journal of Molecular Biology*, Volume 7, Issue 1, Ramachandran, G.N. et al., Stereochemistry of polypeptide chain conformations, pp. 95–99, Copyright © 1963 with permission from Elsevier: http://www.sciencedirect.com/science/journal/00222836

but with no internal hydrogen bonding to stabilize it and requiring at least an additional strand alongside in either a parallel or anti-parallel sense to form inter-strand hydrogen bonds (Ramachandran[17]; see Fig. 13.3). Their results showed:

> Of the 111 tripeptides with two sets of (Φ,Ψ) angles, in 31 instances both sets were in the helical domain… in 33 instances both sets were outside the helical domain, and in 47 instances one value was in the helical domain and the other was outside it.[15]

One year after publication of Wu and Kabat's model the first Fab x-ray structures appeared from Poljak and Davies at a sufficient resolution to specify the structural features of the variable domains (see Chapter 11, references 10 and 15). Wu and Kabat's model was actually not very similar to the x-ray structure, but it was a start. From that time forward an immense activity would take place that would place molecular modelling of antibodies firmly in the structural biologist's toolbox.

Immunoglobulin variable regions: structure-based molecular modelling

In the mid-1970s the technology for carrying out complex protein modelling and displaying the results on computers equipped with molecular graphics software simply did not exist. Crystallographers processed their diffraction data on number-crunching computers, translated that information into physical electron density 'maps', traced the path of the polypeptide chain through the electron density and then built solid models using peptide units made of wire. This was a long, arduous process and could take a number of years for each protein structure. At a Cold Spring Harbor symposium on the 'Origins of lymphocyte diversity' in 1976, 326 scientists gathered to review the state-of-the-art in antibody diversity and the origins of antibody-antigen recognition. Obviously structural information was important to have if detailed answers were to be forthcoming, but, x-ray structures were difficult and time-consuming and the hunger for molecular explanations was insatiable. As David Davies at NIH and David Givol at the Weizmann Institute observed in the introduction to a modelling study, presented by Eduardo Padlan as a joint project between the two groups:

> Since it is clearly impractical to determine by X-ray diffraction the structures of all the interesting antibodies, this model-building method offers an attractive alternative approach when sequence data are available.[18]

Padlan's presentation, which described the first published model of a variable region using information from antibody x-ray structures, was carried out on the VL and VH chain sequences of the myeloma protein MOPC-315. The model was based on the small number of existing x-ray structures and was actually a 'merged' model generated from independent attempts from the two research groups. It essentially used the existing Fab x-ray structural information to build the variable region core beta sheet. An analysis of the structural variability of the variable regions from the known structures had previously been made by Padlan and Davies in 1975 by measuring the average relative displacement (ARD) of each amino acid in the various structures. Their analysis had confirmed that the beta sheet core, or framework, was closely similar between V-domains, even when comparing VH with VL domains, but that the CDRs were as variable in structural position as the original sequence analysis from Kabat and Wu had suggested. Commenting on this Padlan and Davies conclude:

> That significant structural variability occurs only in the hypervariable and carboxy terminal segments is also shown in the ARD plots presented... The agreement between structural variability observed in the ARD plots and the variability obtained from a statistical analysis of sequences... is quite remarkable.[19]

Completion of the 1977 model was achieved by constructing the framework region based on an existing x-ray structure (McPC603) followed by grafting on the CDRs from existing structures. Where these differed from the MOPC-315 sequences, insertions or deletions were made using methods borrowed from the crystallographers. Padlan then maximized the structural stability within the CDRs by forming hydrogen bonds where they seemed reasonable, always ensuring that the phi/psi angles were within allowed ranges. As a final step Padlan maximized the interactions between the CDRs:

> ... leaving no large holes in the domain interior, while minimizing steric hindrance between groups.[18]

Essentially this was model building based on x-ray crystallographic methods but without the benefit of having an electron density map to verify any CDR positions. It was less primitive than the methods used four years earlier by Kabat but it was not yet a set of methods that could be used more generally and as the authors admit in their discussion of the approach, the small database of antibody structures used did not allow them to make specific statements about the nature of the hypervariable surface.

By 1977 Padlan and Kabat had independently continued to analyse the hypervariability of CDRs to try to pinpoint positions in the CDRs that might be most likely to form antigen interactions. Padlan's approach was to essentially repeat Kabat's sequence diversity analysis of VH and VL regions but using a 'structural diversity' metric based on amino acid dissimilarity. Padlan argued that by taking account of the physico-chemical properties of the amino acids a better correlation of the observed variability is obtained, concluding:

> ... structural hypervariability at certain positions appears to be correlated with the involvement of these positions in ligand binding. This suggests that the technique presented might be useful in predicting which residues are potential ligand-contacting residues.[20]

Kabat took a slightly different route, concentrating on the preponderance of 'unusual' amino acids in the CDRs. By analysis of all known sequences (more than 600 light or heavy chains, either completely or partially sequenced) the frequency of occurrence of different amino acids at each CDR position was logged. Low variation was taken to imply structural importance, confirmed by inspection of the x-ray structures, while high variability in a particular position would imply a likely antigen contact role. Kabat was fully aware that even small insertions or deletions in a CDR could influence the accuracy of this contact attribution, drawing attention to one of the fundamental problems in modelling external 'loop' regions, as he pointed out in a later study with Wu and Bilofsky:

… much of the variation in the structure of antibody-combining sites is determined by the insertions or deletions in the CDR… Thus, even the insertion of a single residue… in the light chain may make for substantial differences as to which residues in the site determine specificity.[21]

Up to this point the activities of the main antibody structural and sequence laboratories were focused on identification of trends in antibody structural features as they emerged, essentially the building of a 'knowledge database' that might at some point give clues allowing general algorithms for variable region modelling to be developed. But the field was not there yet. The development of computer graphics, enabled by the digital computer revolution, was dramatically announced to the world of molecular structure analysis as a result of the creative talents of David Evans and Ivan Sutherland, computer science professors at the University of Utah. Their ground breaking visionary advances allowed pictures to be drawn, manipulated, and stored on computers (see Fig. 13.4).

Some of the first applications of this technology, commercialized as the 'Evans and Sutherland Picture System', in protein structure analysis were reported in the mid-1970s but the first use for antibody modelling was reported in 1981 by Richard Feldmann at the NIH for the variable region of an IgA, J539, a galactan-binding myeloma antibody. Using 'grafting with insertions or deletions' methods, essentially as used in previous

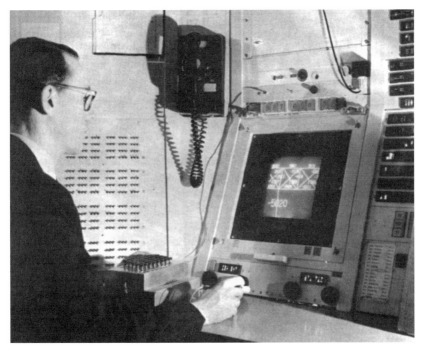

Fig. 13.4 Ivan Sutherland using the product of his thesis entitled Sketchpad: A Man Machine Graphical Communication System, 1963.

Reproduced with permission from Ivan Sutherland.

studies, Feldmann was able to use the graphics display in combination with computer programmes to explore the joins arising from insertions or deletions in a more systematic way during the CDR construction. A limitation of the computer method was that manipulation of individual amino acids could only be carried out 'one at a time' so that any coordinated or linked effects of changing one amino acid position on neighbouring amino acids could not be investigated. Since Feldmann actually changed the positions of as many as 14 amino acids, any conformational interdependence would not have been accounted for. Manipulation of the ensemble of residues would become possible with the computational advances made by Brooks and Karplus,[22] Levitt,[23] and others that would allow a whole section of structure to be subjected to coordinated movement (e.g. by molecular dynamics simulation) in which interactions between all amino acids in a protein could be optimized in a coordinated fashion. Energy minimization methods would then adjust the final structure to improve atom-atom contacts, provided the changes in position were small. Feldmann's model, which included attempts to locate the CDR contacts for the antigen (an oligosaccharide consisting of six linear galactose molecules) within a groove that appeared in the hypervariable region after the modelling, was less an example of providing a definitive structure for J539 than a prediction of how computer graphics allied with sophisticated computer-modelling programmes could take the field forward. Feldmann refined the model three years later using CHARMM (*C*hemistry at *HAR*vard *M*olecular *M*echanics)[22] developed by Martin Karplus at Harvard, an advanced computer programme for macromolecular modelling with the capability of minimizing the energies of modelled proteins as one of its features. This was an important advance since it was believed that the native protein structure was at a minimum energy compared with all other possible conformations the protein chain could adopt. Notwithstanding this improvement and however sophisticated the computational techniques, exploring the structural space available to CDRs where only small conformational changes are allowed required that the starting CDR conformation was very close to the actual native structure. Methods were not yet good enough to be sure of that. In the event, when the crystal structure of J539 emerged the variation in positions of CDR atoms in the model compared with the actual structure was quite large—main chain atoms had RMS deviations of between 1.1Å and 4Å while an all-atom comparison showed values between 2Å and 6.5Å.[24] Note: Close to identical x-ray structures should have an RMS deviation of 1Å or less although independent structures of the *same* protein can often have RMSD values of ~0.5Å.

During 1984–86 a similar path was being taken by Rees and colleagues at Oxford. In their studies of antibody responses to peptide antigens, models for five different monoclonal antibodies raised against the same peptide antigen were generated by 'homology (or comparative) modelling'.[25] The framework cores of the variable domains were taken from existing x-ray structures after consideration of the sequence and structural similarity between the anti-peptide antibodies and the known structures. Of particular concern was the need to conserve amino acid types at the VL-VH interface to avoid a shift in orientation of the VH and VL domains or worse, an inability to form a correct interaction. In this respect the analysis of Novotny in 1983[26] was critically important. The CDRs were modelled by taking CDRs from other x-ray structures that matched the number of amino acids (length) and maximized sequence identity. Insertions or deletions were dealt with by the standard methods used by Feldmann and others and the final conformation subjected to 'energy optimization' by the method of Levitt[23]—the premise here was that the native conformation would normally have the lowest energy compared with all other possible conformations of the polypeptide chain. Out of this study came a set of observations on modelling CDRs and on antigen interactions:

> The overall conclusions are: (i) that CDR length, in particular that of L1 and H3, is an important factor in determining the size and architecture of the combining site and that this effect is modulated by differences in residue volume; (ii) that an extensive region of the surface of the combining site is involved in the interaction including residues from all CDRs; (iii) that electrostatic interactions may be important in establishing the initial orientation between antibody and antigen, followed by adjustment to maximise stereochemical complementarity, perhaps strongly influenced by the high proportion of aromatic residues in the combining sites … ; iv) that extensive contacts are made with the polypeptide backbone of the epitope; (v) that conformational changes may be necessary in either antibody or antigen, or both, in order to optimise interactions when an anti-peptide antibody combines with the native protein antigen.[25]

The study also attempted to predict those CDR residues that might interact with the antigen. These predictions could then be subjected to test by an experimental procedure outlined by Rees and de la Paz in the same year[27] and employing the new methods of 'protein engineering' (see Chapter 14). It was clearly important for the credibility of the modelling community to verify models either by reference to x-ray structures determined after the models were completed, or by mutation of predicted antigen contact residues and measurement of the effect on antigen binding. Both approaches would be taken by different research groups.

Later the same year Cyrus Chothia and Arthur Lesk plus a 'Who's Who' of structural luminati published the results of a model for the Fab of antibody D1.3 and its comparison with the crystal structure.[28] Four of the six CDRs were correctly predicted. In this approach Chothia and Lesk identified a small number of amino acids in particular positions in the CDRs that had the potential to determine a given CDR conformation even when the remaining residues in the sequence varied. This had some resonance perhaps with the CDR analyses carried out earlier by Kabat in which low variation at particular CDR positions was taken to imply structural importance.[21] Chothia and Lesk's approach was a significant advance on the ideas of Rees and de la Paz and would soon be extended, resulting in an important CDR conformation 'rulebook'. The first version of the rulebook emerged in 1987 when Chothia, again working with Arthur Lesk, published a breakthrough paper that brought antibody modelling to new heights. In an exhaustive analysis of Fab and VL fragments of antibodies Chothia and Lesk identified:

> … the relatively few residues that, through their packing, hydrogen bonding or the ability to assume unusual φ, ψ, or ω conformation, are primarily responsible for the main chain conformations of the hypervariable regions.[29]

Of the six CDRs, five were described well by these rules with CDR H3 the exception. Within each CDR type there were multiple classes differing in the key residue or residues that were present and giving rise to different loop backbone structures. These 'base' conformations were named 'canonical structures' and became widely used in construction of antibody models. As an example of how the algorithm worked, Chothia and Lesk gave an example for CDR L1 where its conformation would be defined by checking the match with the canonical residue set for this CDR at sequence positions two, 25, 29, 30, 33, and 71. If the residues matched, the structure for that CDR would be defined whatever the nature of the residues at the other positions in the CDR. This example illustrates an important aspect of the canonical hypothesis. In the above list only positions 29 and 30 are within the CDR itself while residues two, 25, 33, and 71 are within the beta sheet framework and form a packing cavity into which the key residues at position 29 (kappa light chains) or 30 (lambda light chains) penetrate. When these criteria are met the CDR will adopt the canonical structure predicted. The 'Chothia rules' as they became known were refined and tested by Chothia and Lesk in a blind study on four new crystallographic Fab structures in 1989 involving a large multi-author team from eight different laboratories in Europe, USA, and Australia. The results were spectacular compared with previous attempts although the authors were circumspect in their opening abstract, suggesting that 'these hypotheses are now supported by reasonably successful predictions...'.[30] However, in conclusion, the utility of the canonical approach was clearly stated: if the canonical method was followed it:

> ... should allow, for many immunoglobulins, the prediction of the structure of five of the hypervariable regions with accurate local conformation and errors in position of 2Å or less.[30]

Despite its methodological successes the canonical method only worked for five of the CDRs with CDR H3, the most variable genetically and arguably the most critical provider of antigen interactions, out on a limb. H3 turned out to be the most hypervariable CDR both in length and in sequence and its promiscuous conformational tendencies made it impossible to locate positions with confidence that tied this CDR to one particular structure or another. To complete the antibody combining-site picture other approaches for H3 would be necessary. Those would come initially from the biophysicists, exploiting the increasing effectiveness of computational methods in exploring all available conformations open to a CDR, computing the overall energy of each candidate conformation and then selecting the structure with the lowest energy.

In 1986, Cyrus Levinthal and his team at Columbia University, applying the methods of Brooks, Levitt, Karplus, and others developed a protocol for modelling CDRs using a 'molecular dynamics simulation' method in which sequences were allowed to adopt all possible conformations in the computer and then applying 'smart' energy-based methods to rank the large number of conformations, arriving at one or a small number of low-energy candidates for the model.[31] The results from this study were 'mixed', with short CDRs giving good results while longer CDRs (e.g. L3 with nine amino acids and H3 with eleven amino acids) were less well predicted. The computer power necessary to generate all conformations of the longest CDRs (L1 at 17 and H2 at 17 amino acids respectively) was insufficient in 1986 to even attempt the simulation. On the question of how a polypeptide chain can find its native structure from an unfolded linear chain given so many degrees of freedom at each peptide unit, it is worth noting that in 1969 Cyrus Levinthal gave a talk at a small conference in Monticello, Illinois in which he posed this question during presentation of the paper 'How to Fold Graciously' and suggested a rather interesting conundrum. For a protein of 150 amino acids:

> … there would be 10^{300} possible configurations in our theoretical protein. In nature, proteins apparently do not sample all of these possible configurations since they fold in a few seconds…[32]

This has since become known as 'Levinthal's Paradox'. Without knowing the real folding pathway Levinthal and others, in attempting to find the minimum energy conformation, would need to explore as many of these conformations as possible. With the computer power then available they would be able at best merely to scratch the surface of this conformation landscape. As the computer hardware got better this approach would gain some traction but the Achilles heel would always be in the ranking of the conformations generated. Nature does not have time to sift through a large number of possible conformations until it gets it 'right' and must therefore explore only a limited number of paths to the correct structure. How does it do it? To simulate nature's process would require a solution to the protein folding problem which in 2014 is still one of the central unsolved problems in biology.

A way of approaching the 10^{300} problem was developed by Martin Karplus and Bob Bruccoleri in 1987. In this approach all possible conformations are generated by systematic variation of the peptide dihedral angles (phi and psi) and the side-chain dihedral angles (omega) in a tree search—the computer programme was called CONGEN. Tree searches have a habit of growing exponentially, particularly when the number of degrees of freedom in the search increases. This means that CONGEN as conventionally used for long CDRs ran into the same computer power limitation as the molecular dynamics approach of Levinthal. Bruccoleri got over this problem by employing some clever 'tricks' that reduced the number of conformations generated as the algorithm worked its way through a sequence. A year after describing the method, Bruccoleri, Haber, and Novotny published their first significant foray into CDR modelling. The results were impressive, with RMS deviations from the crystal structures for the two antibodies modelled of 0.6–2.6Å for the peptide backbone atoms and 1.7–4.1Å for all atoms (1.7–3.1Å if the worst CDR model is removed). However, the painful ranking issue reared its head again. Bruccoleri noticed that the correct (nearest to actual structure) CDR conformation was not always the lowest energy. Since for an unknown set of CDRs energy was the only metric that could be used for selection, this raised some doubts about the 'generality' of this approach.

Whatever its shortcomings, this was a big improvement on previous methods and suggested that a conformational search algorithm of this sort might be an important part of the modeller's armory. There was another question however that needed to be considered. By essentially randomizing all the CDRs during this type of procedure was this not throwing away nature's own conformational 'knowledge' embedded in existing antibody CDRs and there to be mined from the crystal structure database, as had been elegantly demonstrated by Chothia and Lesk?

In 1989, Andrew Martin combined the knowledge-based and conformational search approaches and arrived at a 'combined algorithm' (CAMAL for combined antibody modelling algorithm) that took advantage of existing antibody structure information where it was appropriate but addressed CDR models by a conformational search method when no useful database information was available.[33] Using this hybrid method, RMS backbone deviations on two different antibodies of 0.5Å–2.5Å (HyHEL-5) and 0.63Å–1.53Å (Gloop 2) and all atom RMS deviations of 1.42Å–3.71Å (HyHEL-5) and 1.01Å–3.19Å (Gloop 2) were achieved. As the authors state the utility of this method is at its best for CDRs that do not have a defined canonical structure and for modelling the multiplicity of conformations likely to be met for CDR H3. This development now allowed all six CDRs to be modelled in the same exercise. While an improvement on methods that were strictly focused on generating random conformations for all CDRs and then attempting to select the correct one, the combined algorithm was just a start. The relative merits and limitations of the available methods were brought into sharp focus by a critical methodology review in 1991 from Martin, Cheetham and Rees that proposed a combination of the canonical CDR method of Chothia and Lesk in combination with the combined algorithm for non-canonical CDRs.[34] Of these, the particular conformational variability of CDR H3 attracted a great deal of attention through the 1990s.

In 1994, Webster, Henry, and Rees proposed a classification of hypervariable region surface 'topographies' (see Fig. 13.5).[35] This classification also proposed a 'finger-type' structure for CDR H3s with long sequences that would enable it to penetrate into deep pockets in a large protein antigen or complex of antigens, as in viruses for example. What was clear was that this was just the beginning of a classification that would soon be seen to be just the tip of the iceberg. In 1996 Martin, now working with Janet Thornton at University College London, developed a clustering method that automatically assigned CDRs to one or another canonical class. When tested on a large number of antibodies the canonical classification held up in >88% of cases. [36] There were however 'rogue' CDRs that were not defined easily by the 'key residue' method. Some of these were single example CDRs for which the criticality of particular defining residues could not be established unless further members of the same class became available. Other CDRs simply had no defining canonical features and would require new class rules to extend the generality of the modelling procedures. H3 remained a particular problem, partly because its relationship to the framework region to which it was attached played an important role in respect of its 'orientation' on the framework platform. As Martin observed:

> We have applied the method to antibody CDR-H3 loops… The fact that well-saturated clusters have not been observed for these loops… may suggest that the canonical hypothesis cannot be applied to this loop.[36]

But the search for H3 classification rules also saw new players enter the field of antibodies. In 1996, Hiroki Shirai in the group of Haruki Nakamura at BERI in Osaka published the results of an analysis of 55 H3 CDRs from crystal structures which allowed the authors to derive what they described as 'several remarkable rules'. Shirai's rules essentially divided H3 CDRs in two classes (kinked and extended) which differed in the C-terminal portions of the CDR depending on certain residue requirements near the C- and N-terminus of the CDR sequence.[37] Similar rules with some extensions that took into account H3-H1 interactions were proposed by Morea[38] working

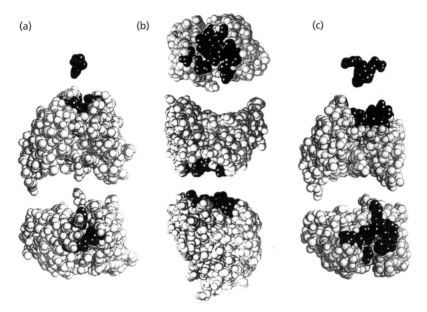

Fig. 13.5 Topographic classes of antibody combining site: (a) cavity type, exemplified by anti-fluorescein antibody 4-4-20; (b) groove type, exemplified by anti-peptide
(myohemerythrin) antibody B13 12; (c) planar type, exemplified by influenza virus N9
neuraminidase-NC41 complex. The antigen is shown in dark grey at the top of the figure.
The antibody variable region has been pulled apart from the antigen and is the centre
image. Amino acids which lie within 4Å of any atom in the antigen are coloured dark
grey. The bottom image shows the antibody variable region rotated through 90° to highlight the centre of the antigen binding site. Details of the antibodies referred to can be
found in reference 35.

Reprinted from *Current Opinion in Structural Biology*, Volume 4, Issue 1, Webster, D.M. et al.,
Antibody-antigen interactions, pp. 123–129, Copyright © 1994 with permission from Elsevier: http://www.
sciencedirect.com/science/journal/0959440X

in Chothia's research group, leading to the statement that the 'torso' of the CDR could
be predicted with reasonable confidence while the 'head' (usually the apex of the CDR
that may form the critical antigen interactions) was not always as straightforward.
Oliva and Sternberg[39] used a conformation clustering approach coupled with a search
for sequence rules but few clear, concise motifs emerged and those that did required
broadening of the definitions as additional Fab x-ray structures entered the database. In
all of these methods some of the H3 examples tested for their conformity with the rules
proposed were well predicted but some were not. In their analysis of the multitude of
approaches to modelling H3 regions, Whitelegg and Rees concluded in 2004 that apart
from the kinked and extended classifications of Shirai which were useful:

> … there are too many exceptions to the other proposed rules to be able to construct any-
> thing resembling a clear, canonical-style set of rules for H3 conformation.[40]

Like all good hypotheses, extensive testing and verification is essential if improvements are to be made to the algorithms or methods under development. In 2000 Whitelegg and Rees launched a web-based online antibody-modelling service, WAM (for web antibody modelling; much of its core modelling routines were derived from the earlier modelling version, CAMAL, developed by Andrew Martin) freely available to all academics, which opened up an opportunity for a large user group validation. For the CDRs the algorithm used a search for canonical CDRs as a first step followed by conformational search and later side-chain placement methods using either conformation search (CONGEN) or an alternative method adapted from the work of Lasters,[41] the 'dead-end elimination' algorithm. The software was updated in 2004 by Whitelegg and Rees to include the classes defined by Shirai and a much larger number of new quasi-canonical classes defined for all six CDRs, including an extensive analysis of H3 regions and algorithms for side-chain building.[40] At the time of writing WAM has been used by a large number of institutions with many hundreds of antibody variable regions modelled from around the world.

In solving scientific problems, the passing of time generates new ideas and new generations of problem solvers. Haruki Nakamura was one of such new age structural biologists. After his initial attempts to classify H3 CDRs in 1996 and 1998, Nakamura made a considerably more comprehensive attack on the problem and in 2008 produced what is arguably the most effective H3 'rules' algorithm yet developed. In this new rules-based approach, a success rate of 89.7% was achieved for H3 models from 314 different antibody crystal structures. Perhaps the word 'remarkable' should have been reserved for this study. Nakamura did not stop there however and addressed the sometimes difficult modelling of CDR L3 one year later. In this study Nakamura described new canonical structures for L3 but more importantly identified key interactions between H3 and L3 that influenced the conformations of both CDRs. In a show of confidence in the method Nakamura created a web server at which anyone can generate an H3 classification by submission of the sequence.[42]

In 2008 Anna Tramontano at Sapienza University in Rome, who previously worked with Chothia and Lesk in Cambridge, UK, described an automatic antibody-prediction programme named PIGS (Prediction of Immunoglobulin Structure).[43] This approach basically applied the canonical structure rules to variable region structure prediction using the Chothia rules for L1–3, H1, and H2, and for H3 the class definitions of Shirai,[37] Morea,[38] and Whitelegg.[40] The method was made available via the web[44] and is also free for academic users. The following year Sivasubramanian and colleagues at Johns Hopkins released a new protocol called Rosetta modelling[45] which had some resemblance to the CAMAL algorithm of Martin published 20 years earlier and the WAM method from 2000.

In the Rosetta method the framework is constructed first using information from a large number of crystal structures to achieve the best VH-VL interface fit and relative orientation. This is followed by grafting using the conformations of those CDR loops that have database 'homologues' from the BLAST search (typically L1–3, H1, and H2), modelling of H3 using fragment insertion plus a novel algorithm for closing the CDR loop, refining the entire variable region allowing the non-H3 and framework positions to change while keeping H3 static to optimize the H3 interacting contacts, and finally repacking of the side-chain positions. The VH-VL orientation is adjusted during the procedure to avoid steric clashes across the inter-domain interface that might arise as the sequence to be modelled is 'threaded' into the chosen beta barrel framework template. Interestingly these authors do not rely on canonical CDRs but rather on the correspondence between loop length and conformation, first proposed by de la Paz in 1986 and developed more stringently by Whitelegg and Rees in 2004. As the Rosetta authors point out, referring to the Whitelegg analysis:

> … with limited exceptions, there is essentially a one-to-one correspondence between loop length and the canonical class assignment. Because of the evidence that the loop length is an appropriate surrogate for the canonical class, we have chosen to identify the correct loop template based on the length alone…[45]

The performance of Rosetta in the authors' own analysis was impressive, with global non-H3 CDR predictions having accuracies of 1Å or better, equivalent to that of canonical CDR methods. For H3 CDRs the accuracies were between 1.25Å and 2Å, again impressive. However, the acid test of any predictive method is a blind prediction assessed independently. In the blinded Centocor modelling competition in 2011[46] a number of methods including Rosetta and PIGS obtained very good backbone accuracies of ~1.2Å while H3 prediction only had accuracies of 3–4Å and in some instances considerably larger deviations of up to 5Å were seen, highlighting the difficulty of modelling this CDR. Since only a handful of antibody-modelling research groups participated in this exercise it is difficult to know how close other methods may have been. The participants of the competition, who allowed their methods to be exposed to a demanding public assessment, commented:

> … as the protein modeling field progresses and more computational power becomes more easily available, it is expected that refinements in enhanced protein prediction methods will be incorporated in antibody modeling packages. For instance, H3 modeling could benefit from protocols demanding more computational power and/or including more sophisticated algorithms that take into account the environment of the loop. This could complement the increase in the number of structures as a rich source of information to generate knowledge-based rules to improve antibody modeling methods.[46]

In 2012, Seth Pincus and colleagues in New Orleans carried out a further comparison between the three publicly accessible (via the Internet) modelling methods Rosetta, PIGS, and WAM.[47] In this study the models produced by the three methods were compared to a single Fab crystal structure at 1.9Å resolution (high resolution). This study concluded that there was no statistically significant difference between the accuracy of the three methods although Rosetta and in particular PIGS showed typically lower RMSD values.

Reprise

The development of antibody modelling using *ab initio* methods such as conformational search or molecular dynamics has often been hampered by the lack of computer power to take every amino acid in the variable region in the presence of an external 'box' of water and allow simultaneous movement of all atoms until an energy minimum has been reached. This is partly to do with the sheer magnitude of the computational operations required to explore all of the three-dimensional space open to the molecule but also with the completeness of the 'force fields' which dictate the preferred conformations of individual peptide units, select the energetically most favourable interactions between elements of the peptide chain, and also take into account the interactions between atoms of protein and the solvent. The use of existing structural information, the knowledge-based approach, is only effective when CDR structural or sequence homologues are present in the database. Combining the two approaches works well when non-canonical CRDs are short or have simple structural motifs. The limitations of the *ab initio* methods are still with us. When that is resolved, entire antibodies will be modelled from sequence alone. In 2014 we are still waiting.

The prerequisites for therapeutic antibodies are defined

The development of a treatment for syphilis, captured in the apotheosis of its discoverer, Paul Ehrlich, in the 1940 film 'Dr Ehrlich's Magic Bullet', is often quoted as the birth point of targeted therapeutic intervention. Ehrlich's bullet was actually a small molecule (Salvarsan) for treatment of syphilis and as we have seen in earlier chapters his observation that certain chemical dyes had affinity for particular cell types or tissues spawned the idea of tissue targeting. It became evident in the years after the purification of γ-globulins that antibody species with the right specificity had the potential for therapeutic applications, the capacity to become 'magic bullets' if also carrying a toxic payload. The scientific proof of concept was conceived in the Hôpital Hérold in Paris by Georges Mathé (see Fig. 13.6), Tran Ba Loc, and Jean Bernard in 1958 using chemistry developed by Karl Landsteiner some ten or so years earlier. Using Landsteiner's diazo method, Mathé conjugated the anti-metabolite amethopterin (methotrexate) to an immune γ-globulin fraction that had been prepared from the immune serum of hamsters injected with murine leukaemia cells in two exposures seven days apart.

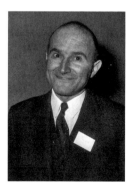

Fig. 13.6 Georges Mathé (1922–2010).
Reproduced with permission from Rue des Archives and IBL Bildbyrå, Sweden.

Using appropriate controls Mathé demonstrated a remarkable improvement in survival of animals treated with the amethopterin-globulin conjugate over animals either non-treated or treated with conjugates made with non-immune γ-globulin.[48] Thus, in this small hospital in Paris the first 'magic bullet' construction using antibodies was carried out and the first *in vivo* demonstration was completed with a remarkable therapeutic result, remarkable that is, given the primitive state-of-the-art in immunotherapy at that time. Mathé's closing words announcing this new development were quite poignant:

> *Une nouvelle méthode générale de chimiothérapie semble ouverte: transporter électivement par des γ-globulines de sérum immune, des agents chimiques actifs jusqu'à l'agent pathogène ou aux cellules malade . . .*[48]

> [A new general method of chemotherapy appears to have opened up; selectively carried by immune serum gamma globulin, chemical agents active against pathogens or diseased cells . . . (author's translation)]

The following year Mathé would carry out the first bone-marrow transplant, on six Yugoslav physicians who had been exposed to radiation.[49] Four of them survived.

Small molecule 'bullets' in antibody conjugates were interesting but a large quantity of 'drug' was typically required to be delivered to each cell or tissue to initiate cell death. This was not so for some of the potent plant or bacterial toxins on which many immune response studies in the first part of the twentieth century had focused, molecules such as diphtheria toxin and the potent ricin toxin from castor beans. In the early 1960s extensive studies were in progress on the mechanism of cell toxicity induced by diphtheria toxin, exemplified by the front line research of Alwin Max Pappenheimer Jr. at Harvard University who showed that it required only about 25–50 molecules of the toxin per cell to bring about complete cellular shut-down.[50] The available methodology for purification of the toxin allowed Moolten and Cooperband at Boston University School of Medicine to demonstrate the first cellular proof of the efficacy of antibody-toxin conjugates. Using mumps-virus infected monkey kidney cells they showed impressive cell killing (see Fig. 13.7) by an anti-mumps virus antibody conjugated to diphtheria toxin.[51]

Moolten's antibody and toxin were chemically conjugated by a rather non-specific method causing some loss of effectiveness of the diphtheria toxin. In later work the same group used anti-SV40 (a sarcoma virus) rabbit antibody-diphtheria conjugates and demonstrated specific killing effects *in vivo* in virally infected hamsters, specifically a reduction in tumour incidence after treatment of animals with a single dose of antibody-toxin conjugate and simultaneously challenged with SV40-transformed sarcoma cells. In some cases prolongation of the life-spans of hamsters that developed tumours was seen while treatment of established sarcomas was ineffective.[52]

Significant improvements in this chemical methodology were made a few years later by the group of Philip Thorpe at the Chester Beattie Research Institute in London. Thorpe reasoned that one of the reasons for the marginal effectiveness of previous studies was that the methods used to conjugate toxins to antibodies were chemically promiscuous leading to cross-links within the toxin molecules themselves and in addition formation of toxin polymers. This would have been inimical to the effectiveness

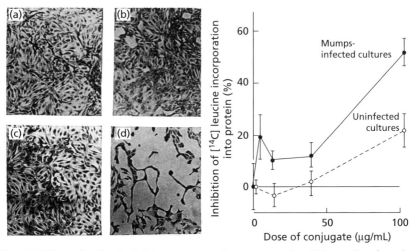

Fig. 13.7 Effect of antibody-diphtheria toxin conjugate on monkey kidney cells infected with mumps virus. (a) Top left, normal kidney cells; (b) top right, uninfected kidney cells after exposure to conjugate for 24h; (c) bottom left, normal kidney cells after six days infection with mumps virus; (d) bottom right, infected kidney cells treated with conjugate for 24h.

From Moolten, F.L. and Cooperband, S.R., Selective Destruction of Target Cells by Diphtheria Toxin Conjugated to Antibody Directed against Antigens on the Cells, *Science*, Volume 169, pp.68–70, Copyright © 1970, reprinted with permission from AAAS.

of diphtheria toxin or ricin which have two subunits (A and B) only one of which (the A subunit) penetrates the cell and exerts the toxic effect. The B subunit mediates attachment of the toxin to the cell surface. Thorpe's approach was to use a more controlled method of conjugation that avoided formation of toxin polymers or cross-linking of subunits. When targeted to human lymphoblastoid cells by a horse anti-lymphocyte antibody, the cytotoxic effect of the conjugate was 1000 times more potent than diphtheria toxin alone.[53] Further improvements in the toxin approach were made three years after Thorpe's results by the group of Hubert Vidal, Bernard Pau, and others in Montpellier, France. Vidal and Pau conjugated only the toxic A-subunit of the ricin toxin to an anti T-cell antigen (Thy-1) monoclonal antibody. The authors observed both *in vitro* and *in vivo* killing effects although apparent issues of non-specific adsorption of the conjugate *in vivo* militated against the expected level of killing based on the high activity level of the injected toxin conjugate.[54] Nevertheless, this was real progress and over the next decades more sophisticated chemistry allied with recombinant DNA technology and supported by the identification of new toxic drugs and toxins would take this approach into a significant number of clinical trials. Despite the interesting history of the area of antibody drug conjugates, further elaboration is beyond the scope of this book and the reader is directed to an excellent perspective on the subject published in 2013 by a Pfizer oncology research unit.[55]

While the approach of toxin targeting was exciting the issue for *in vivo* antibody therapy was really one of immunogenicity of non-human antibodies in humans. For toxin conjugates the immunogenic potential of the toxins themselves would somewhat overshadow any immune response to the antibody that might reduce its lifetime in the circulation and hence its efficacy. For therapeutic approaches using antibodies alone however this was a potential major issue since any anti-antibody response would significantly reduce the circulating lifetime of a heterologous therapeutic antibody and with that its efficacy. The structural information available from Fab crystal structures and the ability to generate models of variable regions coupled with molecular biology techniques that allowed antibody gene manipulation and production of the modified antibody in mammalian host cells, was a powerful combination that would change the direction of molecular immunology by endowing it with the ability to evolve antibodies in the 'test tube'. This would have two powerful effects on the treatment of human disease. Firstly, if appropriate methods could be developed it would prepare a foreign (e.g. murine) antibody for human treatment by reducing its immunogenicity and secondly, it would allow improvements in affinity and/or selectivity to avoid or minimize unwanted cross-reactivity. In the 1980s both developments would occur while at the end of that decade a new approach to immunogenicity prevention would arrive that would revolutionize human immunotherapy.

Monoclonal antibodies were produced either from murine or less commonly rat spleens. Production of human monoclonal antibodies was, to understate the situation, problematic. Knowledge of the domain structure of antibodies enabled early attempts to make murine antibodies less murine by fusing the genes encoding VL and VH domains to human light and heavy chain constant regions. In more or less simultaneous reports a collaborative effort in 1984 between Sherrie Morrison at Columbia, Leonard Herzenberg at Stanford, and Vernon Oi at Becton Dickinson described the construction of a mouse variable region from an anti-phosphocholine IgA fused to the constant regions of either IgG1 or IgG2 human immunoglobulins,[56] while in Toronto, Gabrielle Boulianne, Nobumuchi Hozumi, and Marc Shulman fused the variable region genes from an anti-trinitrophenyl IgM to the κ and μ constant regions from a human IgM.[57] In both constructions the 'chimeric' antibodies were fully functional and illustrated the utility of an approach that enabled human constant regions to be selected at will and spliced to murine variable regions of choice. This was an important lesson in 'effector engineering' that would allow different immunoglobulin isotypes to be joined to variable regions of interest depending on the type of effector activity required. Both sets of authors were positive if circumspect with regard to their constructions exhibiting reduced immunogenicity although Shulman stepped a little further backwards from scientific caution by stating:

> We have no reason to expect the mouse variable region would in this form be more immunogenic than a human variable region of the same specificity.[57]

While the focus on methods for reducing immunogenicity would change in the coming four years, the chimeric antibody technology would have its day in the clinic. Today the mouse–human chimeric antibody Rituximab, targeted to the antigen CD20 on lymphocytes, has had remarkable success in the treatment of B-cell non-Hodgkin's lymphoma.

But the murine variable region was from a mouse and until it was shown that murine V-regions were non-immunogenic in humans there would still be the lingering doubt about taking such constructs routinely into the clinic. Two years after Morrison's and Boulianne's chimeric papers, Greg Winter's laboratory at the MRC in Cambridge published what was a major breakthrough in antibody technology. Winter's group took an IgM antibody with specificity for the hapten NP-cap (4-hydroxy-3-nitro-phenylacetyl caproic acid), and constructed an artificial gene for the heavy chain variable domain in which the CDR sequences from the IgM (Kabat designation) were incorporated into the heavy chain variable region framework sequence of the human myeloma NEWM. The new heavy chain which was constructed using an ε-constant region was then transfected into a myeloma cell line that was already producing a λ-light chain known to form a suitable binding partner for this particular hapten recognition. The resulting antibody was then a hybrid of mouse CDRs contained in an IgE antibody that was otherwise completely human. The authors described this process as 'antibody humanization' and the cutting and pasting procedure as 'CDR grafting', definitions that are now written into the dogma of antibody technology. This idea, allegedly suggested by Cesar Milstein, revolutionized the development of antibodies for human therapy.

As to Schulman's prediction of the low immunogenicity of murine variable domains, Winter (see Fig. 13.8) established that some idiotopes (antigenic sites associated with or close to the antigen binding sites of antibodies) present on the murine heavy chain

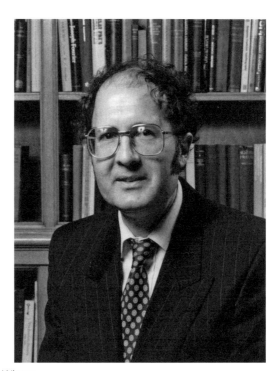

Fig. 13.8 Greg Winter.

Image IM/004972, Copyright © Royal Society. Reproduced by permission of The Royal Society, London, UK.

variable domain were absent on the humanized domain and further that these idiotopes had been removed without affecting hapten binding suggesting that idiotypic antibodies may interact not just with CDRs but also with framework amino acids. While some recognition was retained when tested with a rabbit polyclonal anti-idiotypic antiserum the authors were prepared to conclude that:

> ... antibody retains hapten binding but has lost idiotypic determinants, indicating that the immunoglobulin uses different sites to bind hapten and idiotypic antibodies. It appears, therefore, that both FR and CDR side chains form the binding site for these anti-idiotopes, but mainly CDR side chains interact with hapten.[58]

Surprisingly, the *Nature* issue in which this paper appeared did not consider the work important enough to include in its 'News and Views', despite the British experience with monoclonal antibodies. In this instance however, Winter and the MRC were commercially smart enough to patent the process before publication.

In a follow-on study two years later the Winter group extended their CDR grafting to include all six CDRs, transplanted from a rat monoclonal antibody that recognized the antigen CAMPATH 1 (CD52), a strongly expressed marker on lymphocytes and monocytes.[59] In this study the strategy involved selection of two different human antibodies to supply the heavy and light chain variable domain frameworks plus some amino acid changes to address a concern about CDR-framework packing in the heavy chain domain, enabled by visualization of the crystal structure and by molecular modelling. The CAMPATH antigen selected was not a purely accidental choice since the original rat monoclonal antibody had already been used to deplete T-cells from bone marrow *in vitro* to reduce graft versus host disease by Waldmann and colleagues,[60] also in Cambridge. Early in 1987 the humanized version, bearing an IgG1 isotype to give greater effectiveness in both complement and cell-mediated killing, was administered to two patients with non-Hodgkin's lymphoma.[61] The results of this first therapeutic administration of a humanized monoclonal antibody were immensely exciting from an immunotherapy perspective (the author recollects the numerous conferences he attended in which Greg Winter put up the clinical data on slides to the amazement of the audiences) but also provided important information about the potential for reduced immunogenicity using humanized antibodies. In Fig. 13.9, CT scans of the two patients are shown before and after treatment with the humanized CAMPATH antibody. The effects were dramatic. Eighteen days after treatment of patient one, lymphoma cells were cleared from the blood, the spleen volume decreased by eight-fold, and during the following four months normal lymphocytes appeared in the blood. After splenectomy and further antibody treatment the patient had close to normal blood cell counts although with reduced lymphocyte levels. In the second patient who had stage IVA grade I lymphoplasmacytoid non-Hodgkin's lymphoma similar results were obtained.

In the discussion the authors stated:

> The remissions achieved in these two patients show that it is possible to clear large numbers of tumour cells with small amounts of an unmodified monoclonal antibody.... The selective lysis of lymphoma cells with recovery of normal haemopoiesis during the course of treatment was an important advantage...[61]

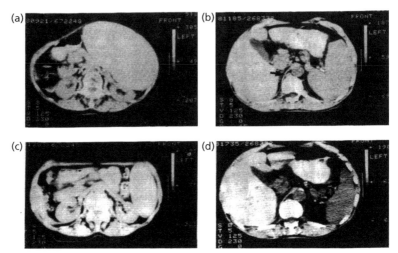

Fig. 13.9 (a) = patient one before treatment with CAMPATH-1H; (b) = patient one on day 57; (c) = patient two before treatment with CAMPATH-1H (retrocrural node arrowed); (d) = patient two on day 51.

Reprinted from *The Lancet*, Volume 332, Issue 8625, Hale, G., Clark, et al., H. Remission induction in non-Hodgkin's lymphoma with reshaped human monoclonal antibody CAMPATH-1H, pp.1394–1399, Copyright © 1988, with permission from Elsevier: http://www.sciencedirect.com/science/journal/01406736

Neither patient showed evidence of immune responses to the administered antibodies although, as the authors caution, these patients were severely immunosuppressed. However, patient one had previously shown severe reaction to the parent rat monoclonal antibody while no detectable serum globulin response could be detected for the humanized version. This was a clear-cut if slightly premature indication that humanization of rodent antibodies reduces or even abolishes anti-rodent immune responses (for the mouse known as the HAMA response for Human Anti-Mouse Antibody). Since these first experiments, the anti-CAMPATH antibody, now known as Alemtuzamab, has been explored in the clinic in transplantation, rheumatoid arthritis, leukaemia, and even more recently relapsing remitting multiple sclerosis. Here was the first humanized antibody constructed using structure-based modelling, artificially produced in mammalian cells, and showing potential for effective immunotherapy. *Per ardua ad astra*.

When in 1988 and in parallel to the CAMPATH work, Martine Verhoeyen in Winter's team extended the grafting idea to an anti-protein antibody (the anti-lysozyme antibody D1.3) the results required some discussion. CAMPATH is a small surface-bound antigen much smaller than a protein and perhaps behaving more like a hapten with only part of the CDR region required for binding. The anti-lysozyme crystal structure D1.3 showed a much more extensive mutual surface between antibody and antigen, involving potentially all six CDRs. In Verhoeyen's experiments, transferring the CDRs alone caused a ten-fold loss of affinity for the antigen.[62] This had been seen previously in the hapten case but had been analysed by models and critical CDR-framework interactions corrected. In the lysozyme example Verhoeyen suggested that since the reshaped antibody still bound lysozyme this might indicate that some sort of 'induced fit' of antibody and antigen occurred that could neutralize the CDR-framework imperfections in an anti-protein interaction. A year after the Winter publications, Cary Queen and colleagues at Protein Design Labs, Stanford University and the NIH humanized an anti-receptor antibody that blocked the binding of the cytokine interleukin-2 to its receptor on T-cells (named anti-Tac).[63] During the CDR grafting Queen noticed a decrease in affinity for the antigen and was forced to make changes to amino acids that participated in CDR-framework interactions, using much the same procedure as Reichmann had done when constructing the humanized anti-CAMPATH antibody. The therapeutic application of this antibody in graft rejection was approved by the FDA for renal allograft rejection in 1997, under the name Daclizumab and it has since been used in the therapy of T-cell malignancies and certain autoimmune disorders.

Over the years following the Jones and Winter humanization method, many research groups would further develop the methodology and propose rules for selection of the most appropriate framework domains from the antibody structural database, rules for ensuring CDR-framework interactions were taken account of in a systematic way and even algorithms for identifying and removing T-cell epitopes, adventitiously incorporated as murine CDRs, were fused to human framework regions. The story does not quite end there however.

In 1991, Eduardo Padlan at NIH carried out an analysis of the surface-residue differences at each position in the variable region frameworks of a number of human kappa, lambda, and heavy chain sequences.[64] The positions in space of these residues were validated by reference to two Fab x-ray structures, KOL (human) and J539 (mouse). On the basis of this analysis Padlan proposed that mouse antibodies could be humanized by selecting the closest human surface sequence to the murine antibody of interest and then making those substitutions in the mouse variable region. From the data produced it appeared that somewhere between six and 16 replacements (mutations) would have to be made to make the mouse surface look human. Individual examples explored by Padlan suggested this method might require a 'case-by-case' analysis since in some instances residue positions were different between the mouse and human variable region. This was an interesting idea but was not explored further by Padlan for specific humanization applications. In 1990, Jan Pedersen and Stephen Searle in the Rees group, now at the University of Bath (UK) had begun a much larger study of variable regions in which the relationship of surface accessible residues in the light or heavy chain framework regions to VL or VH gene families that were traditionally defined by reference to Kabat V-region families or the heavy chain germ line families of Tomlinson[65] was investigated. To characterize the surface locations, 12 different crystal structures were used to define surface accessibility while all existing mouse and human non-redundant and complete variable domain sequences were taken from the Kabat, OWL, and Genbank databases.[66] Two rather surprising conclusions came out of this analysis. Firstly, almost identical family groupings of VL and VH genes were obtained by consideration of the exposed surface amino acids only, compared with the families defined by the complete V-region sequences. As the authors stated:

> ...the traditional classification of light and heavy chain V-region families... can be reproduced by an analysis of either core framework or surface framework residues... These

results lead to the surprising conclusion that the surfaces of immunoglobulin V- region frameworks are probably at least as conserved as their β-sheet cores.[66]

Surprising because the exposed surfaces of proteins might be expected to accept mutation more frequently than the protein core where even a conservative mutation might lead to structural disruption. The second conclusion, that humanization of murine antibodies could be carried out by a process of 'resurfacing', had already been developed and tested by the time this analysis was published. In a collaboration with the company Immunogen early in 1991, led by the molecular biologist Brad Guild, potential target antibodies for humanization by this approach were proposed, N901 (anti-CD56) and anti-B4 (anti-CD19). These two antibodies were resurfaced by Guild's team from designs generated in the Rees group using two slightly different methods for selection of the donor surfaces and retained full binding affinity for their respective antigens.[67] Furthermore, in a comparative study of the two antibodies N901 and anti-B4, in which antigen affinity was measured after either CDR grafting or resurfacing, it was seen that anti-B4 required 17 changes by CDR grafting to restore affinity while the resurfaced antibodies retained full affinity at the first attempt.[68] One of these resurfaced antibodies, N901 which binds to the adhesion molecule NCAM (CD56), is now (at the time of writing) in clinical trials for a number of cancer indications with the generic name lorvotuzumab and in a further therapeutic construction that contains a conjugated toxic drug, lovotuzumab maytansine (LM).[69] Since the first description of the resurfacing method, five murine monoclonal antibodies have been humanized (C242, Anti-B4, My9–6, DS6, and Anti-CD38) and tested in cancer therapy, either alone (CD38) or as maytansanoid conjugates. In clinical trials of three of these antibody-immunoconjugates, over 200 patients have been treated with no detection of an anti-antibody response.[70,71]

Epilogue

The importance of molecular modelling and the impact of sophisticated computer graphics software on the development of therapeutic antibody constructions has been enormous. From the first rather primitive models of the early 1970s, today's sophisticated modelling methods have reached heights that approach the accuracy of x-ray structures on occasion. This quiet revolution in computational biology was, in its early days, an almost elitist activity due to the specialised biophysical and mathematical knowledge required to make any significant advances in the field. Today, numerous antibody-modelling software packages are available either as stand alone or web-based facilities and computer software for visualizing, comparing, measuring, and displaying antibody variable region structures or models is available for even the average home computer.

In recognition of the enormous contribution to many fields of endeavour in chemistry and biology, the 2013 Chemistry Nobel Prize was awarded to three theoretical chemistry giants, Martin Karplus, Michael Levitt, and Arieh Warshel, 'for the development of multi-scale models for complex chemical systems'.[72]

While the antibody modelling developments were in progress, in a Canadian University in the mid-1980s a different type of development was occurring that would provide an exciting new experimental platform for engineering of antibodies. This development was 'oligonucleotide-directed site-directed mutagenesis' which would turn out to be a revolutionary addition to the already rich tapestry of molecular biology techniques enabling therapeutic antibody discovery. We shall explore that tapestry in the next chapter.

Acknowledgements

Text extracts reproduced from Jirgensons, B., Saine, S. and Ross, D.L., The ultraviolet rotatory dispersion and conformation of Bence-Jones proteins, *Journal of Biological Chemistry*, Volume 241, pp. 2314–2319, Copyright © 1966 The American Society for Biochemistry and Molecular Biology.

Text extract from de la Paz, P. et al., Modelling of the combining sites of three anti-lysozyme monoclonal antibodies and of the complex between one of the antibodies and its epitope, *The EMBO Journal*, Volume 5, pp. 415–425, Copyright © 1986, reproduced with permission of the authors.

Text extract from Almagro, J.C. et al., Antibody modeling assessment, *Proteins*, Volume 79, Issue 11, pp. 3050–3066, Copyright © 2011, reproduced with permission from John Wiley and Sons, Ltd.

References

1. **Perutz, M. F., Rossman, M. G., Cullis, A. F., Muirhead, H., Will, G., and North, A. C. T.** (1960). 'Structure of Haemoglobin.' *Nature*, **185**: 416–21.

2. **Kendrew, J. C., Dickerson, R. E., Strandberg, B. E., Hart, R. G., and Davies, D. R.** (1960). 'Structure of Myoglobin.' *Nature*, **185**: 422–7.

3. **Pauling, L., Corey, R. B., and Branson, H. R.** (1951). 'The Structure of Proteins: Two Hydrogen-Bonded Helical Configurations of the Polypeptide Chain.' *Proc. Natl. Acad. Sci.*, **37**: 205–11.

4. **Eisenberg, D.** (2003). 'The discovery of the α-helix and β-sheet, the principal structural features of proteins.' *Proc. Natl. Acad. Sci.*, **100**: 11207–10.

5. **Pauling, L., and Corey, R. B.** (1951). 'The Pleated Sheet: A New Layer Configuration of Polypeptide Chains.' *Proc. Natl. Acad. Sci.*, **37**: 251–6.

6. **Pauling, L. A.** (1940). 'Theory of the Structure and Process of Formation of Antibodies.' *J. Amer. Chem. Soc.*, **62**: 2643–57.

7. **Anfinsen, C. B.** (1959). 'Some relationships of structure to function in ribonuclease.' *Ann. N.Y. Acad. Sci.*, **81**: 515–23.

8. **Levinthal, C., Signer, E. R., and Fetherolf, K.** (1962). 'Reactivation and hybridization of reduced alkaline phosphatase.' *Proc. Natl. Acad. Sci.*, **48**: 1230–7.

9. **Guzzo, A. V.** (1965). 'The influence of amino acid sequence on protein structure.' *Biophysical J.*, 5: 809–22.

10. **Prothero, J. W.** (1966). 'Correlation between the distribution of amino acids and alpha helices.' Letter to the Editor, *Biophysical J.*, 6: 367–70.

11. **Ptitsyn, O. B.** (1969). 'Statistical Analysis of the Distribution of Amino Acid Residues among Helical and Non-helical Regions in Globular Proteins.' *J. Mol. Biol.*, **42**: 501–10.

12. **Pain, R. H., and Robson, B.** (1970). 'Analaysis of the code relating sequence to seconday structure in proteins.' *Nature*, **227**: 62–3.

13. **Kotelchuck, D., Dygert, M., and Scheraga, H. A.** (1969). 'The influence of short-range interactions on protein conformation, III. Dipeptide distributions in proteins of known sequence and structure.' *Proc. Natl. Acad. Sci.*, **63**: 615–22.

14. **Wu, T. T., and Kabat, E. A.** (1971). 'An Attempt to Locate the Non-helical and Permissively Helical Sequences of Proteins: Application to the Variable Regions of Immunoglobulin Light and Heavy Chains.' *Proc. Nat. Acad. Sci.*, **68**: 1501–6.

15. **Jirgensons, B., Saine, S., and Ross, D. L.** (1966). 'The ultraviolet rotatory dispersion and conformation of Bence-Jones proteins.' *J. Biol. Chem.*, **241**: 2314–19.

16. **Kabat, E. A., and Wu, T. T.** (1972). 'Construction of a Three-Dimensional Model of the Polypeptide Backbone of the Variable Region of Kappa Immunoglobulin Light Chains.' *Proc. Natl. Acad. Sci.*, **69**: 960–4.

17. **Ramachandran, G. N., Ramarkrishnan, C., and Sasisekharan, V.** (1963). 'Stereochemistry of polypeptide chain conformations.' *J. Mol. Biol.*, 7: 95–9.

18. **Padlan, E. A., Davies, D. R., Pecht, I., Givol, D., and Wright, C.** (1977). 'Model-building studies of antigen binding sites: The hapten binding site of MOPC-315.' *Cold Spring Harb. Symp. Quant. Biol.*, **41**: 627–37.

19. **Padlan, E. A., and Davies, D. R.** (1975). 'Variability of Three-Dimensional Structure in Immunoglobulins.' *Proc. Nat. Acad. Sci.*, **72**: 819–23.

20. **Padlan, E. A.** (1977). 'Structural implications of sequence variability in immunoglobulins.' *Proc. Natl. Acad. Sci.*, **74**: 2551–5.

21. **Kabat, E. A., Wu, T. T., and Bilofsky, H.** (1977). 'Unusual Distributions of Amino Acids in Complementarity-determining (Hypervariable) Segments of Heavy and Light Chains of Immunoglobulins and Their Possible Roles in Specificity of Antibody-combining Sites.' *J. Biol. Chem.*, **252**: 6609–16.

22. **Brooks, B. R., Bruccoleri, R. E., Olafson, B. D., States, D. J., Swaminathan, S., and Karplus, M.** (1983). 'CHARMM: A program for macromolecular energy, minimization, and dynamics calculations.' *J. Comput. Chem.*, 4: 187–217.

23. **Levitt, M.** (1974). 'Energy Refinement of Hen Egg-white Lysozyme.' *J. Mol. Biol.*, **82**: 393–420.

24. **Suh, S. W., Bhat, T. N., Navia, M. A., Cohen, G. H., Rao, D. N., Rudikoff, S., and Davies, D. R.** (1986). 'The galactan-binding immunoglobulin Fab J539: an X-ray diffraction study at 2.6-A resolution.' *Proteins*, 1: 74–80.

25. **de la Paz, P., Sutton, B. J., Darsley, M. J., and Rees, A. R.** (1986). 'Modelling of the combining sites of three anti-lysozyme monoclonal antibodies and of the complex between one of the antibodies and its epitope.' *EMBO J.*, 5: 415–25.

26. **Novotny, J., Bruccoleri, R., Newell, J., Murphy, M., Haber, E., and Karplus, M.** (1983). 'Molecular Anatomy of the Antibody Binding Site.' *J. Biol. Chem.*, **258**: 14433–7.

27. **Rees, A. R., and de la Paz, P.** (1986). 'Investigating antibody specificity using computer graphics and protein engineering.' *Trends in Biochem. Sci.*, **11**: 144–8.

28. **Chothia, C., Lesk, A. M., Levitt, M., Amit, A. G., Mariuzza, R. A., Phillips, S. E. V., and Poljak, R. J.** (1986). 'The Predicted Structure of Immunoglobulin D1.3 and its Comparison with the Crystal Structure.' *Science*, **233**: 755–8.

29. **Chothia, C., and Lesk, A. M.** (1987). 'Canonical structures for the hypervariable loops of immunoglobulins.' *J. Mol. Biol.*, **196**: 901–17.

30. **Chothia, C., Lesk, A. M., Tramontano, A., Levitt, M., Smith-Gill, S. J., Air, G., Sheriff, S., Padlan, E. A., Davies, D., Tulip, W. R., Colman, P. M., Spinelli, S., Aölzari, P. M., and Poljak, R. J.** (1989). 'Conformations of immunoglobulin hypervariable regions.' *Nature*, **342**: 877–83.

31. **Fine, R. M., Wang, H., Shenkin, P. S., Yarmush, D. L., and Levinthal, C.** (1986). 'Predicting antibody hypervariable loop conformations. II: Minimization and molecular dynamics studies of MCPC603 from many randomly generated loop conformations.' *Proteins*, 1: 342–62.

32. **Levinthal, C.** (1969). 'How to fold graciously.' In J. T. P. DeBrunner and E. Munck (editors), *Mossbauer spectroscopy in biological systems. Proceedings of a meeting held at Allerton house, Monticello, Illinois*, pp. 22–24. Illinois: University of Illinois Press.

33. **Martin, A. C. R., Cheetham, J. C., and Rees, A. R.** (1989). 'Modelling antibody hypervariable loops: A combined algorithm.' *Proc. Natl. Acad. Sci.*, **86**: 9268–72.

34. **Martin, A. C. R., Cheetham, J. C., and Rees, A. R.** (1991). 'Molecular modeling of antibody combining sites.' *Methods. Enzymol.*, **203**: 121–53.

35. **Webster, D. M., Henry, A. H., and Rees, A. R.** (1994). 'Antibody-antigen interactions.' *Curr. Opin. Struct. Biol.*, 4: 123–9.

36. **Martin, A. C. R., and Thornton, J. M.** (1996). 'Structural Families in Loops of Homologous Proteins: Automatic Classification, Modeling and Application to Antibodies.' *J. Mol. Biol.*, **263**: 800–15.

37. **Shirai, H., Kideral, A., and Nakamura, H.** (1996). 'Structural classification of CDR-H3 in antibodies.' *FEBS Letters*, **399**: l–8.

38. **Morea, V., Tramontano, A., Rustici, M., Chothia, C., and Lesk, A. M.** (1998). 'Conformation of the third hypervariable region in the Vh of antibodies.' *J. Mol. Biol.*, **275**: 269–94.

39. **Oliva, B., Bates, P. A., Querlo, E., Aviles, F. X., and Sternberg, M. J. E.** (1998). 'Automated Classification of Antibody Complementarity Determining Region 3 of the Heavy Chain (H3) Loops into Canonical Forms and its Application to Protein Structure Prediction.' *J. Mol. Biol.*, **279**: 1193–210.

40. **Whitelegg, N., and Rees, A. R.** (2004). 'Antibody variable regions: Toward a unified modelling method.' *Methods Molec. Biol.*, **248**: 51–91.

41. **Desmet, J., de Maeyer, M., Hazes, B., and Lasters, I.** (1992). 'The dead-end elimination theorem and its use in protein side-chain positioning.' *Nature*, **356**: 539–42.

42. **Kuroda, D., Shirai, H., Kobori, M., and Nakamura, H.** (2008). 'H3-rules 2007: Identification of CDR-H3 structures in antibodies.' *Proteins*, 73(3): 608–20. http://www.protein.osaka-u.ac.jp/rcsfp/pi/H3-rules

43. **Marcatilli, P., Rosi, A., and Tramontano, A.** (2008). 'PIGS: automatic prediction of antibody structures.' *Bioinformatics*, **24**: 1953–4.

44. http://circe.med.uniroma1.it/pigs/index.php

45. **Sivasubramanian, A., Sircar, A., Chaudhury, S., and Gray, J. J.** (2009). 'Toward high-resolution homology modeling of antibody Fv regions and application to antibody–antigen docking.' *Proteins*, **74**: 497–514.

46. **Almagro, J. C.**, Beavers, M. P., Hernandez-Guzman, F., Maier, J., Shaulsky, J., Butenhof, K., Labute, P., Thorsteinson, N., Kelly, K., Teplyakov, A., Luo, J., Sweet, R., and Gilliland, G. L. (2011). 'Antibody modeling assessment.' *Proteins*, **79**: 3050–66.

47. **Zhao, Z., Worthylake, D., LeCour Jr, L., Maresh, G. A., and Pincus, S. H.** (2012). 'Crystal Structure and Computational Modeling of the Fab Fragment from a Protective Anti-Ricin Monoclonal Antibody.' *Proteins*, 7: 1–10.

48. **Mathé, G., Lo, T. B., and Bernard, J.** (1958). 'Effect on mouse leukemia 1210 of a combination by diazo-reaction of amethopterin and gamma-globulins from hamsters inoculated with such leukemia by heterografts.' *C. R. Hebd. Seances Acad. Sci.*, **246**: 1626–8.

49. **Mathé, G., Jammet, H., Pendic, B., Schwarzenberg, L., Dupaln, J. F., Maupin, B., Laterjet, R., Larrieu, M. J., Kalic, D., and Djukic, Z.** (1959). 'Transfusions and grafts of homologous bone marrow in humans after accidental high dosage irradiation.' *Rev. Fr. Etud. Clin. Biol.*, 4: 226–38.

50. **Pappenheimer, A. M.** (1969). 'Mode of action of diphtheria toxin VI. Site of action of the toxin in living cells.' *J. Exp. Med.*, **127**: 1073–86.

51. **Moolten, F. L., and Cooperband, S. R.** (1970). 'Selective Destruction of Target Cells by Diphtheria Toxin Conjugated to Antibody Directed against Antigens on the Cells.' *Science*, **169**: 68–70.

52. **Moolten, F. L., Capparell, N. J., Najdel, S. H., and Cooperband, S. R.** (1975). 'Antitumor effects of antibody-diphtheria toxin conjugates. II. Immunotherapy with conjugates directed against tumor antigens induced by simian virus 40.' *J. Natl. Cancer Inst.*, **55**: 473–7.

53. **Thorpe, P. E., Ross, W. C. J., Cumber, A. J., Hinson, C. A., Edwards, D. C., and Davies, A. J. S.** (1978). 'Toxicity of diphtheria toxin for lymphoblastoid cells is increased by conjugation to anti-lymphocytic globulin.' *Nature*, **271**: 752–5.

54. **Blythman, H. E., Casellas, P., Gros, O., Gros, P., Jansen, F. K., Paolucci, F., Pau, B., and Vidal, H.** (1981). 'Immunotoxins: hybrid molecules of monoclonal antibodies and a toxin subunit specifically kill tumour cells.' *Nature*, **290**: 145–6.

55. **Sapra, P., and Shor, B.** (2013). 'Monoclonal antibody-based therapies in cancer: Advances and challenges.' *Pharmacology & Therapeutics*, **138**: 452–69.

56. **Morrison, S. L., Johnson, M. J., Herzenberg, L. A., and Oi, V.** (1984). 'Chimeric human antibody molecules: Mouse antigen-binding domains with human constant region domains.' *Proc. Natl. Acad. Sci.*, **81**: 6851–5.

57. **Boulianne, G. L., Hozumi, N., and Shulman, M. J.** (1984). 'Production of functional mouse/human antibody.' *Nature*, **312**: 643–6.

58. **Jones, P. T., Dear, P. H., Foote, J., Neuberger, M. S., and Winter, G.** (1986). 'Replacing the complementarity-determining regions of a human antibody with those from a mouse.' *Nature*, **321**: 522–5.

59. **Reichmann, L., Clark, M., Waldmann, H., and Winter, G.** (1988). 'Reshaping human antibodies for therapy.' *Nature*, **332**: 323–7.

60. **Waldmann, H., Hale, G., Cividalli, G., Weshler, Z., Manor, D., Rachmilewitz, E.A., Polliak, A., Or, R., Weiss, L., Samuel, S., Brautbar, C., and Slavin, S.** (1984). 'Elimination of graft-versus-host disease by in vitro depletion of allo-reactive lymphocytes using a monoclonal rat anti-human lymphocyte antibody (CAMPATH-1).' *The Lancet*, 2: 483–6.

61. **Hale, G., Clark, M. R., Marcus, R., Winter, G., Dyer, M. J. S., Philipps, J. M., Reichmann, L., and Waldmann, H.** (1988). 'Remission induction in non-Hodgkin lymphoma with reshaped human monoclonal antibody CAMPATH-1H.' *The Lancet*, 2: 1394–9.

62. **Verhoeyen, M., Milstein, C., and Winter, G.** (1988). 'Reshaping Human Antibodies: Grafting an Anti-lysozyme Activity.' *Science*, **239**: 1534–6.

63. Queen, C., Schneider, W. P., Seleck, H. E., Payne, P. W., Landolfi, N. F., Duncan, J. F., Avdalovic, N. M., Levitt, M., Junghans, R. P., and Waldmann, T. A. (1989). 'A humanized antibody that binds to the Interlekin-2 receptor.' *Proc. Natl. Acad. Sci.*, **86**: 10029–33.

64. Padlan, E. A. (1991). 'A possible procedure for reducing the immunogenicity of antibody variable domains while preserving their ligand-binding properties.' *Molec. Immunol.*, **28**: 489–98.

65. Tomlinson, I., Walter, G., Marks, J., Llewelyn, M., and Winter, G. (1992). 'The repertoire of human germline VH sequences reveals about fifty groups of VH segments with different hypervariable loops.' *J. Mol. Biol.*, **227**: 776–98.

66. Pedersen, J. T., Henry, A. H., Searle, S. J., Guild, B. C., Roguska, M., and Rees, A. R. (1994). 'Comparison of surface accessible residues in human and murine immunoglobulin Fv domains.' *J. Mol. Biol.*, **235**: 959–73.

67. Roguska, M. A., Pedersen, J. T., Keddy, C. A., Henry, A. H., Searle, S. J., Lambert, J. M., Goldmacher, V. S., Blättler, W. A., Rees, A. R., and Guild, B. C. (1994). 'Humanization of murine monoclonal antibodies through variable domain resurfacing.' *Proc. Natl. Acad, Sci.*, **91**: 969–73.

68. Roguska, M. A., Pedersen, J. T., Henry, A. H., Searle, S. K. J., Roja, C. M., Avery, B., Hoffee, M., Cook, S., Lambert, J. M., Blättler, A., Rees, A. R., and Guild, B. C. (1996). 'A comparison of two murine monoclonal antibodies humanized by CDR-grafting and variable domain resurfacing.' *Prot. Eng.*, **9**: 895–904.

69. Beck, A., Lambert, J., Sun, M., and Lin, K. (2012). 'Fourth World Antibody-Drug Conjugate Summit, 29 February–1 March, Frankfurt, Germany.' *mAbs*, **4**: 637–47.

70. Tolcher, A. W., Ochoa, L., Hammond, L. A., Patnaik, A., Edwards, T., Takimoto, C., Smith, L., de Bono, J., Schwartz, G., Mays, T., Jonak, Z. L., Johnson, R., DeWitte, M., Martino, H., Audette, C., Maes, K., Chari, R. V., Lambert, J. M., and Rowinsky, E. K. (2003). 'Cantuzumab mertansine, a maytansinoid immunoconjugate directed to the CanAg antigen: a phase I, pharmacokinetic, and biologic correlative study.' *J. Clin. Oncology*, **21**: 211–22.

71. Helft, P. R., Schilsky, R. L., Hoke, F. J., Williams, D., Kindler, H. L., Sprague, E., DeWitte, M., Martino, H. K., Erickson, J., Pandite, L., Russo, M., Lambert, J. M., Howard, M., and Ratain, M. J. (2004). 'A phase I study of cantuzumab mertansine administered as a single intravenous infusion once weekly in patients with advanced solid tumors.' *Clin. Cancer Res.*, **10**: 4363–8.

72. http://www.nobelprize.org/nobel_prizes/chemistry/laureates/2013

Chapter 14

Antibody engineering: Improving on natural immunity

Creation of artificial mutations

During the early 1970s the dissection of genomic DNA to establish sequence-function relationships was most strongly driven by the virologists and bacteriologists. In 1971 Hutchison and Marshall described an approach to the genetic assay of small fragments of bacteriophage DNA. In the abstract of their paper they state:

> The double-stranded replicative form deoxyribonucleic acid (RF-DNA) of bacteriophage ΦX174 was fragmented by pancreatic deoxyribonuclease, and the complementary strand fragments were then annealed to intact viral single strands. When such complexes infected Escherichia coli spheroplasts, some of the progeny virus bore genetic markers derived from the RF-DNA fragments. In this way, genetic markers have been salvaged from DNA fragments less than 50 nucleotides in length. This method is potentially useful as a specific assay to aid in the purification of genetically defined DNA fragments and also as a mechanism for the incorporation of small chemically synthesized DNA sequences into viral genomes.[1]

In their introductory section they further elaborate their idea:

> Our reason for attempting this method of assay was a hope that the annealed ... strand fragment would be enzymatically completed, to produce a complete complementary ... strand, within the infected spheroplast ... The resulting RF molecule would be genetically heterozygous.[1]

This was a remarkably interesting idea—salvaging gene features via DNA fragments. However, for technical reasons it was not an easy system to manage and DNA fragments of less than about 20 nucleotides long were not 'rescued' by this method. The approach was picked up by Michael Smith at UBC, Vancouver who had been working on the use of synthetic oligonucleotides to isolate specific messenger RNA species and genes by affinity separation methods. During a visit to Sanger's Cambridge laboratory in 1975 to learn the recently developed 'plus-minus' DNA sequencing methods he met Clyde Hutchison whose work he was already familiar with. The two of them were part of the team working in the Sanger group on the mammoth task of sequencing the genome of the bacteriophage φX174. As Smith recollects:

> In discussing these issues, Clyde Hutchison (who, also, was spending one year in Fred Sanger's group and whose biological knowledge of φX174 was invaluable to the sequencing project) and I realized that the studies of Kornberg and Goulian ... provided an obvious route to a mutagenic method since they had demonstrated that an oligonucleotide as short as nine nucleotides in length could act as a primer for E. coli DNA polymerase I on a

circular single strand template and that the product could be converted to a closed circular duplex by enzymatic ligation.[2]

After returning to their home institutions Hutchison (University of North Carolina, Chapel Hill) and Smith (University of British Columbia, Vancouver) developed their ideas and published the method that was to cause the field of gene and protein functional analysis to explode.[3] Their method, extraordinarily simple in retrospect, is illustrated in Fig. 14.1. In summary, a short (up to 12 nucleotides) oligonucleotide was synthesized containing a mismatch to the wild type sequence at a single position and then annealed to a wild type φX174 viral single-strand template, acting as a primer for DNA extension. The primer is then extended by the Klenow fragment of DNA polymerase, which lacks the 5'–3' exonuclease activity of DNA polymerase. In the presence of DNA ligase the circle is then closed, creating a duplex DNA with a single mismatch at one position. Any incomplete duplexes are degraded by a single strand-dependent nuclease (shown as S1 in Fig. 14.1) leaving the mismatched duplex only. Transfection into bacterial host cells then resulted in both wild type and mutant strand replication yielding normal and mutant bacteriophages. Here then was the birth of a method that, when applied to any gene of interest, could enable dissection of protein and gene function, amino acid by amino acid or nucleotide by nucleotide.

Following Smith and Hutchison's paper, which was arguably as fundamental an advance as the development of DNA sequencing methods by Sanger, the molecular biologists and protein chemists now had the tools to examine biochemical and genetic mechanisms at the single residue or nucleotide level. In 1982, Alan Fersht and Greg Winter in Cambridge, Mike Smith and Mark Zoller in Vancouver, and Tony Wilkinson at Imperial College London took the first steps together into site-directed enzyme mutagenesis, or 'enzyme engineering', with the mutation of an active site cysteine to serine in the enzyme tyrosyl t-RNA synthetase.[4] This resulted in a change in K_M of the enzyme for its co-factor ATP. This was the first mutated protein of any kind altered by the Smith method. It was an exciting development for enzymologists but it also became clear quite quickly that when making such changes answers are not the only currency delivered; new questions are also raised, as Winter and colleagues commented:

> Why the substitution of serine for cysteine should result in reduced ATP binding is not clear from this experiment alone.[4]

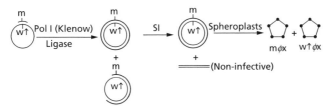

Fig. 14.1 The process of oligonucleotide-directed mutagenesis illustrated for the circular genome in bacteriophage φX174.

The site-directed mutagenesis (SDM) method was soon widely adopted and during the following year or so hundreds of publications appeared, driven by massive improvements in methods for synthesis of pure oligonucleotides required to prime the polymerase copying step.

In 1986 Roberts and Rees applied the SDM technology to antibodies also describing a system for the rapid expression of whole antibody sequences in amphibian oocytes for production of sufficient protein to allow analysis of antigen binding and other functional properties.[5] The target antibody was one of the five anti-peptide antibodies already cloned, sequenced, and characterized by Darsley and Rees in 1985. In 1987, using the oocyte protocol, Roberts and Rees published the results of a site-directed mutagenesis study of this antibody in which CDR residues, identified as potential contact residues in earlier modelling studies, were systematically mutated resulting in a ten-fold increase in affinity of the antibody for its antigen.[6] This affinity increase also appeared to 'mould' the hypervariable surface to fit the avian native protein (hen-egg lysozyme) from which the peptide fragment antigen had derived more closely and to reduce the antibody cross-reactivity with the same protein from related avian species. While this study also raised questions about the accuracy of early modelling methods, it was a start to the development of model-based site-directed mutagenesis of antibodies that would enable affinity and specificity engineering to become routine.

Antibody reductionism

The generation of antibodies *in vitro* in sufficient quantities for full physico-chemical characterization and ideally structure determination by x-ray crystallography required much larger quantities than could be produced by such simple expression systems. Several approaches were taken in the 1980s to facilitate the production of antibodies, culminating in 1988 in development of an antibody form that would become a discovery vehicle of immense utility. During 1984 and 1985 whole IgG and even IgM antibodies were expressed in *E.coli* and yeast cells. The bacterial system developed by Cabilly and colleagues at Genentech and the Beckman Research Institute of the City of Hope expressed the separate heavy and light chain genes (from cDNA) and then recombined the protein products *in vitro* to restore antigen-binding activity.[7] These studies showed that in bacteria, antibody chains require treatment with denaturing agents followed by slow removal of the denaturant whereupon refolding occurs. In contrast to normal mammalian cells, bacteria contain no glycosylation machinery so that no carbohydrate would be attached to the Fc region in this expression system. To circumvent this Boss and colleagues at Celltech (UK) and the Department of Biochemistry at Oxford attempted expression of a λ-light chain, μ-heavy chain antibody construct in the yeast *Saccharomyces cerevisiae*.[8] Yeast was selected since it is a eukaryotic cell that is able to glycosylate secreted proteins and can be grown in large quantities. Unfortunately, although active, soluble antibody both with and without glycosylation was observed, it was produced at very low yield, with considerable amounts of insoluble antibody displaying no activity. This had also been seen in the bacterial system where intracellular 'inclusion bodies' were formed in which insoluble, unfolded antibody accumulated. Similar experiences with yeast secretion were reported by Horwitz and co-workers, at

International Genetic Engineering and Oncogen in the USA, who were able to secrete a mouse–human chimeric antibody and Fab fragment both of which had full binding activity.[9] In these studies the secretion yield was also extremely low (a few hundred nanograms per mL) but the chimeric IgG lacked the expected complement-activating activity, possibly due to the different glycosylation of the Fc region introduced by the yeast cells. For the yeast system the problem seemed to be that intact antibodies contain many disulphide bonds and the complex multi-chain assembly process required was not very efficient within the yeast cell. Another approach was needed.

In 1972 Givol had first shown that the Fab fragment could be proteolytically split into a smaller fragment containing only the VL and VH domains and which showed equivalent binding to the antigen as the full Fab fragment.[10] This was published before the first detailed x-ray Fab structure in 1973 and demonstrated that antigen recognition resided in the 'Fv' (fragment variable) region as Givol named it. Givol surmised, incorrectly as it turned out, that the VL and VH chains were in some manner intercalated since the structure seemed to be stable and resistant to protease digestion. The low-resolution structure of Poljak in 1972 was superficially supportive of this idea showing as it did two 'globular' regions corresponding to the variable and constant parts of the Fab. In 1988 a number of separate teams returned to consider Givol's result and after constructing the genes corresponding to the VH and VL domains, expressed the domains in bacterial and mammalian cells. The Cambridge group of Winter expressed a humanized Fv in myeloma cells which secreted the assembled Fv fragment into the culture medium at high concentration. The activity of the Fv was measured rather crudely but appeared to be fully functional.[11] Skerra and Plückthun described a clever variation on the bacterial expression theme by placing a secretion signal sequence onto the N-terminus of each of VH and VL so that the Fv was transported into the more oxidative environment (required for formation of the intra-domain disulphide bond in both the VH and VL domains) of the bacterial periplasmic space where it folded, assembled, and then passed into the culture medium.[12] In this approach the secreted Fv was fully active. Field and Rees, in collaboration with the UK biotechnology company Celltech, expressed the separate VL and VH chains within the bacterial cell and then reformed the active Fv by solubilization and refolding.[13]

There were two remaining teams who hit on a rather different idea at the same time. Both groups were in commercial environments, illustrating the extraordinary transition that occurred at the turn of the 1980s where cutting-edge research shifted from the long-established monopoly by academic institutions with the creation of powerful discovery research groups within biotechnology companies. Jim Huston and colleagues at Creative Biomolecules in Boston, in collaboration with Harvard University and Massachusetts Hospital, took an Fv structural model and surmised that by joining the C-terminus of one of the domains to the N-terminus of the other they could create a single polypeptide chain that included both VL and VH domains. The linker between the domains would have to be long enough to allow the two domain interfaces to find each other, but if feasible they expected the stability of the Fv to be greatly increased. These constructions were named single chain Fvs (scFvs) and were produced in bacteria as fusion proteins (where the scFv is fused at its

N-terminus to the C-terminus of a protein known to be expressed efficiently in bacterial cells) and then processed by fusion cleavage, solubilization, and refolding. The affinity of the Huston scFv, which had the VH domain followed by linker and then the VL domain, was reduced by about six- to eight-fold when compared to the parent Fab fragment, a small change given the nature of the unusual construction.[14] In the Genex Corporation team, Bird's single-chain construction had the domain order reversed with the VL domain placed in front of the VH.[15] The peptide linkers used were longer and slightly more complicated than the Huston version, containing a mixture of amino acids (Glu-Gly-Lys-Ser-Ser-Gly-Ser-Gly-Ser-Glu-Ser-Lys-Ser-Thr) thought to be necessary to optimize solubility while also being able to span the larger distance from the VL C-terminus to the VH N-terminus. The scFvs constructed were functional in terms of antigen binding although also with some loss of affinity (~eight-fold). Subsequently, extensive use of the scFv technology led to the simpler Huston linker (lacking hydrophobic or charged amino acids thereby reducing the potential for interactions of the linker with the V-domain surfaces) and Huston domain order, VH=>VL, being the most frequently adopted construction. The scFv technology however was not just a curiosity of antibody engineering. As Huston pointed out:

> … their small size may accelerate the pharmacokinetics and reduce the immunogenicity observed for Fab fragments administered intravenously… Further research on the single-chain Fv and related immunoconjugates may lead to biomedical applications that have been heretofore impossible with conventional antibody fragments.[14]

Bird and colleagues echoed the Huston views on the future potential of this technology suggesting that single-chain antibodies:

> … are expected to have advantages in clinical applications because of their small size… should be cleared from serum faster than monoclonal antibodies or Fab fragments. Because they lack the Fc portion… they should be less immunogenic. They may penetrate the microcirculation surrounding solid tumors better than monoclonal antibodies.[15]

In a review of the field some eight years later Huston compared the possible constructions that can lead to a functional scFv, indicating also how effector functions might be engineered into such constructions (Fig. 14.2).[16]

Somewhat unexpectedly, when the linker is reduced in length so that it is unable to span the inter-domain distance, a new dimeric scFv is formed in which two extended VH-VL chains undergo dimerization at their respective VH-VL interfaces to form what were termed 'diabodies' by Hollinger and the Winter group (Fig. 14.3).[17] We shall return to these later.

While the methods for introducing site-directed mutations at individual amino acid positions in the CDRs and even the framework of VH and VL domains for affinity and specificity improvement would continue to develop in sophistication, new extremely powerful technological tools were being forged in the laboratories of the MRC in Cambridge, the Scripps Institute in San Diego, and companies such as Stratagene in La Jolla and Cambridge Antibody Technology (CAT) in the UK. These new developments would in some ways 'trump' the monoclonal antibody technology, would be a

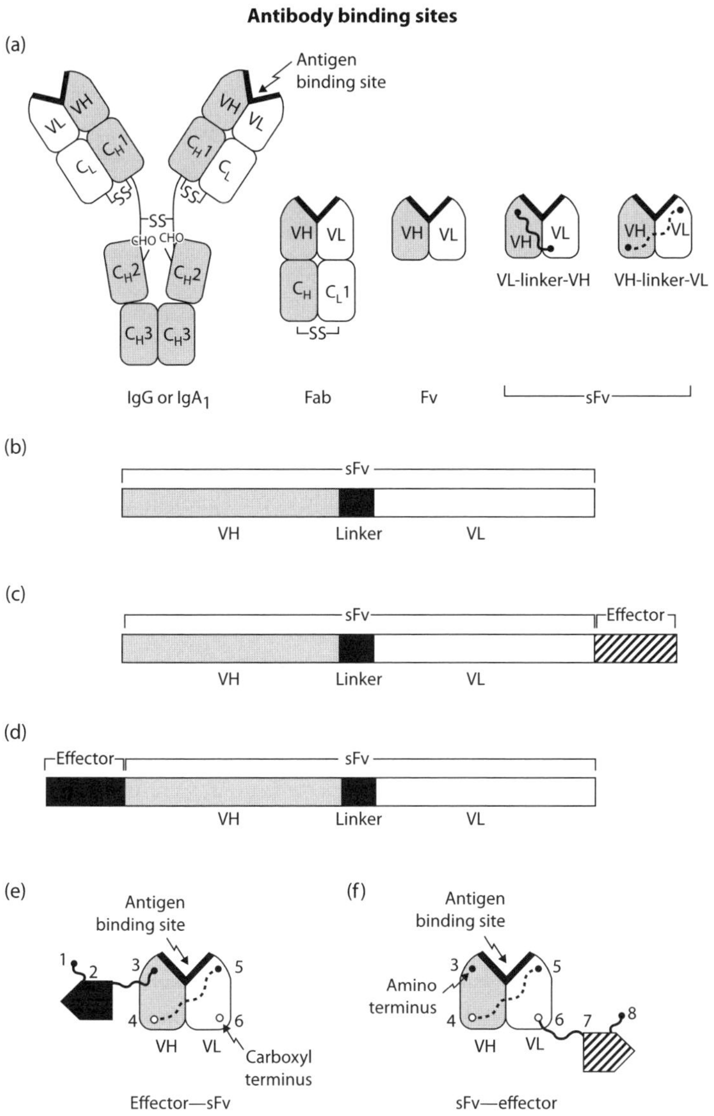

Antibody binding sites

Fig. 14.2 The different antibody-derived sFv constructions are shown in (a). The preferred construction is shown in (b) in which the VH domain is N-terminal to the VL domain. The linker has to span a distance of about 35Å in this format (longer in the VL-VH orientation). A peptide unit is about 3.8Å but to allow for the fact that the distance between the two points of attachment would not be an exact straight line Huston chose a linker of 15 amino acids $(Gly_4-Ser)_3$. Huston also illustrates how effector units (e.g. Fc, toxins etc.) might also be attached (c)–(e).

Reprinted from *Advances in Protein Chemistry*, Volume 49, Huston, J. S. et al., Antibody Binding sites, pp. 329–450, Copyright © 1996 with permission from Elsevier: http://www.sciencedirect.com/science/bookseries/00653233

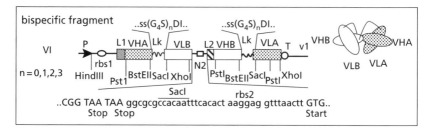

Fig. 14.3 The gene constructions of VH-VL constructs from two different antibody specificities (A and B) with short linkers, forcing the formation of VH-VL dimers, or 'diabodies'.

much faster discovery method, and importantly would eliminate the need for animals to generate new antibody specificities. They would also enable the development and optimization of human antibodies for which the classical monoclonal antibody methods were struggling to find cellular fusion vehicles that matched the effectiveness of the mouse or rat monoclonal systems.

With the arrival of PCR (polymerase chain reaction), VH and VL sequences from mouse and even human lymphocyte populations could be cloned rapidly by turning lymphocyte mRNA into DNA copies (cDNA) and expressing the DNA as either soluble protein Fab or scFv 'libraries' in bacteria. These libraries, which in these early versions might contain up to ten million different variable regions, were 'combinatorial' in the sense that during the cDNA generation the particular VH-VL clonal relationship present in each lymphocyte was lost and any VH domain could be associated with any VL domain during what was now a random recombination. This would bypass the 'one antibody, one cell' requirement for the normal antibody repertoire and could potentially generate all possible VH-VL pairs in a single library.

To 'carry' the respective genes, the cDNAs were either expressed by cloning into bacterial plasmids[18] or efficient viral DNA packaging vehicles such as bacteriophage λ[19,20] a format that could be switched to express the encoded protein on introduction of the phage into bacterial host cells. But screening large numbers (as many as 10^7) of expressed proteins by identifying the bacterial colony expressing that Fab or scFv was time consuming and laborious. What would be ideal was a means of fast screening that also involved antigen selection and isolation of the required VH-VL clone at the same time.

Evolving antibodies *ex vivo*—bypassing immunization

In 1990 John McCafferty and David Chiswell at CAT and Andrew Griffiths and Greg Winter at the MRC made the essential advance that changed from that point on the way new antibodies would be discovered. Rather than introducing the variable domain genes into a phage vector that required protein expression to visualize the

repertoire members, McCafferty embedded the scFv gene into the gene for a surface coat protein of the filamentous bacteriophage, fd.[21] The gene they chose, gene
III, was already used by the phage to attach itself to bacterial cells and hence had
an intrinsic 'binding function'. McCafferty surmised that adding a specific antibody
binding function at the N-terminus of this protein might allow normal assembly of
the phage and expose the additional scFv binding function. The idea was not born
in a vacuum. Earlier studies by a number of groups had used the fd phage to display
peptide epitopes (an epitope is a region of a protein antigen recognized by an antibody) in order to select antibodies for a particular epitope from a population or carry
out epitope 'mapping' in which the specificity profile of a given antibody could be
defined.[22,23] The construction used by McCafferty is illustrated in Fig. 14.4 (in this
cartoon the closely related filamentous bacteriophage, M13, is shown[24]). The process
was simple: introduce the scFv DNA at the 5'end of the gene III DNA sequence and
incorporate it into a suitable vector (a phagemid vector is shown in Fig. 14.4), infect
bacterial host cells and grow the phage with the aid of a 'helper phage', attach protein
antigen(s) to a plastic plate, add the phage particles, incubate and wash, elute those
particles binding to the plate, and optionally further purify by passing the detached
particles through a chromatography column containing the attached antigen. The
'purified' phages could then be analysed by DNA sequencing to identify the particular scFvs that gave rise to the binding.

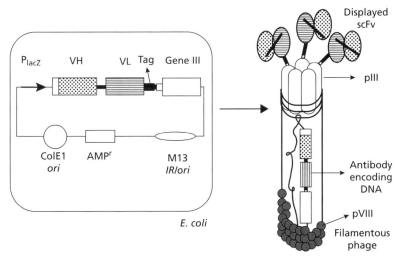

Fig. 14.4 Display of scFv antibodies on filamentous phage. Bacteria harbouring a
phagemid vector (left figure), encoding the VH and VL genes, or preferably the scFv, fused
to gene III of filamentous phage fd, are superinfected with helper phage to drive production of phage particles carrying the scFv, as a fusion product with the phage coat protein
pIII, on the surface, and its encoding DNA inside.

Reprinted from *Advanced Drug Delivery Reviews*, Volume 31, Issue 1–2, Hans de Haard et al., Creating
and engineering human antibodies for immunotherapy, pp. 5–31, Copyright © 1998 with permission from
Elsevier: http://www.sciencedirect.com/science/journal/0169409X

The phage expression technology was simple, elegant, and powerful and would become with further variations the developmental workhorse for most antibody engineers, by-passing monoclonal antibody technology at least for the time being.

During the following year several variations of the technology merit mention. The first was the exploration of a different phage protein as carrier for the antibody constructs. In May 1991, Richard Lerner's group at the Scripps Institute described the use of the more numerous surface protein encoded by gene VIII of bacteriophage M13. In this construction (shown in Fig. 14.5) the Lerner group were able to produce a functional Fab fragment at up to 24 copies per phage. The Fab was assembled by attaching the heavy chain ($V_H + C_H 1$) to the gene VIII protein while the light chain was expressed separately.[25] Attachment of leader sequences to each construct led to their secretion into the periplasm of the bacterium whereupon the 'free-floating' light chain could diffuse and find its phage-associated heavy chain partner, forming an immobilized and intact Fab. The resulting bound Fab would then be packaged into the phage particle.

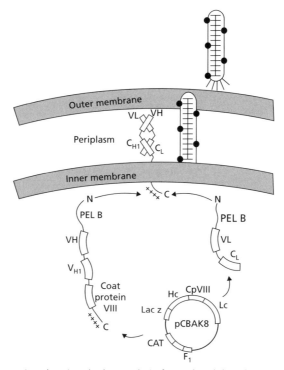

Fig. 14.5 Construction showing the heavy chain formed and directly incorporated into the phage particle while the light chain is expressed separately. The heavy chain is anchored in the membrane whereas the light chain is secreted into the periplasm. The heavy chain in the presence of light chain assembles to form Fab molecules (shown as •).

The advantages of using gene VIII over gene III were presumed by the authors to include both a higher number of binding sites per phage and less interference with infectivity, one of the normal functions of the gene III protein. Furthermore, the use of a Fab fragment would allow its transference onto an appropriate Fc region with ease to produce an intact IgG or any other isotype as required.

The second variation was supplied by the Winter group in August of the same year. In this study, Clackson and team prepared a phage library from the B-cells of a mouse immunized against the small molecule hapten 2-phenyloxazol-5-one (phOx). scFv-bearing phage containing particular VH and VL pairings that bound the hapten were selected in the first hapten screening, separated, and the individual VH or VL domains then re-paired with the entire repertoire of the immunized mouse VH and VL domains to form second order (hierarchical) libraries. This generated new pairings for the original eight VH and seven VL domains selected from the first library. Sequencing of the new libraries identified 14 new partners for the original VH domains and 13 for the original VL domains. Within the second generation libraries scFv antibodies were identified that had both low affinities (characteristic of a primary immune response) but also high affinities (1000 times higher) that would normally only be found in a secondary response.[26] This hierarchical approach also confirmed that particular VH or VL domains could pair promiscuously with many different partners and still retain antigen recognition. In some ways this was a *sine qua non* for the phage approach if it was to become a general discovery vehicle for many different antigens. The weak link however was the finding that all the positive phage antibodies identified contained only minor changes to the CDRs when compared with the germ line sequences. If a large and diverse repertoire was to be derived for isolation of extensively mutated CDRs, some other *in vitro* diversification strategy would be required.

A third and important step, if phage discovery was ever to become a method for generating clinically relevant antibodies, was taken in the autumn of 1991 during a further collaboration between Cambridge Antibody Technology and Winter's group. Jim Marks and colleagues took peripheral blood lymphocytes from non-immunized human donors and using PCR, cloned the VH and VL domains (including both IgG and IgM V-domains) and by random recombination formed a library of about ten million scFv members which were then displayed on the phage surface via gene III, as in McCafferty's earlier construction.[27] When this library was screened against a protein antigen and a small molecule hapten (phOx), scFv candidates were identified that exhibited binding affinities similar to those that could have been expected for an IgM response after immunization. While the affinities were reasonable for a primary antibody response, Marks observed that a number of the VH and VL sequences were of germ line origin and hence not yet subjected to somatic mutation. To reflect a more diversified antibody repertoire and notwithstanding the advantages seen with a 'hierarchical library' approach, the method would require further development in which both sequence complexity and library size would need to be expanded, as the authors speculate:

> … diverse libraries might be constructed by assembling unrearranged V-genes with synthetic D and J elements, or by assembling diverse antigen binding loops on a common structural framework… Larger libraries could be made by improving transfection and

ligation efficiencies and by scale up, or by encoding repertoires of light chains on one vector and heavy chains on another… Alternatively higher-affinity antibodies might be made by mutating the binders and selecting those with improved affinity…[27]

At about the same time Dennis Burton, working in Lerner's group at the Scripps Research Institute, published a fascinating approach in which a human Fab library was prepared using lymphocytes from asymptomatic, HIV-1 positive donors and cloned into the gene III site of the bacteriophage M13.[28] This was a deviation from the earlier gene VIII construction taken by this group and followed the approach of the Winter Cambridge group, although strangely no reference to McCafferty's paper on the initial discovery of antibody phage display was made in the Burton paper. On screening of the phage library against the HIV-1 surface glycoprotein, gp120, a number of different reactive Fab's were obtained all of which had affinities less than ten nanomolar (10nM), representing the typical affinities expected of a moderately mutated germ line population. The clinical potential of the sourcing of B-cells (in this study bone marrow cells) for producing libraries of human antibodies where donors are known to have been exposed to particular antigens was noted by the authors (in this instance focused on HIV):

> The sensitivity of the method in combination with cell enrichment techniques should also allow us to draw upon the 'fossil record' of the antibody response of an individual. This may be important in situations where immunological competence has deteriorated such as in AIDS or aging.[28]

Three years later a hugely impressive body of work was published which achieved both the diversity and size objectives referred to earlier by Marks. The work was carried out in Cambridge by no less than 18 authors. In some ways it was a landmark publication revealing the power of the 'phage technology' for human antibody discovery, at the same time introducing artificial diversity into certain CDR regions known to be critically important in forming antigen recognition sites both in terms of their influence on overall topography but also on fine specificity. Griffiths and his small army of colleagues, building on the earlier work by Hoogenboom and Winter in which variations were introduced into CDR H3 of 49 human germ line genes in a scFv format,[29] constructed a Fab library in which natural VH and VL genes contained synthetic variations in both CDR H3 and CDR L3.[30] The generation of the library made use of some clever molecular biology 'tricks' that enabled individual bacteria that carried a heavy chain gene within filamentous phage DNA and a light chain gene on a plasmid to 'zip together' the two genes to form a single Fab molecule on the phage. By this highly efficient recombination approach a library of 6.5 x 10^{10} (sixty billion) Fab members was generated. Despite the enormous improvement over previous library sizes this represented just 0.01% of the theoretical library size of 10^{13} (10 trillion) members (10^8 heavy chains x 10^5 light chains) but was it enough to match the normal human or mouse immune repertoire? Griffiths was able to demonstrate Fab fragments in the library that had specificity for a large number of antigens—five haptens, 14 non-human proteins, and 17 human proteins were actually measured. Furthermore, affinities characteristic of affinity matured natural antibodies that had undergone extensive somatic mutation (termed nanomolar affinity antibodies) were delivered. In concluding their work the authors, perhaps unwittingly, drove a stake in the immunological heart of the monoclonal technology:

> We conclude that human antibodies with affinities in the nanomolar range, and specific for protein antigens and haptens, can be derived directly from large and diverse synthetic phage antibody repertoires. The binding affinities are typical of somatically mutated mouse antibodies produced in vivo, and presumably could be improved further through rounds of 'chain shuffling'… or point mutagenesis… to create binding specificities and affinities outside the reach of the immune system.[30]

> Reprinted by permission of Macmillan Publishers Ltd: *The EMBO Journal*, Griffiths, A.D., et al., Isolation of high affinity human antibodies directly from large synthetic repertoires, Volume 13, Number 14, pp. 3245–60, Copyright © 1994.

Of course, the size of a phage library required to generate all possible theoretical VH-VL combinations would be beyond the physical capability of any laboratory method to generate. For example, if there are 10^{10} different antibodies in a normal human immune repertoire that contains a fixed VH-VL pairing then random recombination of every separated VH with every VL would require a library of 10^{20} phage-bearing antibodies to have all members of the library represented. Just to put this in context, if each phage was generated at only one microgram of total protein this would require a system that could generate 10^{11} kilograms of phage in order to have every member accounted for. While not all combinations would be possible or even functional it would still become a challenge for the phage engineers to sample even a fraction of the recombination landscape. But would that actually be necessary? Macken and Perelson pointed out in 1989 that even in a normal *in vivo* immune response:

> … antibodies will not reach a local optimum by the end of an immune response but will only have evolved to a high fitness. Thus, the observation that somatic hypermutation generally leads to an order of magnitude increase in affinity… but not to very high affinities… may be explained either by the attainment of a low fitness optimum or by the response terminating before a sufficient number of variants are tested.[31]

Perelson's fitness model for antibody-antigen recognition was based on the notion of 'shape space' and the ability of a finite number of antibodies to cover the shape space of all possible antigens, a paradox recognized by Ehrlich, Koch, Landsteiner, and others some 60 years earlier.

In a review of the application of 'fitness landscapes' to immune network models, Perelsen derived a simple function that described the probability that an epitope on an antigen would not be recognized by some antibody, as follows:

$$P = \exp\left(-N_{Ab} \cdot V\epsilon / V\right)$$

P, the probability, is a function of the total antibody population, N_{Ab}, multiplied by the fractional volume, $V\epsilon$, of total shape space, V, occupied by a given antibody operating within some threshold affinity. $V\epsilon$ assumes that each antibody in the population can recognize a 'family' of antigens closely related in structure, that is antigens having shapes within some shape 'set' sufficiently close to the most 'fit' shape to be considered as a single antigen recognition unit. Perelsen then takes some empirical data from Klinman and Press indicating that something like one in 10^5 B-cells respond to a given epitope. From the above equation $V\varepsilon/V$ is then approximately $1/10^5$ or 10^{-5}. For a library (repertoire) of size 10^5 antibodies (as in the earlier phage libraries) the probability of an antigen having no antibody partner is:

$$P = \exp-\left(10^5 \cdot 10^{-5}\right)$$
$$= \exp-(1) = 0.37$$

This leads to the prediction that ~37% of epitopes would have no matching antibody. When the library size is expanded beyond 10^6, $P = \exp-(10) \approx 0$ and essentially all epitopes are covered. In Griffith's study 10^{10} members were present which should have saturated Perelsen's antigen landscape if all or most antibodies in the population had different sequences. However, the reality is not that simple when higher affinity antibodies are required. The frequency of B-cells having a nanomolar or higher affinity for an antigen may be much less than $1/10^5$. As Perelsen points out, if the frequency drops to one in 10^7 B-cells as the affinity threshold climbs then library sizes of 10^8 different antibodies would be required. If even higher affinity antibodies are sought then much larger repertoire sizes would be required. Griffiths and co-workers were mindful of this issue and commented that larger libraries would be necessary to identify high affinity antibodies. Of course, random recombination of VH and VL chains would more than likely result in some redundancy and possibly non-functional partnering, effects that would also need to be factored into any model.

But 'static' repertoire size was not the only way to generate high affinity antibodies. Hoogenboom's and Griffith's studies had shown that artificial expansion of the CDR sequence space could increase the frequency of high affinity antibodies. This was the equivalent in effect of raising the frequency of high affinity B-cells in a normal immune system population, something that cannot be controlled or perhaps even known.

Acknowledging the distinction between the framework and CDR regions of an antibody variable region Perelsen and Macken extended their 1989 study in 1995 to take account of the fact that proteins may have multiple domains that differ in their mutation acceptance. Antibody variable regions were an obvious case in point since the framework was known to be much less tolerant to mutation than the CDRs. To take account of this structural heterogeneity they proposed a 'block' model in which the random walks to a particular point in the fitness landscape would be different for the framework and CDR regions.[32] For the framework region the assumption was made that it has already evolved to a high starting fitness while a much lower starting fitness was assigned to the CDRs reflecting the lower affinity typical of a germ line or close to germ line sequence. In Perelsen's model the average length of walks to a local optimum was found to be 11.4 ± 3.1 steps with around five mutations in the FW and six in the CDRs. As an example of the correlation of the model prediction agreement with experimental data, Perelsen cites a study of phosphocholine antibodies that experienced around 3.3 and 5.3 mutations in FW and CDRs respectively during the memory response to a small molecule hapten, as measured in 21 antibodies. While the model may have had some limitations, particularly in dealing with 'additive mutation effects' within a defined block and even between blocks (for example it was known that FW changes could also impact antigen affinity) it would have been reassuring to the phage antibody community that walking an antibody to a local optimum in the affinity landscape by randomly mutating the CDRs would not require large numbers of mutations. The key question would be however where those mutations should be targeted to have maximum impact.

Clinical opportunities for antibody fragment technologies

The power of molecular biology in the creation of new protein designs is tempered only by the imagination of the protein engineers and the rules governing protein structure and stability. By the mid-to-late 1990s a multitude of antibody constructions appeared that had the potential to take many different biological roles, including *in vivo* imaging, targeted drug delivery, immunotoxin therapy, blockade of inflammatory ligands, neutralization of toxins, or plain and simple improvements in ADCC or CMC effects. In a review in 1998 Hoogenboom graphically summarized the results of the design activities at that time (see Fig. 14.6).[33]

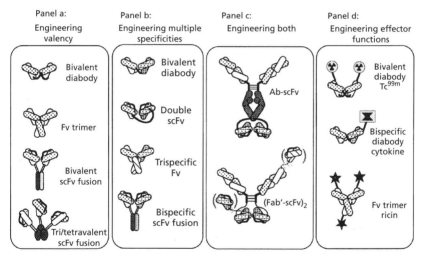

Fig. 14.6 Engineering technologies. Antibodies may be made multivalent using a variety of different formats (panel a), or may be made multi-specific antibodies (panel b), or both (panel c). This will create antibodies that are able to bridge two different epitopes (chelating antibodies) or cross-link cells. Dependent on the clinical use, different effector functions may be introduced (panel d), for instance, for imaging, for indirect stimulation of the immune system, or for delivery of cytotoxic molecules.

The first human *in vivo* application of the scFv technology was applied in 1996 to tumour imaging, exploiting the small size of the scFv molecule and its associated pharmacokinetic behaviour. Richard Begent and colleagues at the Royal Free Hospital School of Medicine in London identified a scFv antibody (MFE-23) against carcinoembryonic antigen (CEA) by screening a phage library prepared from B-cells of a mouse that had been immunized with CEA. After labelling with iodine-123, the MFE-23 was given to nine patients with colorectal cancer and one with breast carcinoma. One hour after administration the radiolabelled scFv began to localize in tumour tissue while over

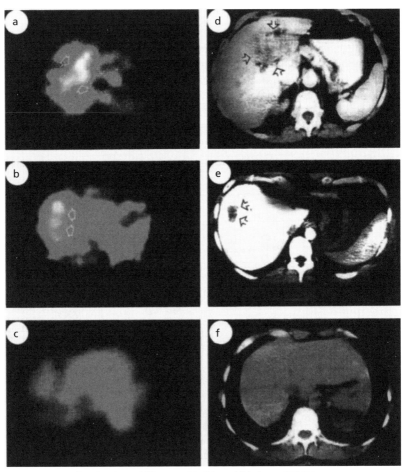

Fig. 14.7 Tumour localization of ^{123}I-MFE-23. (a) and (b) show SPECT gamma camera images of liver metastases in two patients with colon carcinoma; (d) and (e) show the corresponding CT scans confirming the tumour presence (arrowed); (c) and (f) are SPECT and CT scans of a patient with no tumour.

the same time period rapid fractional clearance from the blood was observed—tissue half-lives of 0.42h and 5.32h respectively. The remarkable targeting effect of this miniaturized antibody was demonstrated by SPECT imaging (see Fig. 14.7) with optimum images being obtained four hours after injection.[34] This study opened up an entirely new field of antibody diagnostics and provided the first clinical evidence of what was up to that point a speculative hope from the discoverers of the scFv technology.

Four years after this study Begent and clinical colleagues reported a Phase One clinical study using the same radiolabelled scFv (but this time using ^{125}I) as a guiding image for colorectal cancer surgery.[35] This technique, called RIGS (radioimmunoguided surgery), was initially described using whole antibodies in 1984[36] and again in 1991[37] by Aitken, Hinkle, and colleagues. However, full-sized antibodies are cleared slowly and these studies suggested that a long interval (up to four weeks) between administration of labelled antibody and surgical resection was necessary to enable proper discrimination between normal and tumour tissue. With the scFv, construction scanning and detection of tumour deposits was possible within 24–72 hours after injection of reagent allowing a more rapid surgical resection process. In Begent's study the overall accuracy of the scan results compared with histology was 84%. As Begent comments:

> The short interval between injection and operation, the lack of significant toxicity, and the relatively simple production in bacteria make MFE-23-his scFv suitable for RIGS... the data also support the use of MFE-23 as a targeting moiety of therapeutic molecules.[35]

Realizing the therapeutic targeting applications of scFv technology, as suggested by Begent, were set to become more of a challenge than perhaps first contemplated by Huston and Bird at the time of their 1988 discovery. The original concept of a small, penetrative molecule that would have enhanced tumour localization was certainly proven for diagnostic imaging. However, scFv molecules had a short serum half-life and furthermore tended to accumulate in the kidney en route to the outside world. This was not the set of specifications one would have written for an ideal biologics therapeutic. Nonetheless, spurred by the excitement of a novel technology, numerous research groups, many in biotechnology companies, would explore the scFv construction as a therapeutic drug in its own right or as a vehicle for magic bullet delivery either using small molecule drugs or protein toxins or enzymes that could activate prodrugs at the tumour target, and even using constructions that had normal antibody effector domains engineered onto the scFv. Like Topsy, the scFv construction landscape seemed to grow out of nowhere with divalent diabodies, triabodies, or tetrabodies formed using short VH-VL linkers where the di-, tri-, or tetra-body non-covalent formation was determined by linker length, inter-domain location, and/or sequence;[16,38] divalent versions involving scFvs linked end-to-end (tascFvs for tandem scFv); or having two different specificities each exhibiting the identical activity to the parent scFvs (bis-scFvs for bi-specific scFvs);[39] and even tetravalent scFvs generated by use of linkers that joined two scFvs together which then formed non-covalent tetramers.[40] The explosion of antibody engineering in the 1990s was accompanied by a great deal of expectation, particularly from the financial investment community, a significant amount of hype,[41] definite clinical promise, but also some cautionary tales.

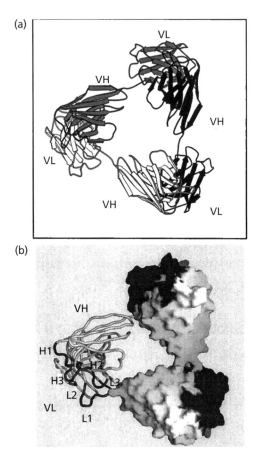

Fig. 14.8 The overall structure of the triabody. (*a*) Three polypeptides in one triabody are related to each other by crystallographic symmetry and are rendered in different shades of grey. The triabody has three Fv heads, each consisting of a VH domain from one polypeptide paired with the VL domain from a neighbouring polypeptide. (b) A view of a triabody with the molecular surface superimposed on two of the Fv heads in the triabody and the third Fv head shown in worm representation. The CDRs of each Fv head are shaded dark grey.

Reproduced with permission from Pei, X.Y. et al., The 2.0-Å resolution crystal structure of a trimeric antibody fragment with non-cognate VH–VL domain pairs shows a rearrangement of VH CDR3, *Proceedings of the National Academy of Sciences*, Volume 94, Number 18, pp. 9637–42, Copyright © 1997 The National Academy of Sciences, USA.

In 1997, Xue Pei and colleagues from the MRC Cambridge determined the x-ray structure at 2Å resolution of one of such scFv constructions, a VH-VL scFv in which no linker is present between the domains forcing the scFv to form a trimer in a head-to-tail configuration (see Fig. 14.8).[42] While this structural study confirmed the models commonly used to explain these constructions, it also threw up an unexpected result. During switch of the VL domain from a kappa to a lambda chain, the VH CDR3 underwent a dramatic conformational change. The authors speculated that this type of conformational 'plasticity' on association of heavy chains with different light chains in normal antibody pairing may operate as a further diversifying mechanism in the natural immune system. However, it should also have been a warning to antibody engineers that tinkering with antibody structures that have been optimized over millions of years may have unexpected consequences, both for stability and specificity.

Notwithstanding the uncertainties associated with unnatural and in many cases untested antibody fragment constructions, pre-clinical and clinical development programmes began in earnest from the mid-1990s. By 2005 Holliger and Hudson reviewed the status of ten scFv-like antibodies,[43] one of which, Pexelizumab—a complement C5 inhibitor for coronary bypass indication (Alexion Pharmaceuticals)—was in Phase Two/Three, and CC49, a murine tetra-scFv anti-TAG-72 construct carrying streptavidin and used as a pre-targeting agent followed in by ^{90}Y-biotin (Neorx and University of Alabama), was in Phase One. Eight other constructions were in pre-clinical studies for various indications focused on cancer therapy (five) or imaging (three). An additional scFv ('Aurograb', Neutec and Novartis) not included in the Holliger review and targeted to a membrane transport protein in MRSA, entered Phase Three clinical trials in 2004. By 2007 clinical development of CC49 had been discontinued and in 2008 Aurograb had also been discontinued due to lack of efficacy. Of course, it was unknown if this was due to the nature of the antibody constructs or the target antigen biology. Nevertheless, it was not an encouraging start for antibody fragment technology. By contrast, all three antibody fragments that had been approved by the FDA were Fab fragments, one mouse–human chimeric and two humanized. None of the three were for cancer indications but were used as treatments for cardiovascular (ReoPro), ophthalmic (Lucentis), and immunological (Cimzia) indications.

While scFv molecules were small, when conjugated with other molecules such as effector domains or immunotoxins the aggregated size might start to approach that of an intact antibody. For example, two scFv molecules linked together to form a tascFv could have a size more than 50% greater than a Fab fragment,[44] challenging somewhat the original scFv concept of 'small size equals improved access' to tumours or other tissues. Addition of constant domains to such constructs might begin to defeat the miniaturization objective of the technology. Could further reduction of a binding region be feasible to allow an engineering start from a smaller fragment? In 1964 Utsumi and Karush gave the first hints that a single antibody chain could reproduce the antigen binding of the full antibody by separating the heavy chain of a rabbit IgG and showing it retained 87% of the binding for a small molecule hapten (the dye molecule p-dimethylaminobenzeneazophenyl-a-lactoside, or Lac dye) as the intact antibody.[45] Of course, these experiments were primitive and too early to make any prediction about heavy versus light chain contribution to antigen recognition, even though the authors elected to do so. The notion that either a VH or VL domain could operate independently as an antigen recognition unit was not further explored until 1989 when Sally Ward and colleagues, working in Winter's laboratory in Cambridge, cloned and secreted from *E. Coli* a library of VH domains.[17] The VH domains (termed Dabs for domain antibodies) were cloned from mice that had been immunized with two different proteins and the binding of the isolated VH domains to these proteins then measured. Affinities similar to those seen for intact antibodies were reported although significant debate ensued in conference discussions (as this author recollects) after the reported results questioning whether isolated VH domains, which were as the authors themselves point out 'sticky', were binding to protein surfaces with the true specificity of an antibody or merely through hydrophobic or charge 'patch' interactions. After all, as interested antibody engineers might have supposed at the time, a VH domain does not normally exist independently of its 'sticky' VL partner. Or does it? As we have seen in Chapter 11, the antibody form that consists solely of heavy chains, found in camelids and cartilaginous sharks in 1993, was an obvious answer to the stickiness problem. Since the VH domain antibodies were 'partnerless' the equivalent surface to that engaged in VL interactions in 'normal' antibodies had acquired an amino acid composition typical for a protein surface exposed to aqueous environments. The development of VHH (*v*ariable *h*eavy domain of *h*eavy chain antibodies) domain antibodies as therapeutics and diagnostics (part of the so-called third generation antibody fragment therapeutics) has been behind the curve compared with other more mature formats but may yet find its therapeutic or diagnostic niche. In 2009 Nelson and Reichert reported that five 'third-generation' fragments had entered clinical development, all within commercial environments.[46] Whether heavy chain Dabs will exhibit greater efficiency in tissue penetration than other fragment constructions remains to be seen although it is interesting that the most advanced study so far, publicly known, involves use of a dimeric VHH format in a blocking function operating in the systemic circulation. The molecule, ALX-0082 or Caplacizumab, is under development by Ablynx (who calls these Dab constructs 'Nanobodies') for treatment of TPP (thrombotic thrombocytopenic purpura) by binding to von Willebrand factor and inhibiting its activation of the platelet glycoprotein (Gb)1b-IX-V receptor.[47] An international Phase Two study was expected to complete its recruitment by the end of 2013.[48]

Bifunctional antibodies: a game-changing development

Normal antibodies are divalent but monospecific. The two Fab arms carry the identical VH and VL sequences and hence exhibit the same specificity. In the early 1960s experimental forays into 'mixed specificity' antibodies were made by several research groups. In 1961 Alfred Nisonoff described in a 'Letter to the Editor' the results of reassembling Fab' fragments from two different rabbit antibodies into one antibody fragment of mixed specificity.[49] Given the ease with which Fab' fragments could be reoxidized to form (Fab') two fragments and the interest in improving histologic reagents or the formation of precipitating antibodies, this was an obvious if at the time original trick to play with the proteolytic methods Rodney Porter had described. Three years later Nisonoff confirmed the bispecificity of the mixed Fab' arms by coating human and chicken erythrocytes with different antigens and showing agglutination of both sets of red cells by the mixed specificity (Fab') two construct.[50] At the time, speculation was rife on the existence of mixed specificity antibodies in normal antibody populations *in vivo*. In 2007 and again in 2011 groups at the University of Amsterdam reported on the phenomenon of spontaneous chain exchange in human IgG4 molecules, generating chimeras that would presumably operate *in vivo* as natural bispecific antibodies.[51,52] The evidence for and against this phenomenon as an important immunological mechanism has been open to differing interpretations (see Riethmüller's excellent review[53]). Further activity was given a boost by the arrival of monoclonal antibodies. Multifunctional antibodies had been described by Köhler and Milstein in the myeloma–spleen-cell fusion products where each cell was still producing its own antibody chains but as well as the normal heavy and light chain pairings, hybrid chain molecules were seen (see Chapter 12). But this was not a controllable source, either from an antigen specificity—antigens for myelomas were rarely known—or from a 'clean' production point of view. Expression of genetically engineered antibodies was not yet possible and chemical cross-linking was still the method of choice. In 1983 Milstein published results exploiting the hybrid monoclonal approach in the development of more potent histological reagents, also noting that this hybrid approach may have a 'variety of uses in biology and medicine'.[54] Whether that was a trigger for the avalanche of activity that followed is moot since a good number of immunologists would have been aware of the earlier work of Nisonoff and others, notwithstanding the publication of some of that work in less widely read journals.

Two years after Milstein's paper two landmark papers appeared that without engaging in excessive hyperbole, arguably set the stage for all future developments in bispecific antibody biology. The first to appear was a study by Michael Bevan at the Scripps Clinic and Research Foundation and colleagues from Lilly Research laboratories. Bevan's objective was cytotoxic T-cell targeting to tumour cells. First, an antibody able to bind to the T-cell receptor was chemically cross-linked to target lymphoma cells and then exposed to CTLs. Lysis of the lymphoma cells was only seen when the cross-linking had taken place. In follow-on experiments a bispecific antibody was prepared having the dual recognition of the T-cell receptor and the Thy-1 antigen present on lymphoma cells. Mixing of the cells and the bispecific antibody resulted in impressive cell killing. The generality of this approach was clearly stated by the authors:

> The results presented here suggest that it is possible to focus a strong T-cell response to a particular target antigen using hybrid antibodies; this could have clinical significance in the rejection of tumor cells or viral infections.[55]

Three months after the Bevan publication, David Segal and colleagues from the NCI, Bethesda published similar results but this time the antigen was the T-cell receptor-associated protein known as T3. A number of bispecific antibodies were generated where the anti-T3 specificity was common to all constructs while the second specificity was derived from antibodies reactive with different target cell types. In summarizing the results Segal observes:

> … we have now been able to direct Tc cells [cytotoxic T-cells] to lyse every target cell for which we have an appropriate anti-target cell antibody… it is reasonable to suppose that Tc cells could be directed against various pathogenic cells in vivo, for example against tumor cells.[56]

By 1987 several publications exploiting the technology had appeared, including a further study by Bevan in which influenza-virus-infected cells had been killed by the same approach.[57] A different application of the chemical cross-linking approach was taken by Martin Glennie and colleagues working at the Tenovus Laboratory in Southampton, UK. Glennie prepared bispecific (Fab')$_2$ molecules with various combinations of specificity, which included one Fab' arm specific for IgM on leukaemia (L$_2$C) cells and the other Fab' specific for the plant toxin, saporin. Efficient cell killing was observed by specific delivery of the toxin. In a further configuration, the same anti-IgM arm was paired with a Fab' that bound to the Fcg receptor on peripheral blood lymphocytes, recapitulating the observations of Bevan and Segal some two years earlier. Mixing the bispecific with the two sets of cells triggered cell killing of the L$_2$C cells by the PBLs. In the discussion of the results Glennie commented:

> If a bispecific antibody is to target an unwanted cell for killing by an effector cell or a toxin, it must first bind to one or both surfaces, and then remain bound and available until such time as the two surfaces are juxtaposed.[58]

Glennie's statement about surface juxtaposition was fortuitously (or perhaps brilliantly) prophetic since much later it would become clear that for efficient cell killing it may be enough to bring the target cell and killing cell in close enough proximity to form a synapse-like interaction to trigger cytotoxicity.[59]

In the early 1990s a number of studies of chemically cross-linked bifunctional antibodies or fragments continued to appear. While it was not impossible that chemically cross-linked antibodies could find their way into human clinical applications, the most elegant approach would be a cloning method that would allow production of large amounts of protein with a fully controllable specification. In 1993, Griffiths noticed the presence of dimers in scFv preparations secreted from bacteria. Their presence might have been somewhat serendipitous since the linker used was a standard length (~15 amino acids) scFv linker and the normal VH-VL intrachain formation would have been the expected configuration. At this point the authors were not totally seduced by the observation either, concluding that:

> Presumably the dimers are scFv fragments interlocked through the flexible linker joining the heavy and light chains, or with the heavy chain of one scFv molecule associated with the light chain of the other.[60]

The follow-on work by Philipp Holliger cemented the mechanism and cast the model for future development. Holliger investigated different length scFv linkers and established an obligatory diabody formation with linkers of five amino acids or less. Furthermore, by including two different scFv VH-VL chains, hetero-scFvs or 'bi-specific' scFvs were formed containing both specificities of the two starting scFvs. Here was the trigger for a new kind of antibody that could be engineered to have two (or perhaps more) antigen recognition sites within the same molecule. In parallel with Holliger's work, Mallendar and Voss had constructed a bi-specific scFv using a slightly different approach in which the two individual scFv constructs were covalently linked via a separate linker allowing expression of the entire bispecific chain in one linear gene sequence.[61]

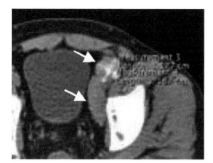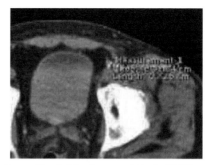

Fig. 14.9 Antitumour activities of T-cell–engaging antibody blinatumomab (called BiTE for bispecific T-cell engager). Computer tomography (CT) images of patient 16 (0.015 mg of blinatumomab/m2 per day) before (left image) and after (right image) eight weeks of treatment. The response of this patient was rated as complete. Arrows indicate two lymph-node tumours in the pelvic area.

From Bargou, R. et al., Tumor Regression in Cancer Patients by Very Low Doses of a T Cell–Engaging Antibody, *Science*, Volume 321, Number 5891, pp. 974–976. Reprinted with permission from AAAS, Copyright © 2008.

New technology is exciting and often persuasive in its claims of clinical potential. The proof of the pudding is in the eating however. By 2008 the earlier ideas of Bevan and Segal were taken to the clinic with outstanding results for such an unproven model in humans. In a collaborative study between the University of Wurzburg, a number of other German universities in Essen, Mainz, Ulm, Munich, and the German company Micromet, used a bispecific scFv carrying specificities for CD19 (a B-cell protein associated with the antigen receptor) and CD3 (T-cell receptor complex and known previously as T3) to treat 38 patients with non-Hodgkin's B-cell lymphoma (NHL) that had relapsed to standard therapies.[62] An example of the patient response to this treatment is shown in Fig. 14.9.

While not all patients were as responsive, the overall results were impressive and provided great promise for this therapeutic approach. A particularly important aspect of this study in comparison with rituximab, the humanized antibody therapy for NHL developed by Waldman and Winter, was the dose required for the therapeutic effect. Blinatumomab effects were seen at doses of 0.015mg/m^2 per day in comparison with rituximab which requires does at 375mg/m^2 per week. This enormous potency difference was attributed to the high lytic potential of cytotoxic T-cells which can engage in serial lysis and can also proliferate at the site of action.

The promise of fragment-based antibody constructs in the treatment of human disease has yet to be fully realized despite the promising early examples. The complexity of establishing relevant single or multi-specificity constructions and then arranging for the fragments generated to be able to engage in normal antibody effector functions such as ADC or ADCC, or carry toxic payloads to specific tissue sites, was always going to be an immense technical barrier to the development of potent, immune-based disease modulators. Two new approaches paved the way for what may be more robust bispecific formats. In 1998, Carter and colleagues from Genentech described a novel construction in which the CH3 domains of two different IgG heavy chains were engineered to contain complementary 'knob and hole' features.[63] On expression of the full-length antibody, assembly of the bispecific antibody heavy chains would be preferred for those chains able to pair via the shape complementarity introduced into the CH3 domains. This technology has advanced to the state where it has been applied for both IgG1 and IgG4 human isotypes with encouraging *in vivo* results.[64]

A more recent approach to the 'antigen binding plus effector function' conundrum was provided by Rüker and colleagues at the Christian Doppler Laboratory for Antibody Engineering in Vienna, in collaboration with the biotechnology company f-star. Rüker surmised that by randomizing the short loops at the C-terminus of the Fc region (the CH3 domain), different antigen recognition sites could be generated. This randomization was carried out using the relatively little used 'yeast display' platform for antibody library construction but which was ideal for surface localization of eukaryotic, disulphide-containing proteins. The assumption with this format required that the CH3 loops (the two heavy chains are identical giving the C-terminus of the CH3 domain a two-fold symmetry and hence two repeated loop regions to be engineered, either separately or in concert) were 'engineerable' without disrupting the Fc structure and that once in place, normal effector functions of the Fc region would remain intact. Remarkably, both requirements were met and Fcabs (Fc antibodies) were born.[65] This approach opened up two obvious applications. Firstly, an antigen-binding fragment was now possible that contained all the Fc functions of an intact antibody. Crucially, Rüker showed that FcRn binding was unimpaired allowing the Fcab to have the same *in vivo* half-life of normal antibodies. Secondly, antigen specificity in combination with effector functions was demonstrated by production of an anti-HER2 Fcab that was able to engage in cell killing via ADCC. The Fcab technology is currently under development but had a further twist in its armamentarium. By replacing the normal Fc of an antibody with a complementary specificity by an engineered Fcab, a fully functional bispecific, or even tri-specific antibody could be produced. Here was the hybrid antibody but in a rather different guise to that anticipated by Milstein. We await the development of this technology with interest.

The bathwater not the baby

The seductiveness of antibody engineering technologies has had and may continue to have a Medusa-like effect on the immunology community and its academic and in particular its commercial sponsors. Not all technologies will end up as successful, clinically approved drugs, as evidenced by the failure of many of the recent development candidates.[45] In parallel with antibody fragment technology, development of non-antibody scaffolds on which to introduce antigen-binding activities has also been actively pursued. Those technologies do not concern us here but should be added to the radar screen by clinicians. Not all approaches however are focused on size reduction. In fact the most successful antibody therapies today come from whole antibodies, albeit modified in various ways. We shall explore the history of two examples of this success in the following chapters.

Particularly important aspects of whole-antibody therapy are the *in vivo* stability of antibodies, reflected in the circulation lifetime, and biological efficacy, influenced both by target antigen relevance and Fc-mediated effector functions. Armed with the knowledge of FcRn-mediated protective recycling, mutations at the site of FcRn binding in the Fc region have enabled half-life increases of two to four times,[66,67] allowing for less frequent dosing and contributing to increased efficacy. Impressively, this approach has been taken to increase the lifetime of the highly effective ADCC- and CDC-mediating isotype, IgG3, which has a short half-life due to the fact that it is out-competed at the FcRn receptor by the much higher concentrations of other IgG isotypes.[68] Other types of modification have been introduced to fine-tune the interaction of the relevant antibody with effector mediators such as C1q or Fcγ receptors by modulating the carbohydrate content and positioning in the CH2 constant domain. As we have seen, the earliest attempts to create multi-specificity were made in the pre-engineering era where protein fragments had to be chemically cross-linked or where in-cell hybrid protein-chain recombination could take place.

In 1995, Lindhofer and colleagues at Ludwig Maximilians University in Munich used a novel variation on the hybrid hybridoma method in which two different hybridoma cells are fused to form 'quadridomas' to produce bispecific whole antibodies. Rather than fusing two mouse hybridomas however, which had proved problematic to purify, Lindhofer fused a mouse with a rat hybridoma, giving the rat-mouse hybrid certain properties that made its isolation and purification simple.[69] This technique was subsequently used by Linke and colleagues at Fresenius Biotech, Munich to develop a bispecific antibody combining an anti-CD3 activity and a second binding activity targeting the epithelial adhesion molecule, EpCAM, expressed on the surface of tumourous

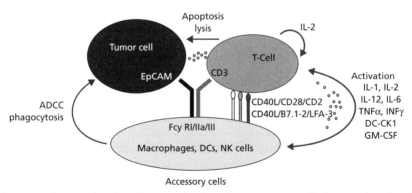

Fig. 14.10 The postulated mechanism of action of catumaxomab: The intact trifunctional antibody catumaxomab accelerates the recognition and destruction of tumour cells by different immune cells. ADCC, antibody-dependent cellular toxicity; DC-CK1, dendritic cell cytokine 1; IL, interleukin; IFNγ, interferon gamma; TNFα, tumour necrosis factor alpha; LFA, lymphocyte function antigen; NK, natural killer; GM-CSF, granulocyte monocyte colony stimulating factor.

epithelial cells in ovarian, gastric, colon, pancreatic, prostate, lung, and endometrial carcinomas but present only on the basolaterial surface of normal epithelia.[70] This antibody, which had a postulated mechanism of action shown in Fig. 14.10, was described by the authors as 'trifunctional' by virtue of its intact Fc-effector functions, a message well understood by the antibody fragment community. It was approved as catumaxomab in Europe for treatment of malignant ascites in 2009.

As of August 2012, 32 monoclonal antibodies were currently on the market according to Buss and colleagues[71], of which 14 were for cancer indications, including a single bispecific antibody. By mid-2014 a further three antibodies had been approved by FDA and another eight antibodies were in review.[72]

Acknowledgements

Text extracts reproduced with permission from Hutchison, C.A. and Edgell, M.H. Genetic assay for small fragments of bacteriophage φX 174 deoxyribonucleic acid, *Journal of Virology*, Volume 8, pp. 181–189, Copyright © 1971 American Society for Microbiology.

Text extracts reproduced from Michael Smith's Nobel Lecture in Chemistry, *Synthetic DNA and Biology*, Copyright © The Nobel Foundation 1993, with permission from Nobel Media.

Text extract reprinted from *The Journal of Molecular Biology*, Volume 222, Issue 3, Marks, J.D., et al., By-passing Immunization: Human Antibodies from V-gene Libraries Displayed on Phage, pp. 581–97, Copyright © 1991 with permission from Elsevier: http://www.sciencedirect.com/science/journal/00222836

Text extract reproduced from Macken, C.A. and Perelsen, A.S. Protein evolution on rugged landscapes, *Proceedings of the National Academy of Sciences*, Volume 86, pp. 6191–95, Copyright © 1989, with permission of the author.

References

1. **Hutchison, C. A., and Marshall, H. E.** (1971). 'Genetic assay for small fragments of bacteriophage φX 174 deoxyribonucleic acid.' *J. Virology*, **8**: 181–9.

2. **Smith, M.** (2013). 'Synthetic DNA and Biology.' Nobel Lecture. http://Nobelprize.org

3. **Hutchison, C. A. 3rd., Phillips, S., Edgell, M. H., Gillam, S, Jahnke, P., and Smith, S.** (1978). 'Mutagenesis at a specific position in a DNA sequence.' *J. Biol. Chem.*, **253**: 6551–60.

4. **Winter, G., Fersht, A. R., Wilkinson, A. J., Zoller, M., and Smith, M**. (1982). 'Redesigning enzyme structure by site-directed mutagenesis: tyrosyltRNA synthetase and ATP binding.' *Nature*, **299**: 756–8.

5. **Roberts, S., and Rees, A. R.** (1986). 'The cloning and expression of an anti-peptide antibody: a system for rapid analysis of the binding properties of engineered antibodies.' *Prot. Eng.*, **1**: 59–65.

6. **Roberts, S., Cheetham, J. C., and Rees, A. R.** (1987). 'Generation of an antibody with enhanced affinity and specificity for its antigen by protein engineering.' *Nature*, **328**: 731–4.

7. **Cabilly, S., Riggs, A. D., Pande, H., Shively, J. E., Holmes, W. E., Rey, M., Perry, J., Wetzel, R., and Heyneker, H. L.** (1984). 'Generation of antibody activity from immunoglobulin polypeptide chains produced in Escherichia coli.' *Proc. Natl. Acad. Sci.*, **81**: 3273–7.

8. Wood, C. R., Boss, M. A., Kenten, J. H., Calvert, J. E., Roberts, N. A., and Emtage, J. (1985). 'The synthesis and in vivo assembly of functional antibodies in yeast.' *Nature*, **314**: 446–9.

9. Horwitz, A. H., Chang, C. P., Better, M., Kellstrom, K. E., and Robinson, R. R. (1988). 'Secretion of functional antibody and Fab fragment from yeast cells.' *Proc. Natl. Acad. Sci.*, **85**: 8678–82.

10. Inbar, D., Hochman, J., and Givol, D. (1972). 'Localization of Antibody-Combining Sites within the Variable Portions of Heavy and Light Chains.' *Proc. Nat. Acad. Sci.*, **69**: 2659–62.

11. Riechmann, L., Foote, J., and Winter, G. (1988). 'Expression of an Antibody Fv Fragment in Myeloma Cells.' *J. Mol. Biol.*, **203**: 825–8.

12. Skerra, A., and Plückthun, A. (1988). 'Assembly of a Functional Immunoglobulin Fv Fragment in Escherichia coli.' *Science*, **240**: 1038–41.

13. Field, H., Yarranton, G. T., and Rees, A. R. (1988). *Vaccines*, pp. 29–34. New York: Cold Spring Harbor Publications.

14. Huston, J., Levinson, D., Mudgett-Hunter, M., Tai, M.-S., Novotny, J., Margolies, M. N., Ridge, R. J., Bruccoleri, R. E., Haberm E., Crea, R., and Oppermann, H. (1988). 'Protein Engineering of Antibody Binding Sites: Recovery of Specific Activity in an Anti-Digoxin Single-Chain Fv Analogue Produced in Escherichia coli.' *Proc. Natl. Acad. Sci.*, **85**: 5879–83.

15. Bird, R. E., Hardman, K. D., Jacobson, J. W., Johnson, S., Kaufman, B. M., Lee, S.-M., Lee, T., Pope, S. H., Riordan, G. S., and Whitlow, M. (1988). 'Single chain antigen-binding proteins.' *Science*, **242**: 423–6.

16. Huston, J. S., Margolies, M. N., and Haber, E. (1996). 'Antibody binding sites.' *Adv. Prot. Chem.*, **49**: 329–450.

17. Holliger, P., Prospero, T., and Winter, G. (1993). ' "Diabodies": Small bivalent and bispecific antibody fragments.' *Proc. Natl. Acad. Sci.*, **90**: 6444–8.

18. Ward, E. S., Güssow, D., Griffiths, A. D., Jones, P. T., and Winter G. (1989). 'Binding activities of a repertoire of single immunoglobulin variable domains secreted from Escherichia coli.' *Nature*, **341**: 544–6.

19. Huse, W. D., Sastry, L., Iverson, S. A., Kang, S. A., Alting-Mees, M., Burton, D. R., Benkovic, S. J., and Lerner, R. A. (1989). 'Generation of a Large Combinatorial Library of the Immunoglobulin Repertoire in Phage Lambda.' *Science*, **246**: 1275–81.

20. Mullinax, R. L., Gross, E. A., Amberg, J. R., Hay, B. N., Hogrefe, H. H., Kubitz, M. M., Greener, A., Alting-Mees, M., Ardourel, D., Short, J. M., Sorge, J. A., and Shopes, B. (1990). 'Identification of human antibody fragment clones specific for tetanus toxoid in a bacteriophage immunoexpression library.' *Proc. Natl. Acad. Sci.*, **87**: 8095–9.

21. McCafferty, J., Griffiths, A. D., Winter, G., and Chiswell, D. J. (1990). 'Phage antibodies: filamentous phage displaying antibody variable domains.' *Nature*, **348**: 552–4.

22. Smith, G. P. (1985). 'Filamentous Fusion Phage: Novel Expression Vectors that Display Cloned Antigens on the Virion Surface.' *Science*, **228**: 1315–17.

23. Parmley, S. F., and Smith, G. P. (1988). 'Antibody-selectable filamentous fd phage vectors: affinity purification of target genes.' *Gene*, **73**: 305–18.

24. de Haard, H., Henderikx, P., Hoogenboom, H. R. (1998). 'Creating and engineering human antibodies for immunotherapy.' *Advanced Drug Delivery Reviews*, **31**: 5–31.

25. Kang, A. S., Barbas, C. F., Janda, K. D., Benkovic, S. J., and Lerner, R. A. (1991). 'Linkage of recognition and replication functions by assembling combinatorial antibody Fab libraries along phage surfaces.' *Proc. Natl. Acad. Sci.*, **88**: 4363–6.

26. Clackson, T., Hoogenboom, H. R., Griffiths, A. D., and Winter, G. (1991). 'Making antibody fragments using phage display libraries.' *Nature*, **352**: 624–8.

27. Marks, J. D., Hoogenboom, H. R., Bonnert, T. P., McCafferty, J., Griffiths, A. D., and Winter, G. (1991). 'By-passing Immunization: Human Antibodies from V-gene Libraries Displayed on Phage.' *J. Mol. Biol.*, **222**: 581–97.

28. Burton, D. R., Barbas III, C. F., Persson, M. A. A., Koenig, S., Chanock, R. M., and Lerner, R. A. (1991). 'A large array of human monoclonal antibodies to type 1 human immunodeficiency virus from combinatorial libraries of asymptomatic seropositive individuals.' *Proc. Natl. Acad. Sci.*, **88**: 10134–7.

29. Hoogenboom, H. R., and Winter, G. (1992). 'By-passing Immunisation: Human Antibodies from Synthetic Repertoires of Germline VH Gene Segments Rearranged in Vitro.' *J. Mol. Biol.*, **227**: 381–8.

30. Griffiths, A. D., Williams, S. C., Hartley, O., Tomlinson, I. M., Waterhouse, P., Crosby, W. B., Kontermann, R. E., Jones, P. T., Low, N. M. Allison, T. J., Prospero, T. D., Hoogenboom, H. R., Nissim, A., Cox, J. P. L, Harrison, J. L., Zaccolo, M., Gherardi, E., and Winter, G. (1994). 'Isolation of high affinity human antibodies directly from large synthetic repertoires.' *EMBO. J.*, **13**: 3245–60.

31. Macken, C. A., and Perelsen, A. S. (1989). 'Protein evolution on rugged landscapes.' *Proc. Natl. Acad. Sci.*, **86**: 6191–5.

32. Macken, C. A., and Perelsen, A. S. (1995). 'Protein evolution on partially correlated landscapes.' *Proc. Natl. Acad. Sci.*, **92**: 9657–61.

33. de Haard, H., Henderikx, P., and Hoogenboom, H. R. (1998). 'Creating and engineering human antibodies for immunotherapy.' *Adv. Drug Del. Rev.*, **31**: 5–31.

34. Begent, R. H. J., Verrhaar, M. J., Chester, K. A., Casey, J. L., Green, A. J., Napier, M. P., Hope-Stone, L. D., Cushen, N., Keep, P. A., Johnson, C. J., Hawkins, R. E., Hilson, A. J. W., and Robson, L. (1996). 'Clinical evidence of efficient tumor targeting based on single-chain Fv antibody selected from a combinatorial library.' *Nature Med.*, **2**: 979–84.

35. Mayer, A., Tsiompanou, E., O'Malley, D., Boxer, G. M., Bhatia, J., Flynn, A. A., Chester, K. A., Davidson, B. R., Lewis, A. A. M., Winslet, M. C., Dhillon, A. P., Hilson, A. J. W., and Begent, R. H. J. (2000). 'Radioimmunoguided Surgery in Colorectal Cancer Using a Genetically Engineered Anti-CEA Single-Chain Fv Antibody.' *Clin. Cancer Res.*, **6**: 1711–19.

36. Aitken, D. R., Hinkle, G. H., and Thurston, M. O. (1984). 'A gamma detecting probe for radioimmunodetection of CEA-producing tumors: successful experimental use and clinical case report.' *Dis. Colon Rectum*, **27**: 279–82.

37. Cohen, A. M., Martin, E. W., Lavery, I., Daly, J., Sardi, A., Aitken, D., Bland, K., Mojzisik, C., and Hinkle, G. (1991). 'Radioimmunoguided surgery using iodine-125 B72.3 in patients with colorectal cancer.' *Arch. Surg.*, **126**: 349–52.

38. Dolezal, O., de Gori, R., Walter, M., Doughty, L., Hattarki, M., Hudson, P. J., and Kortt, A. A. (2003). 'Single-chain Fv multimers of the anti-neuraminidase antibody NC10: the residue at position 15 in the VL domain of the scFv (VL–VH) molecule is primarily responsible for formation of a tetramer–trimer equilibrium.' *Prot. Eng.*, **16**: 47–56.

39. Mallender, W. D., and Voss, E. W. (1994). 'Construction, expression and activity of a bivalent bispecific single-chain antibody.' *J. Biol. Chem.*, **269**: 199–206.

40. Wittela, U. A., Jaina, M., Goela, A., Chauhana, S. C., Colcherb, D., and Batraa, S. K. (2005). 'The in vivo characteristics of genetically engineered divalent and tetravalent single-chain antibody constructs.' *Nucl. Med. Biol.*, **32**: 157–164.

41. **Nelson, A. L.** (2010). 'Antibody fragments: Hope and hype.' *mAbs*, **2**: 77–83.

42. **Pei, X. Y., Holliger, P., Murzin, A. G., and Williams, R. L.** (1997). 'The 2.0-Å resolution crystal structure of a trimeric antibody fragment with non-cognate VH–VL domain pairs shows a rearrangement of VH CDR3.' *Proc. Natl. Acad. Sci.*, **94**: 9637–42.

43. **Holliger, P., and Hudson, P. J.** (2005). 'Engineered antibody fragments and the rise of single domains.' *Nature Biotech.*, **23**: 1126–36.

44. **Gall, F., Reusch, U., Little, M., and Kipriyanov, S. M.** (2004). 'Effect of linker sequences between the antibody variable domains on the formation, stability and biological activity of a bispecific tandem diabody.' *Prot. Eng. Selec. Des.*, **17**: 357–66.

45. **Utsumi, S., and Karush, F.** (1964). 'The subunits of purified rabbit antibody.' *Biochemistry*, **3**: 1329–38.

46. **Nelson, A. L., and Reichert, J. M.** (2009). 'Development trends for therapeutic antibody fragments.' *Nature Biotech.*, **27**: 331–7.

47. **Callewaert, F., Naeye, B., Verheyden, G., Thomas, A., Stanssens, P., van de Sompel, A., Holz, J., and Ulrichts, H.** (2013). *In vitro comparability study of the biological activity and target binding of the liquid and lyophilised drug product formulation of the anti-vwf nano-body® caplacizumab.* Ablynx nv: Zwijnaarde, Belgium. http://www.ablynx.com/wp-content/uploads/2013/05/Poster-AAPS-2013_in-vitro-comparability-ALX-0081_FINAL.pdf

48. http://www.ablynx.com/en/research-development/pipeline/

49. **Nisonoff, A., and Rivers, M. M.** (1961). 'Recombination of mixtures of univalent antibody fragments of different specificity.' *Arch. Biochem. Biophys.*, **93**: 460–2.

50. **Fudenberg, H. H., Drews, G., and Nisonoff, A.** (1964). 'Serologic demonstration of dual specificity of rabbit bivalent hybrid antibody.' *J. Exp. Med.*, **119**: 151–66.

51. **van der Neut Kolfschoten, M., Schuurman, J., Losen, M., Bleeker, W. K., Martínez-Martínez, P., Vermeulen, E., den Bleker, T. H., Wiegman, L., Vink, T., Aarden, L. A., de Baets, M. H., van de Winkel, J. G. J., Aalberse, R. C., and Parren, P. W. H. I.** (2007). 'Anti-Inflammatory Activity of Human IgG4 Antibodies by Dynamic Fab Arm Exchange.' *Science*, **317**: 1554–7.

52. **Rispens, T., Ooijevaar-de Heer, P., Bende, O., and Aalberse, R. C.** (2011). 'Mechanism of Immunoglobulin G4 Fab-arm Exchange.' *J. Amer. Chem. Soc.*, **133**: 10302–11.

53. **Riethmüller, G.** (2012). 'Symmetry breaking: bispecific antibodies, the beginnings and 50 years on.' *Cancer Immunity*, **12**: 1–7.

54. **Milstein, C., and Cuello, A. C.** (1983). 'Hybrid hybridomas and their use in immunohisto-chemistry.' *Nature*, **305**: 537–40.

55. **Staertz, U. D., Kanagawa, O., and Bevan, M. J.** (1985). 'Hybrid antibodies can target sites for attack by T cells.' *Nature*, **314**: 628–31.

56. **Perez, P., Hoffman, R. W., Shaw, S., Bluestone, J. A., and Segal, D. M.** (1985). 'Specific targeting of cytotoxic T cells by anti-T3 linked to anti-target cell antibody.' *Nature*, **316**: 354–6.

57. **Staerz, U. D., Yewdell, J. W., and Bevan, M. J.** (1987). 'Hybrid antibody-mediated lysis of virus infected cells.' *Eur. J. Immunol.*, **17**: 571–4.

58. **Glennie, M. J., McBride, H. M., Worth, A. T., and Stevenson, G. T.** (1987). 'Preparation and performance of bispecific F(ab'g)2 antibody containing thioether-linked Fab'γ fragments.' *J. Immunol.*, **139**: 2367–75.

59. **Offner, S., Hofmeister, R., Romaniuka, A., Kufer, P., and Baeuerle, P.A.** (2006). 'Induction of regular cytolytic T cell synapses by bispecific single-chain antibody constructs on MHC class I-negative tumor cells.' *Molec. Immunol.*, **43**: 763–71.

60. Griffiths, A. D., Malmqvist, M., Marks, J. D., Bye, J. M., Embleton, M. J., McCafferty, J., Baierl, M., Holliger, K. P., Gorick, B. D., Hughes-Jones, N. C., Hoogenbooml, H. R., and Winter, G. (1993). 'Human anti-self antibodies with high specificity from phage display libraries.' *EMBO J.*, **12**: 725–34.

61. Mallender, W. D., and Voss, E. W. (1994). 'Construction, expression and activity of a bivalent bispecific single-chain antibody.' *J. Biol. Chem.*, **269**: 199–206.

62. Bargou, R., Leo, E., Zugmaier, G., Klinger, M., Goebeler, M., Knop, S., Noppeney, R., Viardot, A., Hess, G., Schuler, M., Einsele, M., Brandl, C., Wolf, A., Kirchinger, P., Klappers, P., Schmidt, M., Riethmüller, G., Reinhardt, C., Baeuerle, P. A., and Kufer, P. (2008). 'Tumor Regression in Cancer Patients by Very Low Doses of a T Cell-Engaging Antibody.' *Science*, **321**: 974–6.

63. Merchant, A. M., Zhu, Z., Yuan, J. Q., Goddard, A., Adams, C. W., Presta, L. G., and Carter, P. (1998). 'An efficient route to human bispecific IgG.' *Nat. Biotechnol.*, **16**: 677–81.

64. Spiess, C., Bevers, J. 3rd, Jackman, J., Chiang, N., Nakamura, G., Dillon, M., Liu, H., Molina, P., Elliott, J. M., Shatz, W., Scheer, J. M., Giese, G., Persson, J., Zhang, Y., Dennis, M. S., Giulianotti, J., Gupta, P., Reilly, D., Palma, E., Wang, J., Stefanich, E., Scheerens, H., Fuh, G., and Wu, L. C. (2013). 'Development of a human IgG4 bispecific antibody for dual targeting of interleukin-4 (IL-4) and interleukin-13 (IL-13) cytokines.' *J. Biol. Chem.*, **288**: 24935.

65. Wosniak-Knopp, G., Bartl, S., Bauer, A., Mostageer, M., Woisetchläger, M., Antes, B., Ettl, K., Kainer, M., Weberhofer, G., Wiederkum, S., Himmler, G., Mudde, G. C., and Rüker, F. (2010). 'Introducing antigen-binding sites in structural loops of immunoglobulin constant domains: Fc fragments with engineered HER2/neu-binding sites and antibody properties.' *Prot. Eng. Des. Selec.*, **23**: 289–97.

66. Hinton, P. R., Johlfs, M. G., Xiong, J. M., Hanestad, K., Ong, K. C., Bullock, C., Keller, S., Tang, M. T., Tso, J. Y., Vásquez, M., et al (2004). 'Engineered human IgG antibodies with longer serum half-lives in primates.' *J. Biol. Chem.*, **279**: 6213–16.

67. Hinton, P. R., Xiong, J. M., Johlfs, M. G., Tang, M. T., Keller, S., and Tsurushita, N. (2006). 'An engineered human IgG1 antibody with longer serum half-life.' *J. Immunol.*, **176**: 346–56.

68. Stapleton, N. M., Andersen, J. T., Stemerding, A. M., Bjarnarson, S. P., Verheul, R. C., Gerritsen, J., Zhao, Y., Kleijer, M., Sandlie, I., de Haas, M., et al (2011). Competition for FcRn-mediated transport gives rise to short half-life of human IgG3 and offers therapeutic potential.' *Nature Communications*, **2**: 599.

69. Lindhofer, H., Mocikat, R., Steipe, B., and Thierfelder, S. (1995). 'Preferential Species-Restricted Heavy/Light Chain Pairing in Rat/Mouse Quadromas: Implications for a Single-Step Purification of Bispecific Antibodies.' *J. Immunol.*, **155**: 219–25.

70. Linke, R., Klein, A., and Seimitz, D. (2010). 'Catumaxomab: clinical development and future directions.' *mAbs*, **2**: 129–36.

71. Buss, A. P. N. S., Henderson, S. J., McFarlane, M., Shenton, J. M., and de Haan, L. (2012). 'Monoclonal antibody therapeutics: history and future.' *Curr. Opin. Pharmacol.*, **12**: 615–22.

72. http://www.antibodysociety.org/news/approved_mabs.php

Therapeutic antibodies Case study I: Prevention of respiratory syncytial virus illness

Background

Respiratory syncytial virus (RSV) is a member of the single-stranded RNA virus family *Paramyxoviridae*. Parainfluenza, mumps, and measles viruses are members of the same family. RSV is a medium-sized pleomorphic enveloped virus within a separate genus *Pneumovirus*. It is a non-segmented, negative sense RNA virus and has ten genes coding for ten different proteins in the coding sequence order 3'-NS1-NS2-N-P-M-SH-G-F-M2-L-5'. Two important proteins expressed as transmembrane proteins are the G protein which is heavily glycosylated and important for infectivity and the F or fusion protein, important for viral fusion with host cells and subsequently host-cell–host-cell fusion in the formation of syncytia.

RSV was discovered relatively recently when Blount and his colleagues Morris and Savage in 1956, physicians at the Walter Reed Army Institute of Research, Maryland, USA, isolated a cytopathogenic agent from a colony of 20 chimpanzees that were suffering from acute respiratory infection. They named the infectious agent chimpanzee coryza agent (CCA).[1] Applying Koch's postulates they were able to induce the same illness in non-immune chimpanzees, coincidentally infecting a laboratory worker at the Institute as demonstrated by the presence of anti-CCA antibodies and upper respiratory tract symptoms similar to those of the chimpanzees. In the same year Robert Chanock and colleagues at the NIH and Children's Hospital, District of Columbia isolated the same agent from two different infants with pneumonia and bronchiolitis in Baltimore, Maryland. The identity of Chanock's isolate with the CCA agent was confirmed by microscopy and histology although proof of its direct association with the observed respiratory syndromes was only circumstantial at this point.[2] Chanock observed that when human cells in tissue culture were infected with the agent, syncytia or pseudo giant cells were formed leading him to suggest the name respiratory syncytial (RS) virus. In 1961, during a presentation at the 89th meeting of the American Public Health Association symposium in Detroit (published the following year),[3] Chanock summarized the properties of the viral agent he had isolated (see Box 15.1).

In the same article Chanock's conclusions were clear if leavened with some caution, as expected from a practicing physician:

> RS appears to be responsible for a considerable proportion of the severe respiratory illness which afflicts infants and small children. The virus has sharply limited periods of widespread dissemination in the community every year and represents a recurring threat to

the pediatric population. Serologic studies indicate that most children become infected by age four… Reinfection can occur later in life and is probably associated in a proportion of instances with a mild respiratory illness.[3]

Conclusive evidence for the association of Chanock's RSV agent with human respiratory disease soon followed from studies by Marc Beem in Chicago[4] and Chanock's own investigations[5,6] that extended the reach of RSV to respiratory illness in adults (Fig. 15.1).[5,7] During 1963 to 1965 numerous reports appeared from different parts of the world confirming the earlier observations and firmly establishing the RSV aetiology of upper respiratory tract illness in children. In 1965, the WHO published a summary of the prevalence of antibodies to RSV in 14 different countries and concluded:

CF antibodies to RS virus appear early in life. Maternal antibody has been detected in infants under 4 months of age… After the loss of this antibody, titers rise in the next few months of life, but between 6 months and 2 years the percentage of positive sera is still relatively low. In Pennsylvania, USA… 6% of children aged 6-11 months and 16% of those one year old had antibody; in Manchester, England, 38 %-41 % of children between the ages of 7 months and 2 years had antibody…[8]

The WHO comments highlighted some fundamental issues with this condition. While antibodies to the virus would have been passed to the foetus during materno-foetal transmission, their relatively short half-life (~28 days) would have

Box 15.1 Properties of respiratory syncytial virus

1. Growth in (a) continuous human and (b) primary human and monkey cell cultures, the former more sensitive for virus isolation.
2. Characteristic cytopathic effect in tissue culture is formation of syncytium or 'Pseudo Giant Cell' in which eosinophilic cytoplasmic inclusions are prominent.
3. Infectious virus first detected ten hours after inoculation of HEP-2 tissue culture cells.
4. Specific antigen, first detected by fluorescent antibody technic ten hours after inoculation of HEP-2 cells, restricted to cytoplasm throughout growth cycle.
5. Virus size of 90–120mµ [nm].
6. Complement-fixing antigen smaller than virus particle and separable from it by centrifugation.
7. Inactivated by 20% ether.
8. Does not grow in eggs.
9. Haemagglutination not demonstrable.
10. Not pathogenic for mouse, guinea pig, or rabbit.

Reproduced with permission from Chanock, R.M. et al., Respiratory syncytial virus, *American Journal of Public Health*, Volume 52, pp. 918–925, Copyright © 1962 The American Public Health Association.

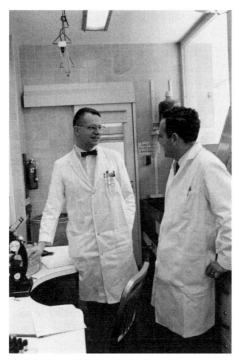

Fig. 15.1 Robert Chanock (left), NYT (Laurence K Altman).
Reproduced with permission from TT Nyhetsbyrån, Stockholm.

conferred limited protection during the six months postpartum and infants after the maternal antibody decline would be at risk until their own antibody responses had developed. A particularly important high-risk group would be pre-term infants born before significant build-up of maternal antibody levels had completed. Further, any innate immune response to the virus would not necessarily have induced 'protective' antibodies, an obvious conclusion given the prevalence of RSV-associated illness in infants. An observation that called into question the effectiveness of natural immune responses to the virus in protecting infants from the more serious consequences of RSV was made by Beem in 1967.[9] Antibody titers in children that had experienced re-infection by RSV in successive seasons of virus prevalence, shown by isolation of the virus and profiling using anti-RSV strain ferret serum, showed no correlation between the onset of repeated symptomatic disease and the level of neutralizing antibodies in their sera. Antigenic variation within the RSV strain as an explanation for non-protection was discounted. This apparent lack of antibody protection led Beem to suggest that 'factors associated with specific resistance by R.S. virus remain to be identified.'[9] By 1979 a significant ten-year study had been completed by Henderson and colleagues at UC North Carolina, Chapel Hill in which infection rates were measured in children experiencing multiple infections. The infection rate decreased from 98% to 75% by the second infection but a third exposure to the virus only reduced the rate of infection to 65%. While the severity of the infection was considerably reduced by the third exposure, Henderson concluded that the best that could be expected from an immunoprophylactic treatment was amelioration rather than prevention of infection.[10] However, there were too many uncertainties to make this a clear-cut prognosis.

By 1981, Ogilvie had established a relationship between maternal anti-RSV antibodies and infection rates in newborn infants. Of the 100 infants studied, 29 showed infection while 31 exposed to an RSV epidemic season were not infected. Ogilvie's summary of this study was:

> Mean titer of maternal IgG antibody to RSV was significantly higher (P less than 0.001) in those mothers whose babies remained uninfected than in those whose babies had proved RSV infection before 6 months of age. Babies born to mothers with high levels of IgG antibody to respiratory syncytial virus were protected against infection with this virus during the first months of life when the risk of severe disease was greatest.[11]

The immune protection picture became clearer when Merz, Scheid, and Choppin published a study in 1980 on the protective effect on cells in culture of antibodies to the two major transmembrane proteins, G (for extensively glycosylated) and F (for fusion), present in the membrane envelope of paramyxoviruses. Their study was actually on the related parainfluenza virus. The results were compelling. Anti-F antibodies were able to completely prevent spread of the virus by blocking cell-to-cell fusion while antibodies to the G protein were only effective under conditions of low cell fusion activity.[12]

After a small clinical study in 1987 by Hemming and associates in which IVIG, given at very high doses (2g/kg), was shown to be well tolerated by RSV-infected infants but with no reduction in hospitalization,[13] Kazel, Taber, and Glezen at Baylor College of Medicine, in collaboration with Walsh at the University of Rochester School of Medicine and Frank at the University of Illinois College of Medicine, carried out a comparative study of antibody titers against the G and F proteins from RSV and the severity of respiratory illness in 34 children followed from birth up to three years of age. The results demonstrated that the principal protective effect against RSV infection was associated with the presence of high titers of anti-F IgG.[14] The authors suggested that such information was relevant to the development of a vaccine against RSV but in fact another approach would turn out to be more effective. Today, there is still no effective RSV vaccine and in some instances, vaccines have been developed that, peculiarly, have enhanced the infectivity of RSV.

Two years after Kasel's work was published, Kathleen van Wyke Coelingh at the NIH reported a detailed epitope-mapping study of the RSV F-protein, the significance of which would only become visible about ten years later. Coelingh had prepared 18 different monoclonal antibodies to the F protein and used different A-group strains of RSV as well as monoclonal antibody-resistant mutants of RSV to identify the antigen sites associated with the fusion function of F-protein.[15] A number of these epitopes were shown to be highly conserved across all subgroup A and B RSV clinical strains examined. This was in contrast to antibodies to the G protein which exhibited strain-to-strain epitope variation.

By 1991 it had become clear that the presence but also the level of anti-RSV antibodies in the sera of infants exerted a protective effect, if only in reducing the severity of seasonal RSV infection. However, infants with cardiopulmonary disease and pre-term infants were a known high-risk group for severe pulmonary disease. Based on the results of several animal experiments in which prophylactic injection of intravenous pooled immunoglobulin (IVIG) containing anti-RSV antibodies exerted a significant protective effect on challenge with RSV, a clinical safety study of 23 high-risk infants was carried out in Colorado, Washington D.C., New York, and Bethesda, Maryland. In this study IVIG was administered monthly with a follow-up period of two years. The results were reported by Jessie Groothuis at the University of Colorado School of Medicine in 1991.[16] Despite the commercial IVIG preparation having a relatively average RSV titer (~1:1000) after infusions at 750mg/kg a target RSV antibody level in the infant group of ≥1:100 was achieved. While such levels may be effective when IVIG is administered prophylactically, to treat established infection it was considered that higher serum titers must be achieved. At titers of 1:1000 extremely large and inappropriate doses of IVIG would be required. In an attempt to define more effectively donor antibody with higher RSV neutralizing-antibody levels, Siber and colleagues developed a microneutralization screen that better predicted high protective activity in RSV-infected mice, the IVIG antibodies selected having a five-fold improvement in RSV neutralization than unscreened IVIG.[17,18] One observation made by Siber and colleagues, perhaps somewhat puzzling based on the results of Coelingh, was that the best neutralizing IVIG may have contained antibodies against other RSV antigens in addition to the G and F proteins. This approach was used to screen human plasma donors to identify high titer 'neutralizing antibodies' for potential human therapy. The first trial of a 'high titer' anti-RSV IVIG came from Groothuis in 1993 but this time in a large multicentre trial involving nine paediatric or infectious disease departments in the USA. In this study 249 infants of a mean age of eight months were treated, 102 of whom presented with bronchopulmonary dysplasia due to prematurity, 87 with congenital heart disease, and 60 with prematurity alone. The results of this clinical study were impressive and provided impetus for more effective antibody therapy than donor IVIG. In particular the high-dose regime led to a reduction by 63% of RSV-associated hospitalization, a similar reduction in the number of days of hospitalization, and a huge (93%) reduction in the number of days in the intensive care unit.[19] In concluding, Groothuis suggested that further improvement should be seen with the use of monoclonal antibodies, although the antibody chosen would need to match the neutralizing efficacy of the human donor polyclonal IG that would have contained antibodies against multiple antigens and epitopes within those antigens. The monoclonal approach would soon enter onto the scene accompanied by Groothuis' move from an academic to a biotechnology environment.

By June 1994 a more extensive clinical trial was published by the PREVENT Study Group, this time as a centrally randomized double-blind, placebo-controlled trial at 54 different centres in the USA during the 1994–95 RSV season and involving 510 children with similar risk profiles to those in the Groothuis trial. The children were given five monthly doses of RespiGam, an FDA-approved (January 1996) respiratory syncytial virus-immune human globulin and marketed by MedImmune, at dose levels of 750mg/kg. The conclusions from this study, which were similar to the Groothuis study, were stated as:

> Monthly administration of 750 mg/kg of RSV-IGIV was safe and well tolerated and was effective in reducing the incidence and total days of both RSV hospitalization and overall respiratory hospitalization in infants with a history of prematurity or bronchopulmonary dysplasia or both.[20]

In 1997, MedImmune, Virion Systems, the Uniformed Services University of the Health Sciences, and Pathology Associates Internal, all based in Maryland, USA published the humanization of an antibody from the original set of murine anti-RSV monoclonal antibodies developed by Coelingh in 1989. The antibody, MEDI-493, was a humanized version of antibody Mab 1129 and was one of three antibodies in development[21] at MedImmune. MEDI-493 was directed to a conserved epitope, the A site, on the fusion protein of RSV. The antibody was humanized by Johnson and co-workers using a CDR-grafting approach that included molecular modelling to guide the human chain selection and to identify murine residues that should be retained to ensure structural integrity of the binding site. The humanized and murine antibodies had identical antigen affinities and further equivalence was demonstrated in all *in vitro* cellular assays. The joint Maryland groups led by MedImmune also carried out an *in vivo* study of the humanized antibody in cotton rats and showed a 99% reduction in RSV lung titers at 2.5mg/kg (see Table 15.1; note that polyclonal IVIV doses had been at ~750mg/kg), corresponding to a circulating antibody concentration of ~25–30µg/mL.[22]

The suggestions from previous IVIG studies that a specific monoclonal antibody directed to the right neutralizing epitope should be an improvement on a donor

Table 15.1 Prophylaxis of RSV infection in cotton rats by intravenous administration of MEDI-493.

Compound, dose	n	Concentration of human IgG µg/mL(mean ± SE)	RSV titer, pfu/g (mean $\log_{10}$ ± SE)
Bovine serum albumin 10mg/kg	18	0	5.11 ± 0.06
MEDI-493, mg/kg			
0.312	7	2.67 ± 0.6	4.67 ± 0.18
0.625	17	5.27 ± 0.27	4.44 ± 0.1
1.25	18	10.1 ± 0.29	3.52 ± 0.15
2.5	17	28.6 ± 2.15	2.98 ± 0.17
5	15	55.6 ± 3.43	2,12 ± 0.09
10	18	117.6 ± 5.09	< 2.0

[pfu = plaque-forming units; n = number of experiments]

Table 15.2 Summary of analysis of RSV hospitalization

	Placebo	Palivizumab	% Reduction (95% CI)	P value
Primary analysis (incidence of RSV hospitalization)	52/500 (10.6%)	48/1002 (4.8%)	55% (38, 72)	<.001
Alternative analysis (Kaplan Meier)	53/500 (10.6%)			
Sensitivity analysis				
Dropout before 150 days and no endpoint	53/500 (10.6%)	49/1002 (4.9%)	55% (38, 72)	<.001
Respiratory hospitalization but no RSV test done	56/500 (11.2%)	54/1002 (5.4%)	52% (35, 69)	<.001
Primary inclusion populations				
Premature (no BPD)	19/234 (8.1%)	9/506 (1.8%)	78% (66, 90)	<.001
BPD	34/266 (12.8%)	39/496 (7.9%)	39% (20, 58)	.038

[RSV = respiratory syncytial virus; CI = confidence interval; BPD = bronchopulmonary dysplasia]

polyclonal preparation was more than realized in the humanized monoclonal antibody results, but this was only a cotton rat. While these studies were in progress, a massive clinical trial had commenced during the 1996–97 RSV season with the very same antibody humanized by Johnson and colleagues. Part of the humanization study was reported by MedImmune scientists at a Keystone symposium, Lake Tahoe, in March 1994 (at which this author was present), so that the development and production of MEDI-493 was likely well advanced by late 1996. The pivotal study that established the safety and efficacy of MEDI-493, renamed palivizumab, was carried out by the IMpact-RSV Study Group in 139 centres in the USA, UK, and Canada and involving 1502 high-risk children.[23] The patient groups consisted of prematurely-born children (≤ 35 weeks) and ≤ six months old at the time of the study or had bronchopulmonary dysplasia and ≤ 24 months of age, randomized 2:1 to receive five monthly injections of palivizumab at 15mg/kg or placebo, respectively. The primary endpoint was reduced RSV hospitalization with secondary endpoints relating to the characteristics of the RSV hospitalizations. Children were followed 150 days for the primary endpoint of hospitalization due to RSV infection. The results of this study with respect to the primary endpoint, published in 1998, are shown in Table 15.2.

Based on the success of this study, which demonstrated a 55% reduction in RSV hospitalization in children at high risk for RSV infection, palivizumab was licensed in the USA (as Synagis®) and in other world markets in June 1998 (for the prevention of serious lower respiratory tract disease caused by RSV).

In a follow-on post-marketing study the safety of palivizumab was examined in children with haemodynamically significant congenital heart disease (CHD), a cohort not studied in the IMpact-RSV study. In a study of 1287 children with haemodynamically significant CHD, the palivizumab group showed a 45% reduction in RSV hospitalization rate compared with placebo.[21] As a result of this study, palivizumab was licensed in September 2003 for prevention of serious lower respiratory tract disease caused by RSV in children with haemodynamically significant CHD.

Subsequent to the IMpact studies, several retrospective and prospective studies were conducted in Europe and North America. In reviewing epidemiological aspects of RSV disease, Resch, Kurath, and Manzoni, from the Medical University of Graz and the Anna Hospital in Turin, commented:

> In general, the incidence of RSV-related hospital admissions after palivizumab prophylaxis in post-marketing surveillance studies was lower than the reported rates of the IMpact study.[24]

In attempting to explain the differences and drawing attention to a significant treatment compliance limitation, Resch further observes:

> Adherence to the monthly injections scheme of palivizumab prophylaxis remains a major problem. Parnes et al… noted lower re-hospitalization rates in infants with higher adherence to this scheme, and they observed that approximately half of RSV-related hospitalizations occurred between the first and second injection. Similar findings were also reported by Manzoni et al… consistent with the trends of serum palivizumab levels that may still be inadequate and not fully protective after the first monthly dose… Missed or delayed palivizumab injections resulted in an increase of RSV-related hospitalizations from 2.4 % to 4.4 % (p = 0.02).[24]

Resch concludes that a vaccine is needed but that until a vaccine is developed that can be safely delivered to at-risk infants at birth, prophylactic treatment (e.g. by anti-RSV antibody) is mandatory.

While palivizumab was a big advance on the earlier IVIG treatments, the requirement to administer injections (intramuscular) monthly was seen by MedImmune and the clinical community at large as a limitation, typical of a passive antibody therapy protocol. Mindful of this and aware of the limitations of palivizumab, MedImmune began evaluation of a modified and improved version of this antibody (motavizumab) in clinical studies. At the same time, MedImmune scientists developed a longer-lasting antibody (MEDI-557) by engineering an increased affinity of the IgG1 Fc region (common to both palivizumab and motavizumab) to the neonatal FcRn receptor. Testing in cynomolgus monkeys showed a four-fold increase in serum half-life and bioavailability compared with motavizumab.[21] Despite the theoretical advantages of an antibody engineered to exhibit lifetime improvement, MedImmune, now part of Astra Zeneca, announced in a press release on 21 December, 2010 that it had withdrawn the BLA application of motavizumab and discontinued the development of MEDI-557.

Notwithstanding the mythological skills of Panakeia, daughter of Asclepius and healer of all ills, an immunological panacea for all RSV-induced illnesses may be more

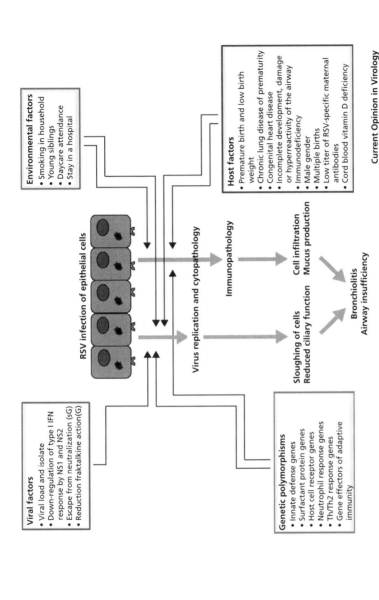

Viral factors
- Viral load and isolate
- Down-regulation of type I IFN response by NS1 and NS2
- Escape from neutralization (sG)
- Reduction fraktalkine action(G)

Environmental factors
- Smoking in household
- Young siblings
- Daycare attendance
- Stay in a hospital

RSV infection of epithelial cells

Virus replication and cytopathology

Immunopathology

Cell infiltration
Mucus production

Sloughing of cells
Reduced ciliary function

Bronchiolitis
Airway insufficiency

Genetic polymorphisms
- Innate defense genes
- Surfactant protein genes
- Host cell receptor genes
- Neutrophil response genes
- Th/Th2 response genes
- Gene effectors of adaptive immunity

Host factors
- Premature birth and low birth weight
- Chronic lung disease of prematurity
- Congenital heart disease
- Incomplete development, damage or hyperreactivity of the airway
- Immunodeficiency
- Male gender
- Multiple births
- Low titer of RSV-specific maternal antibodies
- Cord blood vitamin D deficiency

Current Opinion in Virology

Fig. 15.2 Factors influencing the pathogenesis and clinical disease caused by RSV infection in infants and young children. Reprinted from *Current Opinions in Virology*, Volume 2, Issue 3, Van Drunen, S. et al., Pathogenesis of respiratory syncytial virus, pp.300–305, Copyright © 2012 with permission from Elsevier: http://www.sciencedirect.com/science/journal/18796257

difficult than can be achieved by a single monoclonal antibody administration. In a short review of RSV in 2012, van Drunen, van den Hurk, and Watkiss reminded the scientific community of the complex interplay of factors that play a role in RSV disease pathogenesis (see Fig. 15.2).[25]

One of the key requirements for increasing our understanding of RSV and the mechanisms that give rise to the multiple pathogenic effects is the existence of an effective animal model. While the murine model is still widely used, van Drunen gives two stars for 'outstanding interest' in her reference to a newborn lamb model published by Sow and colleagues in 2011[26] that exhibits a much closer resemblance to the human airway structure and pathology of RSV than other animal models. We await future developments with anticipation.

From this short case study of RSV prophylaxis in neonatal infants by monoclonal antibodies, the power of antibody technology in the prevention of human RSV disease has been demonstrated with consummate elegance. Pioneering studies by Chanock in the late 1950s led to the observation that RSV antibodies are present in both infants and all the way through adulthood but that multiple exposures to RSV were required to confer effective protection. The low fraction of truly neutralizing antibodies in early responses opened up a clear path for passive antibody treatment targeted to key antigenic sites that interrupt virus fusion. The current antibody treatments available have significantly reduced the risk of health-challenged infants to the severe pathologies arising from RSV infection. Long may such antibody-based therapeutic approaches continue to be developed.

Acknowledgements

Text extract reproduced with permission from Chanock, R.M., et al. Respiratory syncytial virus, *American Journal of Public Health*, Volume 52, pp. 918–925, Copyright © 1962 The American Public Health Association.

Text extract reproduced with permission from Doggett, J.E. Antibodies to respiratory syncytial virus in human sera from different regions of the world, *Bulletin of the World Health Organization*, Volume 32, pp. 849–853, Copyright © 1965 World Health Organization.

Text extract reproduced with permission from Ogilvie, M.M., et al. Maternal antibody and respiratory syncytial virus infection in infancy, *Journal of Medical Virology*, Volume 7, Issue 4, pp. 263–271, Copyright © 1981 Wiley-Liss, Inc., A Wiley Company.

Text extracts reproduced with permission from Resch, B., Kurath, S. and Manzonie, P., Epidemiology of respiratory syncytial virus infection in preterm infants, *The Open Microbiology Journal*, Volume 5, Supplement 2, pp. 135–143 Copyright © 2011 Bentham Science Publishers.

References

1. **Morris, J. A., Blount, R. E., Jr., and Savage, R. E.** (1956). 'Recovery of Cytopathogenic Agent from Chimpanzees with Coryza.' *Proc. Soc. Exper. Biol. and Med.*, **92**: 544–9.

2. **Chanock, R. M., Roizman, B., and Myers, R.** (1957). 'Recovery from Infants with Respiratory Illness of a Virus Related to Chimpanzee Coryza Agent (CCA). I. Isolation, Properties and Characterization.' *Am. J. Hyg.*, **66**: 281–90.

3. **Chanock, R. M., Parrott, R. H., Vargosko, A. J., Kapikian, A. Z., Knight, V., and Johynson, K. M.** (1962). 'IV. Respiratory syncytial virus.' *Amer. J. Public Health*, **52**: 918–25.

4. **Beem, M., Wright, F. H., Hamre, D., Egerer, R., and Oehme, M.** (1960). 'Association of the Chimpanzee Coryza Agent with Acute Respiratory Disease in Children.' *New England J. Med.*, **263**: 523–30.

5. **Chanock, R. M., Kim, H. W., Vargosko, A. J., Deleva, A., Johnson, K. M., Cumming, C., and Parrott, R. H.** (1961). 'Respiratory Syncytial Virus. I. Virus Recovery and Other Observations during 1960 Outbreak of Bronchiolitis, Pneumonia, and Minor Respiratory Diseases in Children.' *J.A.M.A.*, **176**: 647–53.

6. **Parrott, R. H., Vargosko, A. J., Kim, H. W., Cumming, C., Turner, H., Huebner, R. J., and Chanock, R. M.** (1961). 'Respiratory Syncytial Virus. II. Serologic Studies over a 34-Month Period of Children with Bronchiolitis, Pneumonia, and Minor Respiratory Diseases.' *J.A.M.A.*, **176**: 653–7.

7. **Johnson, K. M., Bloom, H. H., Mufson, M. A., and Chanock, R. M.** (1962). 'Natural reinfection of adults by respiratory syncytial virus: Possible relation to mild upper respiratory disease.' *New Eng. J. Med.*, **267**: 68–72.

8. **Doggett, J. E.** (1965). 'Antibodies to respiratory syncytial virus in human sera from different regions of the world.' *Bull. World Health Org.*, **32**: 849–53.

9. **Beem, M.** (1967). 'Repeated infections with respiratory syncytial virus.' *J. Immunol.*, **98**: 1115–22.

10. **Henderson, F. W., Collier, A. M., Wallace, A. C. Jnr., and Denny, F. W.** (1979). 'Respiratory-syncytial-virus infections, reinfections and immunity—A prospective, longitudinal study in young children.' *New Eng. J. Med.*, **300**: 530–4.

11. **Ogilvie, M. M., Vathenon, A. S., Radford, M., Codd, J., and Key, S.** (1981). 'Maternal antibody and respiratory syncytial virus infection in infancy.' *J. Med. Virol.*, **7**: 263–71.

12. **Merz, D. C.**, Scheid, A., **and Choppin, P. W.** (1980). 'Importance of antibodies to the fusion glycoprotein of paramyxoviruses in the prevention of spread of infection.' *J. Exp. Med.*, **151**: 275–88.

13. **Hemming, V. G., Rodriguez, W., Kim, H. W., Brandt, C. D., Parrott, R. H., Burch, B., Prince, G. A., Baron, P. A., Fink, R. J., and Reaman, G.** (1987). 'Intravenous Immunoglobulin Treatment of Respiratory Syncytial Virus Infections in Infants and Young Children.' *Antimicrob. Agents. Chemoth.*, **31**: 1882–6.

14. **Kasel, J. A., Walsh, E. E., Frank, A. J., Baxter, B. D., Taber, L. H., and Glezen, W. P.** 'Relation of serum antibody to glycoproteins of respiratory syncytial virus with immunity to infection in children.' *Viral Immunol.* 1987/1988, **1**: 199–205.

15. **Beeler, J. A., and van Wyke Coelingh, K.** (1989). Neutralization epitopes of the F glycoprotein of respiratory syncytial virus: Effect of mutation upon fusion function.' *J. Virol.*, **63**: 2941–50.

16. **Groothuis, J. R., Levin, M. J., Rodriguez, W., Hall, B. C., Long, C. E., Kim, H. W., Lauer, B. A., Hemming, V. G., and The RSVIG Study Group** (1991). 'Use of Intravenous Gamma Globulin To Passively Immunize High-Risk Children against Respiratory Syncytial Virus: Safety and Pharmacokinetics.' *Antimicrob. Therap.*, **35**: 1469–73.

17. **Siber, G. R., Leszczynski, J., Pena-Cruz, V., Ferren-Gardner, C., Anderson, R., Hemming, V. G., Walsh, E. E., Burns, J., McIntosh, K., Gonin, R., and Anderson, L. J.** (1992). 'Protective Activity of a Human Respiratory Syncytial Virus Immune Globulin Prepared from Donors Screened by Microneutralization Assay.' *J. Infect Dis.*, **165**: 456–63.

18. **Siber, G. R., Leombruno, D., Leszczynski, J., McIver, J., Bodkin, D., Gonin, R., Thompson, C. M., Walsh, E. E., Piedra, P. A., Hemming, V. G., and Prince, G. A.** (1994). 'Comparison of Antibody Concentrations and Protective Activity of Respiratory Syncytial Virus Immune Globulin and Conventional Immune Globulin.' *J. Infect. Dis.*, **169**: 1368–73.

19. **Groothuis, J. R.**, et al (1993). 'Prophylactic administration of respiratory syncytial virus immune globulin to high-risk infants and young children.' *New Eng. J. Med.*, **329**: 1524–30.

20. **The PREVENT Study Group** (1997). 'Reduction of Respiratory Syncytial Virus Hospitalization Among Premature Infants and Infants With Bronchopulmonary Dysplasia Using Respiratory Syncytial Virus Immune Globulin Prophylaxis.' *Pediatrics*, **99**: 93–9.

21. **Groothuis, J. R., Hoopes, J. M., and Hemming, V. G.** (2011). 'Prevention of serious respiratory syncytial virus-related illness. II: Immunoprophylaxis.' *Adv. Therapy*, **28**: 110–25.

22. **Johnson, S., Oliver, C., Prince, G. A., Hemming, V. G., Pfarr, D. S., Wang, S.-C., Dormitzer, M., O'Grady, J., Koenig, S., Tamura, J. K., Woods, R., Bansal, G., Couchenour, D., Tsao, E., Hall, W. C., and Young, J. F.** (1997). 'Development of a Humanized Monoclonal Antibody (MEDI-493) with Potent In Vitro and In Vivo Activity against Respiratory Syncytial Virus.' *J. Infect. Dis.*, **176**: 1215–24.

23. **The Impact-RSV Study Group** (1998). 'Palivizumab, a Humanized Respiratory Syncytial Virus Monoclonal Antibody, Reduces Hospitalization From Respiratory Syncytial Virus Infection in High-risk Infants.' *Pediatrics*, **102**: 531–7.

24. **Resch, B., Kurath, S., and Manzonie, P.** (2011). 'Epidemiology of respiratory syncytial virus infection in preterm infants.' *Open Microbiol. J.*, **5** (Suppl 2.M3): 135–43.

25. **van Drunen, S., van den Hurk, L., and Watkiss, E. R.** (2012). 'Pathogenesis of respiratory syncytial virus.' *Curr. Opin. Virol.*, **2**: 300–5.

26. **Sow, F. B., Gallup, J. M. Olivier, A., Krishnan, S, Patera, A. C., Suzich, J., and Ackerman, M. R.** (2011). 'Respiratory syncytial virus is associated with an inflammatory response in lungs and architectural remodeling of lung-draining lymph nodes of newborn lambs.' *Am. J. Physiol. Lung Cell. Mol. Physiol.*, **300**: L12–L24.

Chapter 16

Therapeutic antibodies
Case study II: Targeting
breast cancer

Background

Understanding the mechanisms by which normal cells become malignant took a massive leap in the early 1970s with the discovery of genes present in the family of RNA transforming retroviruses that were able to confer a malignant phenotype on normal cells. The molecular genetics breakthrough came in 1970 when Peter Duesberg and Peter Vogt noted the absence of a particular RNA subunit 'class' (class *a*) in the non-transforming derivatives of avian retroviruses, which included the well-studied Rous sarcoma viruses (RSV). Duesberg and Vogt speculated that the class *a* RNA contains the genetic information necessary for malignant transformation.[1] This discovery was revolutionary at the time and propelled both Duesberg and Vogt into the scientific limelight. By 1974, it was known that the non-transforming mutants of RSV were deletion mutants lacking about 10–20% of the viral genome. At a Cold Spring Harbor meeting on tumour viruses in the summer of 1974, Wyke, Bell, and Beamand announced the arrival of the 'oncogene' by presenting results from analysis of transformation-defective mutants of RSV. These mutants contained a single gene, *sarc*, that appeared to be superfluous for viral replication but essential for maintenance of the malignant state.[2] In 1976, Michael Bishop, Harold Varmus (both would share the Nobel Prize in 1989 for their discovery of retroviruses), and Peter Vogt took the puzzle of transformation to new heights when they took cDNA prepared from the RNA sequence of the *sarc* gene, used it to probe normal chicken cells, and observed homology between the viral gene and normal DNA sequences.[3] Furthermore, this homology was absent from normal mammalian DNA. In their concluding comments on this important step forward, Vogt and co-authors made the following anticipatory observation:

> We anticipate that cellular DNA homologous to cDNA$_{sarc}$ serves some function which accounts for its conservation... and could represent either structural or regulatory genes. But the function of those genes is unknown. We are testing the possibilities that they are involved in the normal regulation of cell growth and development...[3]

A key to the 'function' puzzle was provided in 1983 when two simultaneous reports appeared from Doolittle at UCSD along with Hood from Caltech, Aaronson from NCI, and Antoniades from Harvard,[4] and Waterfield at ICRF, Heldin from Uppsala, and Duel from the University of Washington.[5] Both groups described a direct sequence relationship between a 28kDa protein produced by the Simian sarcoma virus (SSV) and the naturally occurring platelet-derived growth factor (PDGF). PDGF is a potent mitogen stored in the alpha granules of platelets until released during blood clotting. Here then was a logical connection. Once infected by the transforming virus, a virally encoded growth factor would be constitutively produced that would override normal paracrine controls present for normal tissues. However, this mechanism would rely on the presence of an active receptor to transduce the PDGF signal in target cells, conferring a tissue specificity *parri passu* for successful virus transformation. Weiss observed in the *Nature* 'News and Views' accompanying the Waterfield paper that those human tumours expressing the cellular homologue of the SSV transforming gene, *sis*, were sarcomas and gliomas, both cell types deriving from mesenchymal tissues known to be sensitive to the PDGF. Weiss also suggested, based on the observation that the product of the *sarc* gene and the *sis* gene both gave rise to protein phosphorylation on tyrosine residues, that the product of the *sarc* gene was also a growth factor.[6] Of course, it was also possible that the PDGF molecule had been altered during viral evolution to possess a receptor-independent activity. All such mechanisms were up for consideration. But the transformation picture was more complicated than that and one year later Waterfield, Ullrich, Schlessinger, and team added a new scene to the script. Purification of the receptor for epidermal growth factor (EGF) showed that it had 'close similarity' to the sequence of the v-*erb*-B gene present in yet another retrovirus, avian erythroblastosis virus (AEV). However, the receptor was not identical to the normal human receptor. V-*erb*-B contained only the transmembrane sequence attached to the intracellular domain normally associated with the tyrosine phosphorylation activity and lacked the sequence encoding the extracellular domain required for binding to EGF. As Waterfield suggests:

> The absence of the EGF binding domain might remove the control generated by ligand binding and the result could be continuous generation of a signal equivalent to that produced by EGF, causing cells to proliferate rapidly.[7]

The uncertainty of this suggestion was drawn attention to by Peter Newmark of *Nature* magazine, who reminded the oncogene community that so far no tyrosine phosphorylation activity had yet been seen by the *erb*-B truncated receptor.[8] Three months after the Waterfield paper, Ullrich and colleagues published the full sequence of the EGF receptor obtained from the cDNAs of both normal human placenta (the c-*erb*-B gene) and the epidermoid carcinoma cell line A431, renowned for its excessive number of EGF receptors at around ten to 50 times that of normal cells. This study confirmed the partial sequence data of Waterfield and demonstrated that A431 cells have an amplified EGF receptor gene and in addition produce elevated mRNA levels of a smaller rearranged EGF receptor consisting only of the extracellular domain. With customary scientific honesty Ullrich and his team had no explanation for the mechanism by which A431 cells might utilize its EGF receptors and their truncated versions.[9] These data were confirmed in parallel reports showing that A431 cells have both normal length and truncated amplified EGFR genes,[10] and in addition secrete high levels of the truncated receptor containing only the extracellular domain into the culture medium.[11] It seemed to Ullrich that A431 cells might represent a mechanistic cul-de-sac.[9]

It has been said that on the other side of complexity lies simplicity. In 1984 the findings so far suggested that the complexity of cell transformation was a deep crater, perhaps appropriately in that particular year, on an Orwellian scale. But science thrives on complexity and its insatiable appetite was to be further fed by a new twist. At the end of this extraordinary year Robert Weinberg, Mark Green, and colleagues presented results on the discovery of an *erb*-B related gene found in a series of rat neuro/glioblastoma cell lines derived from chemically induced tumours. They named this oncogene gene, which had four independently activated allelic forms, *neu*. When the *neu* gene was introduced into normal fibroblasts the transformed cells were capable of producing tumours in mice. Antibodies produced by the mice precipitated a 185 000 dalton phosphorylated protein (p185) from *neu*-transformed fibroblasts.[12] This protein was not detected in normal fibroblasts nor in cells transformed by other oncogenes such as *ras* (a mutated and oncogenic GTPase isolated from rat sarcomas). Weinberg's analysis went further. It appeared that *neu* was related to the *erb*-B gene, determined by its cross-reactivity with anti-EGFR sera. But, the two proteins were of different sizes and based on additional serology data Weinberg proposed that p185 and the EGFR were distinct, if related, gene products. But for now *neu* was an orphan receptor since if it was distinct from the EGFR its cognate growth factor was unknown.

In July 1985, a variation on this developing receptor high-jacking theme was reinforced by the work of Sherr and colleagues showing that the proto-oncogene c-*fms* had identity with the macrophage colony stimulating factor receptor (CSF-R1) and that the oncogenic version of this gene that is present in feline sarcoma viruses (v-*fms*) and absolutely required for transformation has identity with this CSF receptor.[13] A blow for the simplicity explanation was dealt by this study since the oncogene in this instance was a full length receptor containing both the intra- and extra-cellular domains. As Sherr observes, drawing attention to the multiple cellular mechanisms that are open to be exploited during transformation:

> The data argue against the hypothesis that proto-oncogenes are restricted in their expression to cells that act as targets for their viral oncogene counterparts... activated oncogenes appear to be more promiscuous in their function than their proto-oncogene progenitors... alterations... as a result of retroviral transduction can significantly affect their regulation...[13]

By late 1985 the relationship between *neu* and the c-*erb* gene was established in three separate studies. Semba and colleagues from the University of Tokyo examined a human genomic library and isolated the gene related to v-*erb*B that was distinct from the EGF receptor c-*erb*B gene.[14] They named this related gene c-*erb*B-2, established its identity with the rat *neu* oncogene, and further suggested that the gene may be involved in cancer—in examining a human adenocarcinoma of the salivary gland they observed a 30-fold amplification of c-*erb*B-2. Was this a case of QED? At the same time Stuart Aaronson at the NIH described the amplification (five to ten times) of a novel v-*erb*B-related gene in DNA from a human mammary carcinoma.[15] Although this amplification was not seen in ten other mammary carcinomas it was still a key observation. While the Aaronson manuscript was in the proof stage, the results of Semba were seen by the NIH team, confirming the identity of Aaronson's amplified gene with the c-*erb*B-2 gene. The picture was improving in resolution. By December 1985, Ullrich had described the isolation of genomic DNA clones from normal and malignant human cells that revealed the detailed sequence information for the EGFR-related gene *neu* and established its clear distinction from the EGFR gene. Ullrich named this gene HER-2 and confirmed its authenticity by chromosomal analysis (HER-2 on chromosome 17 and EGFR on chromosome seven).[16]

The importance of the discovery of Her-2/*neu*, as it was now designated, became evident in 1987 when Ullrich, Slamon, and collaborators from UCLA School of Medicine and the University of Texas at San Antonio presented the results of an extensive study on the amplification of the gene in primary breast cancer tumours and its correlation with patient relapse and survival. The results were startlingly clear: Her-2/*neu* was as good a prognostic indicator of disease relapse or patient survival as the presence of positive lymph nodes and better than all other prognosticators.[17] While not all patients had amplified Her-2/*neu* (~28% of 189 primary tumours showed amplification), for those that were positive the presence of more than five copies of the gene correlated with significantly shorter disease-free and overall survival times (see Fig. 16.1).

This was an exciting time but the question of how this finding might be exploited in building a therapeutic strategy was some way off. While Her-2/*neu* was known to be a full-length receptor it was still an orphan, lacking a known growth factor. It was also not clear that mammary carcinoma cells bearing this receptor had any need for an externally acting growth factor for cell survival and growth or whether some alteration

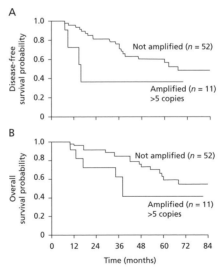

Fig. 16.1 (A) Actuarial curve for relapse in node-positive patients with no amplification versus node-positive patients with more than five copies of HER-2/*neu* and (B) Actuarial survival for node-positive patients with no amplification versus node-positive patients with more than five copies of HER-2/*neu*.

From Slamon, D.J. et al., Human Breast Cancer: Correlation of Relapse and Survival with Amplification of the HER-2/neu Oncogene, *Science*, Volume 235, Issue 4785, pp.177–183, Copyright © 1987. Reprinted with permission from AAAS.

in the receptor sequence had conferred a constitutive 'on' state, for example by permanent activation of the tyrosine kinase domain.

The therapeutic breakthrough

In the spring of 1989 two important steps were taken. As part of their continuing collaboration Slamon and Ullrich, working with several other institutions, addressed the issue of methodology for determining HER-2/*neu* gene status in tumour tissues, a critical element of any clinical diagnostic method that may be developed. This study emphasized the importance of establishing that in tumours being tested methods were used that enabled both gene amplification and over-expression of the protein product to be measured. For example, if a gene is amplified but no mRNA is produced, or mRNA is amplified but no protein is produced, false tumour status will be recorded. The publication also noted that over-expression of the normal HER-2/*neu* gene product may be important for the observed pathology of some tumours. A particularly important finding was that HER-2/*neu* status in ovarian cancers, where prognostic factors for predicting clinical outcome were sadly lacking, showed a similar association between gene amplification/over-expression of p185 and clinical outcome.[18]

The second critical step was taken within the corridors of the Genentech chemistry and biology departments. As part of a normal functional study of the HER-2 protein Ullrich's team prepared monoclonal antibodies by immunizing mice with fibroblasts that had been transfected with the HER-2/*neu* gene and selected for amplified expression of the HER-2 protein. Of those antibodies investigated one murine antibody, 4D5, was able to inhibit the growth of several human breast cancer cell lines but also appeared to increase their sensitivity to the cytokine, tumour necrosis factor alpha (TNFα).[19] 4D5 was not only a potential growth modulator of the cancer cells but was also specific for the HER-2 protein with no measurable cross-reactivity with the related EGF receptor and no apparent reactivity with any other protein expressed by the fibroblasts. At the close of the paper, Ullrich (see Fig. 16.2) and colleagues commented:

> Monoclonal antibodies specific for p185[HER2] may therefore be useful therapeutic agents for the treatment of human neoplasias, including certain mammary carcinomas, which are characterized by the overexpressing of p185[HER2].[19]

As events turned out this was an understatement of gigantic proportions.

Events now moved fast. In 1990 Paul Carter, now a Genentech apostle but once a Winter disciple, together with Len Presta and Mike Shepard, humanized antibody 4D5 by CDR grafting using a parsimonious technique of 'gene conversion mutagenesis', and with the aid of models identified key framework positions that were critical for CDR conformation and in five of those retained the murine amino acid. Surprisingly the best humanized version showed a three-fold higher binding affinity for p185[HER2] and had comparable anti-proliferative activity to the parent mouse antibody. It also displayed ADCC killing activity against target tumour cells in the presence of effector cells but was ineffectual at killing normal epithelial cells.[20] The stage was set, the actors were in place, but would humanized antibody 4D5, trastuzumab, play its part well enough to get through the clinical audition?

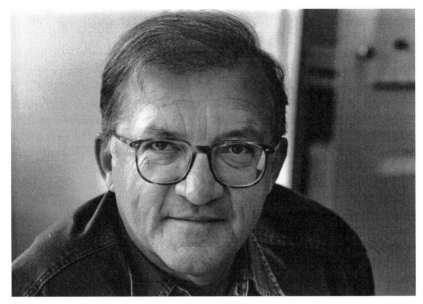

Fig. 16.2 Axel Ullrich.

Reproduced with permission from Axel Ullrich and the Max Planck Institute of Biochemistry, Germany, Copyright © Max Planck Institute of Biochemistry.

In 1992 Genentech filed an IND with the FDA and initiated Phase One clinical trials establishing the dosing regime and safety of trastuzumab. One year later several Phase Two trials were initiated in which trastuzumab was used as first-line therapy or in combination with standard chemotherapy. In the first of these to be completed, a clinical group at the Department of Medicine, Memorial Sloan Kettering Cancer Centre in New York, led by Larry Norton, published the results of a Phase Two study in which 46 patients with metastatic breast cancer who also over-expressed HER2 were treated weekly with trastuzumab alone over a ten week period. While the responses were not demonstrably positive, five out of 43 assessable patients showed objective responses, with one complete remission, and four partial remissions giving an overall response rate of 11.6%. The authors concluded:

> This is evidence that targeting growth factor receptors can cause regression of human cancer and justifies further evaluation of this agent.[21]

This was an extraordinary statement that signalled a change in cancer-therapy thinking for all time to come. Here was a specific, biologically important cellular receptor targeted by a monoclonal antibody for the first time since the monoclonal discovery by Köhler and Milstein some 20 years earlier. A revolution in clinical oncology was about to get under way.

In 1995 Genentech, with the involvement of breast cancer advocates piloted by Frances Visco, President of the National Breast Cancer Coalition (NBCC), began recruitment for a series of Phase Three clinical trials, named 648, 649, and 650.

In his 1998 book, *The Making of Herceptin, a Revolutionary Treatment for Breast Cancer*,[22] Robert Bazell recounts the background to these trials and the method of patient recruitment in which patients who had tested positive for HER2/*neu* and failed other forms of treatment would have their names submitted by their physician to a third-party private company who would select names at random. The trial design also brought into stark relief the ethics of clinical trial designs where patients fighting for their lives might be assigned to a placebo group or a group receiving trastuzumab plus chemotherapy (the pivotal 648 trial) where the proposed chemotherapeutic agent may already have shown little benefit to them. These factors alone clearly played a role in the slow response to enrollment. The interplay between patients, clinicians, feisty breast cancer advocates, and clinical trial designers both inside and outside Genentech, and intense marketing efforts in improving enrollment, including amendment to the trial design to allow chemotherapy with paclitaxel as a replacement for doxorubicin in the 648 trial, which most patients would have received already as the most frequently employed chemotherapy, were just some of the factors that made the clinical breakthrough even more impressive. Add to that the practical difficulties of producing enough Herceptin for a Phase Three trial and a recipe for failure lay close-to-hand. After all, in the mid-1990s Genentech was not a big pharma and clinical trial experience was not yet in its war chest. The sometimes heart-rending personal stories surrounding this frenetic period and the earnest involvement of driven clinical believers such as Dennis Slamon, Melody Cobleigh, Larry Norton, and others are explored in sleuth-like, dramatic detail by Bazell. By dint of hard work and some good fortune, 648 enrolment towards the target of 450 women improved and data started to arrive. By early 1998 the clinical leads involved in the three trials presented the results at the May meeting of the American Society of Clinical Oncology in Los Angeles. The response of the audience has been described as 'staggering'. Trastuzumab therapy had arrived.

In parallel with the Phase Three enrollment a number of Phase Two studies were in progress. At St Lukes's Medical Centre in Chicago, 220 women were enrolled who exhibited HER2-overexpressing metastatic breast cancer and whose disease had progressed after several chemotherapy treatments. Weekly treatment with the antibody at 2mg/kg generated eight complete responses and 26 partial responses giving an objective response rate of 15%, as determined by a blinded response evaluation committee. Melody Cobleigh, who was also involved in the Genentech Phase Three trials, concluded in the published report of this clinical trial in 1999 that trastuzumab produced durable responses and was well tolerated by the patient group.[23] A clinically significant adverse event seen in the study was cardiac dysfunction occurring in 4.7% of patients. This would also be seen in later studies. In a smaller trial, led by Dennis Slamon at UCLA who was also involved in the Phase Three trials, trastuzumab was used in combination with the well accepted chemotherapeutic agent, cisplatin (which binds to DNA during replication or transcription and induces cell death). Of the 37 patients enrolled, all with over-expression of HER2/*neu* and presenting advanced metastatic disease and who had already received extensive chemotherapy, nine achieved a partial response, with a further nine showing a minor response or stable disease while the remaining

19 showed disease progression. This was an impressive result for such a high-risk patient group and showed improved responses over either cisplatin or trastuzumab alone.[24]

In May1998, on the back of results from the still ongoing Phase Three trials, Genentech submitted a biological license application to the FDA for trastuzumab. FDA approval was obtained in September of the same year as a 'Fast Track' product for the treatment of metastatic breast cancer in women who over-express the HER2/*neu* protein. The antibody was marketed under the name Herceptin. In 2000 Herceptin was approved in Europe.

But just what was trastuzumb doing to the cancer cells? Within the Genentech research and development corridors a smart molecular oncology team was seeking the answers. Led by Mark Sliwkowski, the trastuzumab mechanism story was being pieced together. Phenotypic effects were observed at the level of HER-2 receptor expression accompanied by various intracellular modulatory effects. The combined result was an inhibition of cell growth that appeared to be due in part to induction of protein signalling molecules essential for cells to move through the S-phase (a necessary synthesis phase before a cell can divide into two daughter cells).In addition to its direct receptor binding effects, trastuzumab was effective in ADCC mediated by its Fc region.[25] Sliwkowski noted that trastuzumab was more effective when given in conjunction with chemotherapeutic agents, an observation that would become a theme for future Genentech product developments.

In 2001, Slamon had completed and published a clinical study in which Herceptin was combined with a chemotherapeutic agent in comparison with chemotherapy alone, involving 235 and 234 patients respectively, all of whom had metastatic breast cancer. The choice of agent in the combined therapy was based on the chemotherapeutic-agent history of the women enrolled. The results were all the more impressive when, during the study, cross-over therapy was initiated. As Slamon and team concluded:

> We found that trastuzumab-based combination therapy was effective in that it reduced the relative risk of death by 20 percent at a median follow-up of 30 months. Few studies of metastatic breast cancer have demonstrated a survival advantage of this magnitude in association with the addition of a single agent… Particularly noteworthy is that two thirds of patients who were initially assigned to receive chemotherapy alone began, after disease progression, to receive open-label trastuzumab alone or with chemotherapy. Such a crossover design would generally reduce the likelihood that a survival advantage would be found. Significant increases in the time to disease progression, the rates of response, the duration of responses, and the time to treatment failure were observed in both subgroups that were given chemotherapy plus trastuzumab. These results increased survival, an end point free of ascertainment bias.[26]

> Text extract reprinted with permission from Slamon, D.J., et al. Use of chemotherapy plus a monoclonal antibody against HER2 for metastatic breast cancer that overexpresses HER2, *New England Journal of Medicine*, Volume 344, pp. 783–792, Copyright © 2001 Massachusetts Medical Society.

Slamon also drew attention to the observed cardiotoxicity side effects of trastuzumab, particularly when administered in conjunction with anthracyclines and cyclophosphamide. The mechanism of the toxicity was unknown.

One year before the Slamon report, two new Phase Three trials, sponsored by the National Cancer Institute (NCI) in the USA, began enrollment comparing the use of trastuzumab in combined adjuvant therapy with chemotherapy alone in patients with surgically removed HER2-positive breast cancer. These studies were important for two reasons. Firstly, two separate clinical groups (National Surgical Adjuvant Breast and Bowel Project (NSABP); North Central Cancer Treatment Group (NCCTG)) employed related treatment regimens on a large number of patients (2043 for NSABP and 1633 for NCCTG) in multiple centres. Secondly, as pointed out by Cohen,[27] through unprecedented industry/academic/government collaboration, the results of the two trials were jointly analysed for the comparable groups in each study. In 2005, analyses of the joint studies were published. The absolute difference in disease-free survival between the trastuzumab group and the control group was 12% at three years. Remarkably, trastuzumab therapy was associated with a 33% reduction in the risk of death.[28] By November of 2006 and on the back of the NCCGP and NSABP trial results, the FDA had approved Herceptin for adjuvant treatment of women with early-stage breast cancer. In early 2008, Herceptin was approved as a single agent for the adjuvant treatment of early-stage, HER-2/*neu* positive breast cancer or in patients with node-negative breast cancer who had received multi-modality, anthracycline chemotherapy. By October 2008 Genentech reported that more than 420 000 women had been treated with Herceptin worldwide.[25]

But Herceptin was not a miracle drug. It displayed cardiotoxicity when associated with standard adjuvant agents in a relatively high percentage of patients and furthermore, patients on long-term Herceptin therapy developed resistance to the antibody. In addressing the cardiac dysfunction (CD) issue, Seidman carried out a retrospective analysis of patient records from seven Phase Two and Phase Three trastuzumab clinical trials. The results published in 2002 indicated that patients treated with trastuzumab did have an increased risk of CD. The risk was greatest in patients who were on concurrent trastuzumab, anthracycline, and cyclophosphamide therapy (27%) but substantially lower in patients receiving trastuzumab and paclitaxel (13%) or trastuzumab alone (3–7%). Seidman further concluded that of the patients developing CD, most improved with standard treatment for congestive heart failure.[29] Seidman and colleagues concluded that the benefits of Herceptin therapy outweighed the cardiotoxicity risks.

Second generation antibodies

On the issue of Herceptin resistance, Genentech had been aware of this possibility for some time, in addition to the fact that only around 30% of breast cancers have p185[HER2] over-expression and breast cancer cells with low levels of this protein are unresponsive to Herceptin. Two possible explanations existed. Either breast cancer cells were under the influence of other obligate growth mechanisms or Herceptin was only partially capable of blocking a critically important pathway for cell survival that was mediated by HER-2/*neu* signalling. In 1990 Ullrich's team published the results of a study identifying new monoclonal antibodies that discriminated the EGF receptor and HER-2/*neu*. One of these antibodies, 2C4 would become important as a next generation therapeutic, complementing the activity of Herceptin. By 1998 Yarden, working at the Weizmann Institute, had shown that p185[HER2] was something of a receptor 'passenger' and that its probable contribution to cell growth signalling was reliant on its association with one or more new members of the erbB family known as erbB-3 and erbB-4.[30] The formation of a heterodimeric pair between erbB-2 and erbB-3 and the subsequent activity appeared to be dependent on ligands that may have derived from local mesenchymal tissue. What was suggested by Yarden's study was that individual erbB-2 or erbB-3 receptors were signalling-incompetent and only acquired responsiveness on formation of the heterodimer. This gave an important clue to a possible new therapeutic approach and in 2002, a joint Genentech–academic study, led by Mark Sliwkowski, demonstrated that antibody 2C4 blocked the recruitment of erbB-2 receptor into the dimerized pool and in doing so suppressed the growth of tumour cell lines and tumour xenografts in mice.[31] Two important features of this study were that the suppression of cell growth occurred in tumour cells containing low levels of p185[HER2] and also that the effect was evident in both breast cancer and prostate cancer cells. Furthermore, growth suppression was seen in prostate cancer xenografts. Pre-clinical studies in primates, referred to but not given in detail, suggested that the humanized version of antibody 2C4 displayed similar pharmacokinetics to that of Herceptin. The stage was set. In previewing this work by Sliwkowski and colleagues, José Baselga, who had been involved in the 1996 trastuzumab trial led by Larry Norton, speculated that the way forward was a combined therapy approach:

> Finally, it also provides an opportunity to explore combining these agents in a full-scale anti-ErbB2 war by inducing receptor down regulation and an anti-receptor immune response (Herceptin) by isolating ErbB2 from its trans-activating ErbB partners (2C4) and by eliminating any remaining receptor catalytic activity (small tyrosine kinase inhibitors).[32]

During the period 2002 to 2013, numerous clinical studies of antibody 2C4 (now named pertuzumab) were initiated in breast cancer patients but also for other indications in prostate cancer, non-small lung cell cancer, and ovarian cancer. In a Phase One trial with 21 patients Agus, Sliwkowski, and colleagues established that pertuzumab was well tolerated, had a pharmacokinetic profile typical of antibody therapeutics, and showed clinical activity.[33] Several Phase Two studies were reported in 2006 and 2007 in which trastuzumab and pertuzumab were used in combination or with the addition of chemotherapy. Clinical studies were also carried out with pertuzumab alone. In general the results were mixed, with improved prognoses only seen when the two antibodies with or without chemotherapy were employed. In 2010 a Phase Two study was reported by Beselga for patients whose breast cancer had progressed after trastuzumab therapy. The objective response rate in this study was 24.2% and the clinical benefit rate was 50%. Complete response was seen in 7.6%, partial response in 16.7%, and stable disease ≥ six months in 25.8% of patients.[34] On the basis of this a much larger international, multicentre trial was initiated in 2010, the CLEOPATRA study, in which patients were treated either with trastuzumab, pertuzumab and docetaxel, or with trastuzumab, docetaxel and placebo in place of pertuzumab.[35] In January 2012 the Italian trial, NeoSphere, reported significantly improved patient response rates with the combination trastuzumab, pertuzumab, and docetaxel.[36] In January 2012,

Swain, Baselga, and colleagues in the CLEOPATRA study group reported the interim results of the Phase Three study[40]. In summary, the investigator-assessed median progression-free survival time had increased by 50% for the group receiving both trastuzumab and pertuzumab in combination with docetaxel (18.7 months) compared with the group receiving placebo in place of pertuzumab (12.4 months). Interim analysis of overall survival, though incomplete, showed a strong trend towards prolonged survival. In June 2012 pertuzumab received FDA approval and entered the market under the name Perjeta.

Most recently, after a year of follow-up, overall survival results of the CLEOPATRA study were published[41]. Median overall survival was 37.6 months in the placebo group but had not been reached in the pertuzumab group. The study group conclusion was that significant improvement in overall survival in the group receiving trastuzamab, pertuzumab, and docetaxel was shown, representing a 'substantial improvement in the standard care of breast cancer patients.'

The story of Herceptin and its follow-on partner, Perjeta, is an extraordinary one. It has changed the way clinicians think about treatment of epithelial cancers and has changed the lives of a large number of women for whom chemotherapy with its attendant side effects was the only alternative. The magic bullet of Ehrlich has so far been the anti-toxin itself, but the story has not ended there. In 2008 Sliwkowski reported a study in which a derivative of the microtubule inhibitory drug maytansine, known as DM1, was chemically linked by a stable covalent chemistry, developed by the Boston company Immunogen with whom Genentech were collaborating, to trastuzumab and tested on Her-2 positive breast cancer cells *in vitro* and in rodent *in vivo* tumour models. The antibody conjugate was not only selective for over-expressing Her-2 cells but showed a much greater efficacy in arresting the growth of tumours *in vivo*.[37] As a result of these pre-clinical studies the trastuzumab-DM1 conjugate entered clinical trials. After a series of Phase One and Two studies, in 2011 LoRusso reported initiation of two Phase Three trials, EMILIA and MARIANNE, to evaluate the efficacy of this novel conjugate. In 2012 Barginear reported early encouraging results of the EMILIA trial.[38] In May of 2013 the trastuzumab-DM1 conjugate was approved in the USA under the market name Kadcycla.

Despite the newer Retiarian 'net and trident' approaches as Philip Thorpe had referred to antibody-toxin conjugate therapy 20 years earlier,[39] the race to find a definitive treatment that will lead to disease-free breast cancer patients is still ongoing. The single or even dual therapeutic antibody regimen may not yet be the complete answer but it has been and will continue to be a powerful member of the clinician's armamentarium.

References

1. **Duesberg, P.-H., and Vogt, P. K.** (1970). 'Differences between the Ribonucleic Acids of Transforming and Non-transforming Avian Tumor Viruses.' *Proc. Natl. Acad. Sci.*, **67**: 1673–80.

2. **Wyke, J. A., Bell, J. G., and Beamand, J. A.** (1974). 'Genetic Recombination among Temperature-sensitive Mutants of Rous Sarcoma Virus.' *Cold Spring Harb. Symp. Quant. Biol.*, **39**: 897–905.

3. Stehelin, D., Varmus, H. E., Bishop, J. M., and Vogt, P. K. (1976). 'DNA related to the transforming gene(s) of avian sarcoma viruses is present in normal avian DNA.' *Nature*, **260**: 170–3.

4. Doolittle, R. F., Hunkapiller, M. W., Hood, L. E., Devare, S. G., Robbins, K. C., Aaronson, S. A., and Antoniades, H. N. (1983). 'Simian Sarcoma Virus onc gene, v-sis, is derived from the gene (or genes) encoding a platelet-derived growth factor.' *Science*, **221**: 275–7.

5. Waterfield, M. D., Scrace, G. T., Whittle, N., Stroobant, P., Johnsson, A., Wasteson, Å., Westermark, B., Heldin, C.-H., Huang, J. S., and Deuel, T. F. (1983). 'Platelet-derived growth factor is structurally related to the putative transforming protein p28^{sis} of simian sarcoma virus.' *Nature*, **304**: 35–9.

6. Weiss, R. (1983). 'Oncogenes and growth factors.' *Nature*, **304**: 12.

7. Downward, J., Yarden, Y., Mayes, E., Scrace, G., Totty, N., Stockwell, P., Ullrich, A., Schlessinger, J., and Waterfield, M. D. (1984). 'Close similarity of epidermal growth factor receptor and v-*erb*-B oncogene protein sequences.' *Nature*, **307**: 521–7.

8. Newmark, P. (1984). 'Cell and cancer biology meld.' *Nature*, **307**: 499.

9. Ullrich, A., Coussens, L., Hayflick, J. S., Dull, T. J., Gray, A., Tam, A. W., Lee, J., Yarden, Y., Libermann, T. A., Schlessinger, J., Downward, J., Mayes, E. L. V., Whittle, N., Waterfield, M. D., and Seeburg, P. H. (1984). 'Human epidermal growth factor receptor cDNA sequence and aberrant expression of the amplified gene in A431 epidermoid carcinoma cells.' *Nature*, **309**: 418–25.

10. Merlino, G. T., Xu, Y. H., Ishii, S., Clark, A. J., Semba, K., Toyoshima, K., Yamamoto, T., and Pastan, I. (1984). 'Amplification and enhanced expression of the epidermal growth factor receptor gene in A431 human carcinoma cells.' *Science*, **224**: 417–19.

11. Weber, W., Gill, G. N., and Spiess, J. (1984). 'Production of an Epidermal Growth Factor Receptor-Related Protein.' Science, **224**: 294–7.

12. Schecter, A. L., Stern, D. F., Vaidyanathan, L., Decker, S. J., Drebin, J. A., Greene, M. I., and Weinberg, R. A. (1984). 'The *neu* oncogene: an *erb*-B-related gene encoding a 185,000-Mr tumour antigen.' *Nature*, **312**: 513–16.

13. Sherr, C. J., Rettenmier, C. W., Sacca, R., Roussel, M. F., Look, A. T., and Stanley, E. R. (1985). 'The c-*fms* proto-oncogene product is related to the receptor for the mononuclear phagocyte growth factor, CSF-1.' *Cell*, **41**: 665–76.

14. Semba, K., Kamata, N., Toyoshima, K., and Yamamoto, T. (1985). 'A v-*erbB*-related proto-oncogene, c-*erbB*-2, is distinct from the c-*erbB*-1/epidermal growth factor-receptor gene and is amplified in a human salivary gland adenocarcinoma.' *Proc. Natl. Acad. Sci.*, **82**: 6497–501.

15. King, R., Kraus, M., and Aaronson, S. A. (1985). 'Amplification of a Novel v-erbB-Related Gene in a Human Mammary Carcinoma.' *Science*, **229**: 974–6.

16. Coussens, L., Yang-Feng, T. L., Liao, Y.-C., Chen, E., Gray, A., McGrath, J., Seeburg, P. H., Libermann, T. A., Schlessinger, J., Francke, U., Levinson, A., and Ullrich, A. (1985). 'Tyrosine Kinase Receptor with Extensive Homology to EGF Receptor Shares Chromosomal Location with neu Oncogene.' *Science*, **230**: 1132–9.

17. Slamon, D. J., Clark, G. M., Wong, S. G., Levin, W. J., Ullrich, A., and McGuire, W. L. (1987). 'Human Breast Cancer: Correlation of Relapse and Survival with Amplification of the HER-2/neu Oncogene.' *Science*, **235**: 177–83.

18. Slamon, D. J., Godolphin, W., Jones, L. A., Holt, J. A., Wong, S. G., Keith, D. E., Levin, W. J., Stuart, S. G., Udove, J., Ullrich, A., and Press, M. F. (1989). 'Studies of the HER-2/neu Proto-Oncogene in Human Breast and Ovarian Cancer.' *Science*, **244**: 707–12.

19. **Hudziak, R. M., Lewis, G. D., Winget, M., Fendly, B. M., Shepard, H. M., and Ullrich, A.** (1989). 'p185[HER2] Monoclonal Antibody Has Antiproliferative Effects In Vitro and Sensitizes Human Breast Tumor Cells to Tumor Necrosis Factor.' *Molec. Cell. Biol.*, **9**: 1165–72.

20. **Carter, P., Presta, L., Gorman, C. M., Ridgway, J. B. B., Henner, D., Wong, W. L. T., Rowland, A. M., Kotts, C., Carver, M. E., and Shepard, H. M.** (1992). 'Humanization of an Anti-p185[HER2] Antibody for Human Cancer Therapy.' *Proc. Natl. Acad. Sci.*, **89**: 4285–9.

21. **Baselga, J., Tripathy, D., Mendelsohn, J., Baughman, S., Benz, C. C, Dantis, L., Sklarin, N. T., Seidman, A. D., Hudis, C. A., Moore, J., Rosen, P. P., Twaddell, T., Henderson, I. C., and Norton, L.** (1996). 'Phase II study of weekly intravenous recombinant humanized anti-p185HER2 monoclonal antibody in patients with HER2/neu-overexpressing metastatic breast cancer.' *J. Clin. Oncol.*, **14**: 737–44.

22. **Bazell, R.** (1995). *Her-2: The Making of Herceptin, a Revolutionary Treatment for Breast Cancer.* London: Random House.

23. **Cobleigh, M. A., Vogel, C. L., Tripathy, D., Robert, N. J., Scholl, S., Fehrenbacher, L., Wolter, J. M., Paton, V., Shak, S., Lieberman, G., and Slamon, D. J.** (1999). 'Multinational study of the efficacy and safety of humanized anti-HER2 monoclonal antibody in women who have HER2-overexpressing metastatic breast cancer that has progressed after chemotherapy for metastatic disease.' *J. Clin. Oncol.*, **17**: 2639–48.

24. **Pegram, M. D., Lipton, A., Hayes, D. F., Weber, B. L., Baselga, J. M., Tripathy, D., Baly, D., Baughman, S. A., Twaddell, T., Glaspy, J. A., and Slamon, D. J.** (1998). 'Phase II study of receptor-enhanced chemosensitivity using recombinant humanized anti-p185[HER2]/neu monoclonal antibody plus cisplatin in patients with HER2/neu-overexpressing metastatic breast cancer refractory to chemotherapy treatment.' *J. Clin. Oncol.*, **16**: 2659–71.

25. **Sliwkowski, M. X., Lofgren, J. A., Lewis, G. D., Hotaling, T. E., Fendly, B. M., and Fox, J. A.** (1999). 'Non-clinical studies addressing the mechanism of action of trastuzumab (Herceptin).' *Semin. Oncol.*, **26**: 60–70.

26. **Slamon, D. J., Leyland-Jones, B., Shak, S., Fuchs, H., Paton, V., Bajamonde, A., Fleming, T., Eiermann, W., Wolter, J., Pegram, M., Baselga, J., and Norton, L.** (2001). 'Use of chemotherapy plus a monoclonal antibody against HER2 for metastatic breast cancer that overexpresses HER2.' *N. Engl. J. Med.*, **344**: 783–92.

27. **Cohen, R. L.** (2012). 'Adjuvant trials of targeted agents: the newest battleground in the war on cancer.' *Curr. Top. Microbiol. Immunol.*, **355**: 217–32.

28. **Romond, E. H., Perez, E. A., Bryant, J., Suman, V. J., Geyer, C. E., Davidson, N. E., Tan-Chiu, E., Martino, S., Paik, S., Kaufman, P. A., Swain, S. M., Pisansky, T. M., Fehrenbacher, L., Kutteh, L. A., Vogel, V. G., Visscher, D. W., Yothers, G., Jenkins, R. B., Brown, A. M., Dakhil, S. R., Mamounas, E. P., Lingle, W. L., Klein, P. M., Ingle, J. N., and Wolmark, N.** (2005). 'Trastuzumab plus Adjuvant Chemotherapy for Operable HER2-Positive Breast Cancer.' *N. Engl. J. Med.*, **353**: 1673–84.

29. **Seidman, A., Hudis, C., Pierri, M. K., Shak, S., Paton, V., Ashby, M., Murphy, M., Stewart, S. J., and Keefe, D.** (2002). 'Cardiac dysfunction in the trastuzumab clinical trials experience.' *J. Clin. Oncol.*, **20**: 1215–21.

30. **Pinkas-Kramarski, R., Lenferink, A. E., Bacus, S. S., Lyass, L., van de Poll, M. L., Klapper, L. N., Tzahar, E., Sela, M., van Zoelen, E. J., and Yarden, Y.** (1998). 'The oncogenic ErbB-2/ErbB-3 heterodimer is a surrogate receptor of the epidermal growth factor and betacellulin.' *Oncogene*, **16**: 1249–58.

31. **Agus, D. B., Akita, R. W., Fox, W. D., Lewis, G. D., Higgins, B., Pisacane, P. I., Lofgren, J. A., Tindell, C., Evans, D. P., Maiese, K., Scher, H. I., and Sliwkowski, M. X.** (2002). 'Targeting ligand-activated ErbB2 signaling inhibits breast and prostate tumor growth.' *Cancer Cell.*, **2**: 127–37.

32. **Baselga, J.** (2002). 'A new anti-ErbB2 strategy in the treatment of cancer: Prevention of ligand-dependent ErbB2 receptor heterodimerization.' *Cancer Cell*, **2**: 93–4.

33. **Agus, D. B., Gordon, M. S., Taylor, C., Natale, R. B., Karlan, B., Mendelson, D. S., Press, M. F., Allison, D. E., Sliwkowski, M. X., Lieberman, G., Kelsey, S. M., and Fyfe, G.** (2005). 'Phase I clinical study of pertuzumab, a novel HER dimerization inhibitor, in patients with advanced cancer.' *J. Clin. Oncol.*, **23**: 2534–43.

34. **Baselga, J., Gelmon, K. A., Verma, S., Wardley, A., Conte, P., Miles, D., Bianchi, G., Cortes, J., McNally, V. A., Ross, G. A., Fumoleau, P., and Gianni, L.** (2010). 'Phase II trial of pertuzumab and trastuzumab in patients with human epidermal growth factor receptor 2-positive metastatic breast cancer that progressed during prior trastuzumab therapy.' *J. Clin. Oncol.*, **28**: 1138–44.

35. **Baselga, J., and Swain, S. M.** (2010). 'CLEOPATRA: a phase III evaluation of pertuzumab and trastuzumab for HER2-positive metastatic breast cancer.' *Clin. Breast Cancer*, **10**: 489–91.

36. **Gianni, L., Pienkowski, T., Im, Y. H., Roman, L., Tseng, L. M., Liu, M. C., Lluch, A., Staroslawska, E., de la Haba-Rodriguez, J., Im, S. A., Pedrini, J. L., Poirier, B., Morandi, P., Semiglazov, V., Srimuninnimit, V., Bianchi, G., Szado, T., Ratnayake, J., Ross, G., Valagussa, P.** (2012). 'Efficacy and safety of neoadjuvant pertuzumab and trastuzumab in women with locally advanced, inflammatory, or early HER2-positive breast cancer (NeoSphere): a randomised multicentre, open-label, phase 2 trial.' *Lancet Oncol.*, **13**: 25–32.

37. **Lewis Phillips, G. D., Li, G., Dugger, D. L., Crocker, L. M., Parsons, K. L., Mai, E., Blättler, W. A., Lambert, J. M., Chari, R. V., Lutz, R. J., Wong, W. L., Jacobson, F. S., Koeppen, H., Schwall, R. H., Kenkare-Mitra, S. R., Spencer, S. D., and Sliwkowski, M. X.** (2008). 'Targeting HER2-positive breast cancer with trastuzumab-DM1, an antibody-cytotoxic drug conjugate.' *Cancer Res.*, **68**: 9280–90.

38. **Barginear, M. F., John, V., and Budman, D. R.** (2012). 'Trastuzumab-DM1: A Clinical Update of the Novel Antibody-Drug Conjugate for HER2-Overexpressing Breast Cancer.' *Molec. Med.*, **18**: 1473–9.

39. **Edwards, D. C., and Thorpe, P. E.** (1981). 'Targeting toxins—the retiarian approach to chemotherapy.' *Trends in Biochem. Sci.*, **5**: 313–16.

40. **Baselga, J., Cortés, J., Kim, S. B., Im, S. A., Hegg, R., Im, Y. H., Roman, L., Pedrini, J. L., Pienkowski, T., Knott, A., Clark, E., Benyunes, M. C., Ross, G., Swain, S. M. and the CLEOPATRA Study Group** (2012). 'Pertuzumab plus trastuzumab plus docetaxel for metastatic breast cancer.' *N. Engl. J. Med.*, **12**; 366(2): 109–19.

41. **Swain, S. M., Kim, S. B., Cortés, J., Ro, J., Semiglazov, V., Campone, M., Ciruelos, E., Ferrero, J. M., Schneeweiss, A., Knott, A., Clark, E., Ross, G., Benyunes, M. C., Baselga, J.** (2013). 'Pertuzumab, trastuzumab, and docetaxel for HER2-positive metastatic breast cancer (CLEOPATRA study): overall survival results from a randomised, double-blind, placebo-controlled, phase 3 study.' *Lancet Oncol.*, **14**(6): 461–71.

Chapter 17

Antibodies: The therapeutic future

A Personal Ideology

In a letter to a member of the French National Assembly in 1791 on the subject of the recent revolution in France, the Irishman Edmund Burke, a British politician and philosopher, stated that 'you can never plan the future by the past'. When coupled with the view of Francis Crick that 'chance is the only true source of novelty', molecular immunology is confronted by a serious dilemma. If the future is down to chance, a debatable proposition, what strategy should molecular immunologists employ to create novel therapies that exploit the functional chinks in the tumour-cell armour? Many of the current strategies in cancer research are targeted to molecular elements of cellular growth control pathways. At the 23rd Annual Antibody Therapeutics International Conference in San Diego during 3–6 December, 2012 Professor Dane Wittrup (MIT) commented on the low response rate (~10%) of current antibody therapies in cancer therapy, albeit improved by use of multi-antibody modalities.[1] So are the strategies optimal?

Consideration of these observations raises an interesting and perhaps even profound question about tumours and their ability to respond to the external environment by exploiting a multitude of alternative pathways for survival and growth. In May 2011, a collaborative and provocative set of opinions was posted by groups at Princeton, UCSF, and the Salk Institute which have considerable resonance with the views of this author developed over a number of years. In their *Nature* review article the authors explore the analogy between the evolution of drug resistance in malignant tissues and bacterial communities. In the early 1980s, while teaching Oxford biochemists how bacteria can patch together enzymes from different metabolic pathways to take advantage of atypical nutrient supply, the analogy with changing environments in eukaryotic cell assemblies, in its most exaggerated sense within a tumour mass, was a seductive idea to the author as an amateur cell biologist. The prevailing dogma for some decades has been that cancer cells undergo a number of random mutational changes that confer adaptive survival advantages in a somewhat hostile immunological environment enabling the rebel cells to escape their normal spatio-temporal locales (invasive adaptation) and at the same time evade those default pathways that would normally punish abnormal cellular behaviour (e.g. apoptosis). Lambert and colleagues take a somewhat iconoclastic stance in proposing that random genetic changes are not sufficient to explain the success of the malignant phenotype. The position they adopt is summarized in the opening page of their review:

> The interplay between cells seeking survival under stress activates a survival programme that facilitates evolution and adaptation of malignant and pre-malignant cells.[2]

The presumption that cells 'seek' survival is perhaps a trifle anthropomorphic but the message is clarified a little later in the article when the authors propose that researchers might benefit by:

> … viewing cancer tissues as strongly interacting communities rather than as groups of independent, single-celled organisms.[2]

While the analogy is thought-provoking it is also in certain respects naïve as the authors point out. Mammalian cells exhibit complex compartmentalization that does not exist in bacterial cells and the arrival of a transformed cell may rely on interplay between a number of spatially proximal cell types. Again, the increased complexity of the mammalian genome with its highly evolved mechanisms of epigenetic control will out-gun the regulatory simplicity of the bacterial genotype. Nevertheless, the analogy is compelling in other respects. Targeting cytotoxic drugs to extracellular nutrient receptor or membrane channels or key synthesis pathways on bacterial cells inhabiting a multicellular bacterial community would be unlikely to lead to complete stasis or death of the entire community of cells. As Lambert argues from a base of extensive literature, cell-to-cell communication signals within the community would result in some members of the population rapidly acquiring resistant phenotypes at the expense of their 'altruistic' neighbours, enabling them to escape the downstream impact of drug exposure. The unfortunate reality of this is already well known with the growing severity of antibiotic resistance in pathologically important bacterial strains. If such quasi-organismal behaviour operates in human tumour populations then hitting the outside of the tumour mass with an antibody while causing cell death either directly or through ADCC will merely drive the 'disorganism' to activate escape mechanisms. The strategy of coupled antibody-cytotoxic drug combined therapy is one attempt to block these escape routes. While effective for a time, resistant phenotypes often retaining their invasive capabilities eventually neutralize the therapy regime. To combat this, other approaches that target the tumour microenvironment and its 'supply chain' to the tumour cells are being explored by groups such as those of Kerry Chester at UCL in London, John McCafferty in Cambridge, UK, and others.[3]

All of this suggests that future therapeutic approaches might better be targeted to those key decision points in the cell where multiple pathways converge, much like hitting the final step in a bacterial multi-enzyme pathway where recruitment of alternative route members is always upstream. To enable an antibody or antibody fragments to achieve this will require methods for getting them inside cells. At the San Diego conference a number of groups reported the development of strategies based on 'intracellular' antibodies. Jim Marks in particular has described how to use phage libraries to select for antibodies that internalize into cells.[4] Perhaps the ideal therapeutic approach is to combine antibodies such as Herceptin or Perjeta to begin unravelling the tumour mass, with antibodies that internalize simply to deliver small molecule inhibitor payloads that operate at key convergence points in critical cell proliferation pathways. We should also not forget the powerful 'mutator machine' that we have seen operating in antibody somatic mutation. If unleashed in tumour cells that have uncoupled the controls normally in place in antibody-producing cells its dangerous components could spread mutation in a much less selective fashion. Such a system might be an important target for small molecule inhibitors, delivered by antibodies or not. While the above may seem obvious ideas to the cell and molecular biology cognoscenti, in which case I should be labelled a theologist since as Dawkins allegedly mused 'When has theology ever said anything that is demonstrably true and not obvious?', the thrust of antibody-based cancer research needs a new direction. The ideas of Lambert and colleagues merit serious consideration.

The blood–brain barrier

The entry of antibodies into the brain via the blood–brain barrier (BBB) if it occurs at all spontaneously is a rare, fortuitous event. No IgG transporting (FcRn) receptors are available in the blood => brain direction (although antibodies can exit the brain using the FcRn on the brain side of the BBB) and the tight epithelial-like junctions that form between capillary endothelial cells prevent diffusion from blood to brain of large molecules (with the possible exception of artificially cationized serum albumin). Many approaches have sought to transport small molecule drugs attached to positively charged peptide vectors with some success. These vectors have largely been receptor-independent. For many years William Pardridge (UCLA) has pursued a 'Trojan Horse' construction in which large proteins are carried on the back of recycling receptors, such as the transferrin or insulin receptors, that sit in the endothelial cell membranes of the BBB. Of particular interest is the use of this approach to take antibodies and antibody-conjugates (drugs or toxins) into the brain where treatment of horrifyingly difficult-to-treat cancers such as glioma and degenerative diseases in general may become more effective.[5] A particularly exciting application of this strategy was recently developed by Pardridge using an anti-Abeta amyloid peptide antibody. In the construction, an scFv form of the anti-Abeta antibody was fused to the C-terminus of an IgG1 antibody directed to the transferrin receptor, forming a 'tetrabody'. The scFv was linked to the VH N-terminus using a SER-SER linker to avoid disruption of the VH-VL domain in the scFvs. Using this tetrabody construction the authors carried out a treatment regime in a relevant Alzheimer mouse model and concluded:

> … daily sc administration of the cTfRMAb-ScFv fusion protein to 12–15 month old PSAPP AD transgenic mice results in up to a 57%–61% decrease in the Abeta Amyloid plaque burden in the cortex and hippocampus.[6] [PSAPP AD mice are a transgenic model for Alzheimer's disease]

In addition, the construct showed no effect on plasma concentrations of the amyloid peptide and although infusions were carried out daily no cerebral hemorrhage was seen.

The further improvement of strategies for moving biotherapeutics into the brain is a key area for future research. With the sad statistic that 30% of metastatic breast cancer patients will develop brain metastases that no existing antibody therapies can manage (none of the anti-HER2 antibodies cross the BBB), the neurological disease area calls for more concerted efforts in the development of BBB diffusible therapeutic solutions.

Transplacental foetal therapy

The beginning of foetal life is loaded with uncertainty as the merger of maternal and paternal genes produces a genotype with unknown disease susceptibilities for the unborn, more the result of spinning a genetic roulette wheel than of an optimal design process. Superimposed on this unalterable (except for epigenetic modification during the lifetime of the individual) basic pattern are the phenotypic changes imposed on the foetus by the mother's highly effective placental transport system, contributing viruses, autoantibodies, and other soluble factors to the foetal circulation (see Chapter 10). The benefits of transplacental transfer of humoral immunity are unquestionable. However, the dangers of inducing foetal pathologies by this mechanism are particularly acute with mothers receiving antibody therapy where the antibody is directed to molecules that may be responsible for the pathology in the mother but which are important in foetal development and survival. For example, in the treatment of mothers having inflammatory bowel disease, anti-TNF (tumour necrosis factor) antibody therapy may be employed. Such antibodies (IgG) are transferred to the foetus along with other maternal IgG from the late second trimester on until parturition. TNF has a known involvement in the development of the normal (despite its unfortunate name) foetal immune system. While data are sparse warning signs have appeared in the literature, elevated to importance by such comments as 'We lack definitive information about the effects of these agents on the development of the immune system of the human fetus and the newborn baby'.[7] Reducing risk of foetal effects can often be managed by timing of treatment, as suggested by Djokanovic and colleagues who reported in a study of 300 pregnancy outcomes using registry studies and case reports that anti-TNF therapy in the mother (in this case with infliximab) carried low risk to the foetus during the first two trimesters. Their recommendation however was to discontinue treatment 'early in the third trimester ... in order to minimize late foetal exposure'.[8]

To concentrate on the risks of antibody or vaccine therapy for the foetus is to bias the situation unfairly since many examples of considerable benefits are emerging. In a recent analysis of a clinical study of 3819 mothers vaccinated against the HPV virus strains 6, 11, 16, and 18 with the quadrivalent vaccine, qHPV, levels of anti-HPV antibodies were measured in foetal cord blood and found to correlate well with maternal levels. In a somewhat circumspect but optimistic conclusion the authors (from clinical academic groups and a pharma company) commented on the benefits of maternal HPV vaccination during pregnancy and its potential for preventing conditions such as recurrent respiratory papillomatosis in the newborn.[9]

Often, no medical treatment for certain prenatally diagnosed infections is available. Where treatment for the foetus is possible considerable benefits can result. In a recent Japanese study, immunoglobulin therapy was performed in 12 pregnant women who had symptomatic congenital cytomegalovirus (CCMVI) infection. As a result 41.7% of symptomatic CCMVI infants who had received the Ig therapy showed no or minimal sequelae.[10] Clearly a preliminary study which demands further clinical exploration.

While exceptional advances are being made in immunotherapy of adult diseases, the innocent world of the growing foetus is open to unwitting receipt of everything that might represent a danger to its survival as a result of an extraordinarily effective materno-foetal transport system. The future protection of the unborn should receive greater priority in research than it currently has if the eradication of debilitating diseases is to be achieved. As Isabella Ellinger and Renate Fuchs conclude in their analysis of the protection and threats to the human foetus and newborn, 'specific therapeutic molecules transported by hFcRn might be designed for the fetus only.'[11] We await the results of pharmaceutical and academic research in this area with anticipation.

After all, as Pope John Paul II observed in his 1986 homily:

As the family goes, so goes the nation and so goes the whole world in which we live.[12]

References

1. Klöhn, P.-C., Wuellner, U., Zizlsperger, N., Zhou, Y., Tavares, D., Berger, S., Zettlitz, K. A., Proetzel, G., Yong, M., Begent, R. H. J., and Reichert, J. M. (2013). 'IBC's 23rd Annual Antibody Engineering and 10th Annual Antibody Therapeutics International Conferences and the 2012 Annual Meeting of The Antibody Society.' *mAbs*, **5**(2): 178–201.

2. Lambert, G., Estévez-Salmeron, L., Oh, S., Liao, D., Emerson, B. M., Tisty, T. D., and Austin, R. H. (2011). 'An analogy between the evolution of drug resistance in bacterial communities and malignant tissues.' *Nature Reviews Cancer*, **11**: 375–82.

3. Marquardt, J., Begent, R. H. J., Chester, K., Huston, J. S., Bradbury, A., Scott, J. K., Thorpe, P. E., Veldman, T., Reichert, J. M., and Weiner, L. M. (2013). 'IBC's 23rd Annual Antibody Engineering and 10th Antibody Therapeutics Conferences and the Annual Meeting of The Antibody Society.' *mAbs*, **4**(6): 648–52.

4. Zhou, Y., and Marks, J. D. (2012). 'Discovery of internalizing antibodies to tumor antigens from phage libraries.' *Methods Enzymol.*, **502**: 43–66.

5. Pardridge, W. M., and Boado, R. J. (2012). 'Reengineering biopharmaceuticals for targeted delivery across the blood-brain barrier.' *Methods Enzymol.*, **503**: 269–92.

6. Sumbria, R. K., Hui, E. K.-W., Lu, J. Z., Boado, R. J., and Pardridge, W. M. (2013). 'Disaggregation of Amyloid Plaque in Brain of Alzheimer's Disease Transgenic Mice with Daily Subcutaneous Administration of a Tetravalent Bispecific Antibody That Targets the Transferrin Receptor and the Abeta Amyloid Peptide.' *Mol. Pharmaceut.*, **10**: 3507–13.

7. Arsenescu, R., Arsenescu, V., and de Villiers, W. J. (2011). 'TNF-α and the development of the neonatal immune system: implications for inhibitor use in pregnancy.' *Am. J. Gastroenterol.*, **106**: 559–62.

8. Djokanaovic, N., Klieger-Grossman, C., Pupco, A., and Koren, G. (2011). 'Safety of infliximab use during pregnancy.' *Reprod. Toxicol.*, **32**: 93–7.

9. Matys, K., Mallary, S., Bautista, O., Vuocolo, S., Manalastas, R., Pitisuttithum, D. P., and Saah, A. (2012). 'Mother-Infant Transfer of Anti-Human Papillomavirus (HPV) Antibodies following Vaccination with the Quadrivalent HPV (Type 6/11/16/18) Virus-Like Particle Vaccine.' *Clin. Vaccine Immunol.*, **19**: 881–5.

10. **Japanese Congenital Cytomegalovirus Infection Immunoglobulin Foetal Therapy group** (2012). 'A trial of immunoglobulin fetal therapy for symptomatic congenital cytomegalovirus infection.' *J. Reproduc. Immunol.*, **95**: 73–9.

11. **Ellinger, I., and Fuchs, R.** (2012). 'hFcRn-mediated transplacental immunoglobulin G transport: Protection of and threat to the human fetus and newborn.' *Wien Med. Wochenschr.*, **162**: 207–13.

12. 'Apostolic Pilgrimage to Bangladesh, Singapore, Fiji Islands, New Zealand, Australia and Seychelles.' Homily of John Paul II, Perth, Australia, 30 November, 1986.

Author Index

Page numbers in *italics* refer to illustrations

Subject Index

Page numbers in *italics* refer to illustrations; those in **bold** refer to tables